Medical Education
in the Age of Improvement

Medical Education
in the Age of Improvement

Edinburgh Students and Apprentices
1760–1826

LISA ROSNER

EDINBURGH UNIVERSITY PRESS

Edinburgh University Press
22 George Square, Edinburgh

Typeset in Linotron Garamond 3
by Photoprint, Torquay, and
printed in Great Britain by
Redwood Press Limited, Melksham, Wiltshire

British Library Cataloguing
  in Publication Data
Rosner, Lisa
  Medical education in the age of improvement:
  Edinburgh students and apprentices, 1760–1826.
  I. Title
  610.709411

ISBN 0 7486 0245 3 (cased)

Contents

Tables

Acknowledgements

Many people and institutions helped make this book possible. My initial research was supported in part by stipends from the Department of the History of Science of the Johns Hopkins University, and the Wellcome Trust for the History of Medicine, London. Additional research in Edinburgh, New York and Philadelphia was supported by grants from the Research and Professional Development Committee, Stockton State College.

I am especially grateful to the librarians, curators, and staffs of the following libraries and archives: the Edinburgh University Library Rare Books Collection, the Library of the Royal College of Physicians of Edinburgh, the Library of the Royal College of Surgeons of Edinburgh, the Royal Medical Society, the Scottish Record Office, the New York Academy of Medicine Library, the College of Physicians of Philadelphia, the Historical Society of Pennsylvania, the Library Company of Philadelphia, the American Philosophical Society, and the Historical Collection of the National Library of Medicine.

I would also like to thank John Servos, who first encouraged me to study the History of Science. Owen Hannaway provided both insightful suggestions and unfailingly apt criticism. I am especially grateful for his insistence that, occasionally, I look up from my computer printouts and think about what contemporary words and phrases mean. Margaret Marsh and William C. Lubenow supported and encouraged my work on the latter stages of this project. Kitty and Sidney Michaelson provided me with a home and family in Edinburgh, not to mention a great deal of practical help and advice. Of course, all errors and omissions are my own.

I would also like to thank John Theibault, without whom, though this book would have been possible, it would not have been nearly as much fun.

Finally, I dedicate this book to Henry and Lillian Rosner.

Abbreviations

AUL	Aberdeen University Library
EUL	Edinburgh University Library
RCPE	Royal College of Physicians of Edinburgh
RCSE	Royal College of Surgeons of Edinburgh
RMS	Royal Medical Society
SRO	Scottish Record Office
Edinburgh Evidence	*Evidence, Oral and Documentary: Taken and received by the commissioners appointed by His Majesty George IV, July 23rd, 1826; and reappointed by his Majesty William IV, October 12, 1830, for visiting the Universities of Scotland*, 4 vols (London: H.M. Stationery Office, 1837), vol. 1: *University of Edinburgh*.
Glasgow Evidence	*Evidence* . . . vol. 2: *University of Glasgow*.
St Andrews Evidence	*Evidence* . . . vol. 3: *University of St Andrews*.
Aberdeen Evidence	*Evidence* . . . vol. 4: *University of Aberdeen*

These four volumes are also available in Great Britain. House of Commons. Parliamentary Papers (1837):35–8.

Introduction

> A young man who goes abroad at seventeen or eighteen, and
> returns home at one-and-twenty, returns three or four years
> older than he was when he went abroad; and at that age it is
> very difficult not to improve a good deal in three or four years.
>
> Adam Smith, *Wealth of Nations*[1]

The title of this book, *Medical Education in the Age of Improvement*, contains
a mild pun. The Age of Improvement is an historians' term for the
late eighteenth and early nineteenth centuries in Great Britain, because
the image of improvement – in politics, in agriculture, in industry – was
so pervasive.[2] But improvement was also a general term for education,
defined by George Crabb's *English Synonymes Explained* as 'what is gained
in science or arts'.[3] It especially connoted the pursuit of knowledge by
young gentlemen rather than the 'formation of manners in Youth' which
was Samuel Johnson's definition for education.[4] 'Medical improvement'
was used synonymously with 'medical studies:' when Samuel Cleverly left
Edinburgh in 1797, for example, his certificate from the Edinburgh
Quaker meeting stated that he had been residing 'in this city for the
purpose of medical improvement'.[5] We will encounter the phrase often in
the course of this book. Medical students, then, were literally in the 'age
of improvement', especially since they were often between the ages of
seventeen and twenty-one, when, according to Adam Smith, it was 'very
difficult not to improve a good deal'.[6] Some of the economic connotions
of the word improvement find their way into discussions of education as
well.

I began my investigation of medical education at Edinburgh University
with two contrasting images. One was of Edinburgh professors often
described by contemporaries and historians: the elegant philosopher
lecturing to a crowded hall of 300 students on recent advances in chemistry
or physiology. The other was the focus of my research: the student seated
at the back of that crowded lecture hall, one of 300, less concerned with
his professor's eloquence than in making sure he received his money's worth

of medical education. That student's perceptions, I felt, though not necessarily incompatible with the professor's own, was hardly identical to it; until I understood it, I would not really know what went on in that lecture hall. My own subsequent transition from student to lecturer has only confirmed my opinion.

That image of the crowded lecture hall has determined what this book is and is not. It is intended as a study of the nearly 17,000 men who attended Edinburgh University during the period of their lives that they were medical students.[7] They were an important group, for Edinburgh was one of the most prominent centres for medical education in the period between 1760 and 1826. It was widely acclaimed, both within Great Britain and on the Continent,[8] and provided a model for medical schools in the American colonies as well.[9] I have divided students into groups based on educational categories, and discussed their backgrounds and later practice only insofar as it related to their academic careers. My approach owes a good deal to much of the recent work on education in Early Modern Europe.[10] It is also similar in some respects to that of studies of twentieth-century medical students, in that I am interested in why students went to Edinburgh, what their expectations of medical education were, and how their choices affected the institutions providing that education.[11] Edinburgh students had much more impact than their modern counterparts, however, because there was no national regulation either of medical practice or of medical education. What students did in medical school, therefore, depended much more on what they chose to do than on what was prescribed by faculty, University statute, or law.

When I first began to look at Edinburgh medical students I assumed the curriculum itself — what courses students took, in what order, and what that implied about their concept of medical education — would not engage much of my time. Historians had consistently described the standard eighteenth-century medical curriculum as 'medical sciences being taught first, followed by clinical teaching essentially Hippocratic in approach'.[12] This curriculum had been imported from the University of Leyden, where it had been developed by Boerhaave early in the eighteenth century.[13] From Edinburgh, the account continued, the curriculum was transplanted to the American colonies, especially to the newly-founded University of Pennsylvania.[14] This description of the ideal medical curriculum was based primarily on University statutes for graduates, though supported by evidence from many of the available student letters and diaries, which confirmed that some students had indeed followed the course of study it described. Prior to my analysis of Edinburgh University matriculation records, I had no reason to doubt its accuracy.

What the matriculation records revealed was that though this ideal curriculum existed, it was followed by only a small proportion of the student body. It also showed that other, equally set, curricula existed at Edinburgh, not the less important for not being set out in statute. I found that I could not investigate medical students without finding answers to the questions of what courses students took, in what order, and what that implied about their conception of medical education. The answers ultimately expanded to become the bases of what I call the 'student's-eye view' of medical education, a view which stressed the way in which students' different backgrounds, needs, ambitions, and choices created their differing courses of study. Medical students at Edinburgh University, it turned out, were not a homogenous group. No group of 17,000 men could be, of course, but at Edinburgh the lack of homogeneity – the existence of disparate types of students following different courses of study – was so striking as to be a defining characteristic of the institution. For all practical purposes, administrative as well as educational, there was not one medical school at Edinburgh University, but several: a schematic drawing might look like a Venn diagram, with several distinct, though intersecting, spheres.

As I continued to work on this area I realized that even this more complex interpretation of Edinburgh medical education was only a partial one. However important the students'-eye view might be, Edinburgh students were never in a position to impose their own vision of medical education onto the University directly. They did not have any collective power in the University administration: they could not appoint professors, as medical students did at some Italian universities, nor even vote for Rector, as students at Glasgow University did until the nineteenth century.[15] They did not riot, or hold strikes or demonstrations, like their nineteenth- and twentieth-century counterparts.[16] The power students had came from the economic power they wielded collectively as consumers of medical education. Medical students at Edinburgh paid only a small matriculation fee to the University, which went to the purchase of medical books for the library. They paid fees for classes directly to professors, who received no other salary, or only a nominal one. Students who graduated paid an additional fee to the faculty who examined them but, as we will see, there was no necessity for medical students to graduate in order to set up practice. Student choice as to whether to attend lectures in anatomy or clinical surgery, or whether to graduate at Edinburgh or study in London, could have a powerful impact on the income of professors and outside lecturers, and therefore affected what courses and degrees were offered.

Some groups of students occasionally tried to wield this economic power directly. For example, in 1785 members of the Royal Medical Society, the main student society, petitioned the medical faculty to use their influence to have the regulations of the Royal Infirmary changed to allow more student access to patients. If they did not, the petition warned, students might leave the university, being 'determined . . . to forego advantages, rather than submit to insults'.[17] The faculty did act as mediators in the dispute, and proposed new regulations that satisfied the students' demands. They did so in a way which confirmed both their and the managers' authority, though, pointing out that students did not have any 'right, or ought to have any privilege', inconsistent with the welfare of the patients of the Infirmary, and that in any dispute where patients' welfare was at stake, the faculty would side with the managers.[18] Students resorted to similar threats on other occasions, but the size and diversity of the student body militated against their successfully challenging faculty authority.

Yet even though students did not initiate changes themselves, or speak with a single collective voice, their demand for education was nonetheless what supported the institution.[19] It therefore had to be interpreted by individual professors, or the Faculty acting in concert, or outside professional bodies like the Royal College of Surgeons of Edinburgh, which then offered courses or degrees to fill that demand. Motives for supplying education included desire for profit, for student fees, in Edinburgh and elsewhere, were a good source of income.[20] They also included professional prestige, political patronage, and educational ideals.

That last motive, educational ideals, needs to be stressed, because my use of the economic assumptions so prevalent ever since the eighteenth century may otherwise obscure the fact that in Adam Smith's original formulation they, too, carried clear educational ideals. The image of students as rational economic actors, choosing whichever courses would best serve their educational and professional needs, stems ultimately from Adam Smith. Writing to Professor William Cullen in 1774, Smith attributed the 'present acknowledged superiority' of the Edinburgh medical faculty to the fact that they received no salaries and had no national monopoly over degrees, and had to rely on the 'diligence and success in their profession' to attract students.[21] What this analysis implied is that students would choose to spend their three guineas, the price of admission to most courses, on those offered by the most diligent and successful professors. Smith based his ideas on an image of students which many teachers would call idealistic: 'Where the masters . . . really perform their duty, there are no examples, I believe, that the greater part of the students ever neglect theirs,' he wrote. 'No discipline is ever requisite to force attendance upon lectures which are really worth the attendance.'[22] True to his faith in the informed consumer to make wise choices, Smith assumed that students' and professors' and prospective patients' definitions of 'lectures which are really worth the attendance' would always agree. This had implications for educational policy, for if students, left to their own judgement without regulation, would always attend good lectures, and the better the lectures, the more students who attended them, then making professors dependent on their student audience for fees would result in their offering excellent lectures. If it had been suggested to Smith that professors might abuse this system by offering popular courses with little educational content, he would have replied no doubt that students, as rational and well-informed consumers, would realize that such courses were not in their self interest.[23]

Taken to its extreme – as Smith would have liked to take it – this image of the student suggested the elimination of all regulation of education whatsoever. Smith, indeed, regarded medical degrees based on specific requirements as creating a monopoly and interfering in the free market of medical care.[24] Professors, or other writers who wished to preserve or impose educational requirements juxtaposed an alternative image of students as well-meaning, perhaps, but neither rational nor well-informed enough to fully understand their own interests. As Professor William Cullen wrote,

> When one considers that a young man . . . has always set before him the alternatives of ease wealth and honour on one hand or of dependence beggary and contempt upon the other we should suppose ourselves secure of his diligence in study. But it happens sometimes otherwise. Young men are often too little influenced by these distant views.[25]

Not only did the thoughtlessness harm the student himself, but also his potential patients. It was the duty of educational institutions to safeguard both students and patients by requiring proof of educational attainments. 'As the life and health of their fellow-creatures are so often entrusted to those practicing medicine and depend so much upon their skill,' Cullen later wrote, 'it seems a matter of no small importance for the public interest, that care should be taken to prevent any uneducated or unskillful persons from practising this art.'[26]

What this book describes, then, is the interplay between students'-eye views and other views of medical education, between student demands and interpretations of that demand. The students' perspective is the focus of the first part of the book, 'Students and Their Choices'. It could be subtitled 'Things that stay the same' because my focus in this section is the extent to which educational choices remained stable throughout this period, despite changes in medicine itself. The first three chapters deal with aspects of Edinburgh education which affected all students, the wider British context for medical studies, the conditions and restrictions on student life in Edinburgh, and the available courses. The next three divide the student body into the three categories most important for understanding medical education, the graduates, the apprentices and Fellows of the Royal College of Surgeons of Edinburgh, and the auditors, who had no institutional affiliation beyond attending classes. The seventh chapter analyzes the function of student societies, especially the Royal Medical Society.

Part Two of the book, 'Students and their Regulation', approaches medical education from the point of view of institutions trying to regulate it, especially from the 1790s on. It might be subtitled 'Things that changed', for it describes the new developments affecting medical education in several, sometimes competing institutions within and without Edinburgh: the Royal College of Surgeons of Edinburgh, the Edinburgh University Medical Faculty, and finally the Royal Commission to investigate the Universities of Scotland. These regulations, promoted for very different purposes, all had as their goal a kind of partial rationalization of medical education, making it more systematic and less subject to individual student choice. This rationalization was partial not only because of the persistence of conditions which had led to differences in student course of study, but also because the institutions themselves did not agree on what form educational regulation should take.

My choice of starting date, 1760, is to some extent arbitrary. The medical faculty was founded in 1726, but I wished to begin at a point when it was already a stable institution, when students arriving in autumn would find a set series of courses offered during a standard academic calendar. The matriculation records on which much of the analysis is based provide part of the justification for the starting date, since they began in 1762. This is not merely a historiographical convenience: it is based on the assumption that careful record-keeping was itself a sign of institutional stability.[27] I will occasionally refer to sources prior to 1760 where appropriate. The ending date, in contrast, is very specific: 1826 is the year that the Royal Commission to Investigate the Universities of Scotland was convened. The evidence taken by the Commission is a valuable source for Edinburgh student life, and I refer to it throughout the book.[28] Again, my use of it is not dictated solely by its convenience as a source: the Commission was also the first incursion of the state into regulation of medical education, and can be taken as marking the end of the acceptance of Adam Smith's image of students and the freedom of choice that image had endorsed. Once the need for a more standard curriculum and therefore more regulation was assumed, students' differing backgrounds, needs, ambitions, and choices increasingly became less important in determining their courses of study.

In order to present the quantitative evidence on which this study is based, I have chosen to organize the students according to cohorts based on their first year of medical study at Edinburgh University. The year is the academic year, which began in autumn. 'Students in the cohort 1793', then, would include all students who began taking courses in the autumn of 1793. The advantage of this is that is gives me a common baseline against which to measure differences within the student population, such as the percentage of students per cohort who studied for only one year, or the percentage of students per cohort who graduated. One disadvantage is that my figures are usually not comparable to those available in the historical literature, where scholars have counted the number of students who graduated in a given year, or who took Anatomy in a given year. 'Students in the cohort 1793' are not the same as 'students who graduated in 1793', because students who began taking courses in the fall of 1793 did not graduate by December of that year. 'Students in the cohort 1793 who attended Anatomy' are not all the same as 'students who attended Anatomy lectures in 1793', because students attending the lectures in 1793 could easily have begun their studies in, and thus belonged in the cohorts of, 1792 or 1791 or even 1785.[29]

Another disadvantage is that contemporary observers did not measure students in terms of cohorts, but by the numbers they could see filling up the lecture halls or applying for graduation. Moreover, even a small percentage of students could become highly visible. The percentage of Edinburgh surgeons' apprentices was small, but they had a major impact, as we will see. For that reason I have occasionally referred to other measures of the student population besides cohort.

Finally, I should say what this study is not. It is not a social history of students concentrating on their background, father's occupations, and future careers. Nor is it a history of what the faculty taught at Edinburgh. I give brief descriptions of course content, but readers interested in more extensive analysis should refer to the excellent studies on individual professors.[30] Even less is it designed as a complete history of the Edinburgh University Medical Faculty or the Royal College of Surgeons of Edinburgh. I have presented both these bodies as monolithic entities, oversimplifying the often complicated relationships between members, and paying limited attention to individual professors and surgeons. My justification for these omissions is that it is the students' perceptions that have guided my way through the analysis that follows; I have therefore left out what fell outside their range of vision.

Part One

Students and their choices

1

Medical education and medical practice

> I can never sufficiently thank you for the choise [sic] you have
> made for me in my profession, if it is not the only one that
> could make me happy, it is certainly that one which will make
> me most so, the more I study it, the more I am in love with it.
>
> Samuel Bard to his father, John Bard[1]

Young men became medical students at Edinburgh University in order to
set up medical practice. This apparently trivial statement is actually loaded
with four assertions about the majority of Edinburgh students: first, that
they were men, second, that they were young, third, that their education
was deliberately chosen to enable them to set up practice, and fourth, that
they believed study at Edinburgh would help them do that. Analysis of
the first three assertions is the subject of this chapter; analysis of the fourth
is the subject of the rest of the book.

The first assertion, that medical students were men, requires us to define
a medical student. The most useful definition for our purposes is anyone
who attended medical lectures, whether given by a University professor or
an extra-academical lecturer, and whether he intended to take a degree or
not. This is roughly consonant with contemporary definitions, but not
entirely so. Eighteenth- and early nineteenth-century usage of 'student'
carried with it the connotation of 'gentleman', as is implied by the title
of *A Guide for Gentlemen Studying Medicine at the University of Edinburgh*.[2]
This obviously excluded from being students the women who attended
Professor James Hamilton's extra-academical course on Midwifery. Very
little information on the class exists. Women were not considered part of
the University community: they were not included in matriculation
records, nor mentioned in other student's accounts or in any of the
published guides to courses at Edinburgh. When questioned about his class
by the Royal Commission, Hamilton replied that 'the University do not
recognise it'.[3] There is not even any record of a woman applying for the
degree of MD from a British University, as Dorothea Erxleben did in 1755
from Halle.[4]

Eighteenth-century usage also implied a distinction between some of those attending lectures, who were medical students proper and therefore gentlemen, and others, who were apprenticed to surgeons and therefore not. This distinction was based on the traditional attitude that a gentleman did not work with his hands, which an apprentice surely did, and that a gentleman's education was liberal, and an apprentice's, servile. By 1760, many practitioners would have found this outmoded, since the most progressive forms of medical education, anatomical dissection, some degree of physical diagnosis, and post mortem examinations, all required manual skill. By 1800, many practitioners would have insisted on the utility of some form of surgical training as well. Still, the traditional attitudes persisted in competition with the more progressive well into the 1830s: Sir Henry Halford explained to the Select Committee on Medical Education in 1834 that the Royal College of Physicians of London was justified in excluding anyone who practiced midwifery, because

> it is considered rather as a manual operation, and . . . we should be very sorry to throw any thing like a discredit upon the men who had been educated at the Universities, who had taken time to acquire their improvement of their minds in literary and scientific acquirements, by mixing it up with this manual labour.[5]

This meant that apprentices might or might not be considered students, depending on the point of view of the commentator. Paradoxically, the traditional distinction between literary studies and manual operations was one factor which led to progressive change, for it meant that a literary education conveyed prestige upon the man who had it, whatever his occupation. At Edinburgh University, where there were no entrance requirements to any classes, university study became a ready vehicle for upward social mobility even among surgeons and midwives. By the 1820s all medical neophytes, whether apprenticed or not, came to be regarded as medical students, as we will see.[6]

My second assertion was that medical students were young, usually between sixteen and twenty-three. This was a transitional and frequently awkward age. Young men were free from the restraint of school, or apprenticeship, but 'just entering on the stage of life',[7] neither legally nor financially independent and far from free of parental authority. The tensions common to the age group were expressed by referring to students variously as 'rash, impetuous youth',[8] or young men who had 'arrived at years of discretion'.[9] Students were, of course, both, and though they preferred the latter, their parents did not always agree. The emphasis throughout this book on students' choices should not obscure the fact that, in many cases, the dependant status of the student meant that his father actually chose for him. Educational reformers frequently discussed who should make decisions about a son's profession, the young man himself, who would have to practice it, or his father, who would have to pay for it. There was little suggestion that a young man should be forced to do something he hated or had no talent for, but writers did question whether boys had the experience necessary to choose a profession wisely by the age their education would have to begin. Thomas Alcock gave the example of a young man choosing to be a physician because 'Dr. ——— rides in a fine carriage, and receives a guinea for talking five minutes to a patient'.[10] Not far removed from that hypothetical example was Alexander Lesassier who, at the age of eighteen with almost no formal training, decided after consultation with friends that 'from my earnest desire to settle myself in the world, [and] from my great love of domestic comfort . . . I should if possible commence business in a country place'.[11] He tried to set up practice in Rochdale, but attracted no patients, and was very relieved to be rescued by his uncle who insisted he study at Edinburgh.[12]

Richard Edgeworth, in *Professional Education*,[13] even suggested that children should have no say in what they would become. He believed that the much-vaunted individual genius did not exist; it was therefore up to a wise parent to choose professions for his sons. The title of the book referred not to specific studies, but rather to the steps parents should take to 'form the manners' of the youth so that he would grow up wanting to follow his designated profession.

Edgeworth's *Professional Education* aroused great interest, but even reviewers who praised it did not agree with it entirely. A better, and more usual plan, according to one writer, was for all the young men in a family to have a general education first, and then choose a profession

> at a more advanced period, when a sensible and well-educated youth understands something of his own inclinations, can form some estimate of his own powers, and is not unwilling to listen to the suggestions of prudence with respect to his establishment.[14]

This was the method followed by Professor Robert Christison's family, for he told the Royal Commission

> Until I was of the age of 18, I never thought what profession I was to follow . . . I have no doubt there are many students in the same predicament, particularly among those . . . whose parents' circumstances leave them the power of looking around them before they fix upon a profession.[15]

However, it was Christison's parents' circumstances that gave him that power, and most writers concluded that the final decision on education must be up to the father, who was

> the only competent judge, either of those circumstances which must be taken into the account in a prudential view, or of the real value and meaning of those tastes and dispositions which are sometimes urged in favour of the son's own liberty and choice.[16]

Certainly most of the advice literature is directed at fathers, not sons.

What the discussion on education makes clear is that a son's education was frequently part of family strategy for providing for children's future. Historians have most clearly documented entrance into the professions as one strategy for younger sons of landed families, since they could acquire the lifestyle of their elder brothers, though without the leisure associated with it. Joseph Addison, indeed, bemoaned the prejudice which required younger sons to go into either law, divinity, or medicine rather than trade, attributing it to parents 'who would rather see their children starve like gentlemen, than thrive in a trade or profession that is beneath their quality'.[17] That pattern persisted well into the nineteenth century, however.[18]

Other, non-landed families may have employed similar strategies. Although historians have concentrated on the tendency of physician's sons to become physicians,[19] there is some evidence that they, too, were dispersed throughout the professions, where their fathers could afford it. Only one of Professor William Cullen's sons, Edward, went into medicine; another, Robert, went into law.[20] One of Professor Andrew Duncan senior's sons became his successor as medical professor, but another went into law and a third became a merchant. Even in cases where more than one son became a medical practitioner, there seems to have been some careful planning at work. Professor Alexander Monro *primus'* eldest medical son Donald made a career in the military, while his third son Alexander became his successor as professor;[21] Andrew Skene's elder son, David, took over his practice, while his younger one, George, became a surgeon in the East India Company.[22] For a young man to enter a profession where he could benefit from his father's experience, contacts, and practice made sense on pragmatic grounds, but competing with his brothers to do so did not, since a practice which could support one family in respectability and comfort could not support two or three or four. It was, then, a father's responsibility to suggest, if he did not choose, occupations for his sons, and educate them accordingly. Whether this was done fairly, or amicably, or successfully is another matter. Samuel Bard provides one example of a good match between a father's ambitions and his son's inclinations. He wrote to his father, while studying in Edinburgh, 'I can never sufficiently thank you for the choise [sic] you have made for me in my profession, if it is not the only one that could make me happy, it is certainly that one which will make me most so.'[23]

Once the young man or his father had decided he should practice medicine, he had to decide how to go about studying it. There was no national regulation of medical education in Great Britain, and no national consensus on what it should consist of. There was, however, a general consensus that education in some form was necessary, and that more was better than less: students were anxious to acquire it, and lecturers to provide it. There was a wide range of possibilities. Each of the British 'sister kingdoms'[24] had universities which were founded with the privilege of granting the degree of Doctor of medicine: Oxford and Cambridge in England, Trinity College, Dublin in Ireland, and Edinburgh, Glasgow, St Andrews and Aberdeen in Scotland. Aberdeen University was actually made up two colleges, King's and Marischal, each of which had the privilege of granting degrees. Three of those seven Universities, Edinburgh, Glasgow, and, by 1817, Dublin, offered extensive classes in medical subjects, which could, but need not, lead to a medical degree. Of the three, Edinburgh's requirements for the MD were most rigorous, and the academic reputation of its professors generally higher, though that was disputed by the other two.[25] Lack of medical classes did not invalidate the other four universities as places to graduate. Everyone agreed that the practice of medicine required the study of medicine, and indeed that examination for a medical degree should be a test of medical knowledge, but few would agree that all medical knowledge must be acquired at the place granting the degree. Faculty and graduates of the English universities, capitalizing on their strengths, claimed the true benefit of their education came from what Sir Henry Halford called 'the moral and intellectual discipline they undergo at the English Universities'. Their mastery of classics and literary accomplishments enabled them to acquire their purely professional knowledge anywhere; as Halford told the Select Committee, 'if they have their preliminary education, [t]hey will go and find physic wherever it is to be found, afterwards'.[26] Faculty at St Andrews and Aberdeen argued that their granting degrees to practitioners based on two certificates from physicians enabled many worthy men to acquire professional standing without having to return to the classroom like mere boys, though this argument grew less and less convincing.[27] Even Edinburgh and Glasgow, though insisting on a set number of years of medical study for the degree, required the only one of those years be at the degree-granting university.

Other forms of medical education flourished outside the universities. The cities of Dublin, Edinburgh and Glasgow all had their surgeon's guilds, each of which had a monopoly on the practice of surgery within the town and required a period of apprenticeship for admittance. Outside the cities all kinds of practitioners booked apprentices as well, though this did not lead to admission to a guild or convey a monopoly.[28]

Universities and guilds represented the old loci of medical training, though greatly transformed for use in Georgian Britain. The new locus was the hospital, especially in London, the 'Metropolis of the whole World for practical Medicine', according to Samuel Powell Griffitts, who went there in 1783.[29] The most famous hospitals, St Thomas, Guy's, the

Middlesex, and St Bartholomew's, each developed more or less formally constituted schools, which offered courses on medical subjects in addition to extensive clinical experience. 'Walking the wards' at a London hospital became an established form of medical study. There was no need to attend classes exclusively at any one school, and many students attended courses based on the reputation of the lecturer. However, as the *Medical Calendar* warned, 'each school was at least 2½ miles apart',[30] and so students tended to concentrate their activities on one or another of the hospital schools.[31]

Anywhere, in fact, that there was a hospital, there might be students anxious for clinical experience, and frequently lecturers offering courses on medical subjects to attract them. In Edinburgh the University dominated hospital teaching at the Royal Infirmary,[32] but the Public Dispensary provided clinical lectures, and occasional courses on other medical subjects.[33] In Glasgow the balance was reversed, with the University all but excluded from clinical teaching, since it was offered in the Royal Infirmary under the aegis of the Faculty of Physicians and Surgeons.[34] Even hospitals in towns without any formal medical school provided opportunities for students to walk the wards, and attending physicians and surgeons frequently offered lectures on collateral subjects. Alexander Lesassier wrote wistfully of wishing to become a physician's pupil at the Manchester Infirmary, but did not have the necessary five guineas.[35] By 1823 study under the 'able and philanthropic surgeons of provincial hospitals' must have been common, for Thomas Alcock bemoaned the fact that it was not considered equivalent to study in London.[36]

Students could also go abroad, though that was more expensive. The University of Leyden had been the favourite choice in the early eighteenth century,[37] but by 1760 Paris was the most common destination before and after the Napoleonic wars. Its proximity to Britain made it accessible at moderate cost, and the Paris hospitals gave more opportunities for surgical training and dissection even than London.[38] Students could also combine several different forms of medical education. In the 1790s Professor Andrew Duncan junior, for example, visited Germany and Italy after graduating at Edinburgh and spending a winter in London.[39] Thirty years later Francis Augustus Bonney combined lectures in Edinburgh with hospital attendance and dissection in Paris.[40]

Of course all of these choices were not equally available to everyone. One limiting factor was religion, since graduation at Oxford and Cambridge was limited to members of the Church of England. Another was cost, both of the training itself and the time between its completion and when the young practitioner could expect to earn a living. Oxford, Cambridge, and Dublin required students to spend up to seven years for a BA degree, then an additional four years before obtaining the MD. Even though these did not all have to be spent in residence at the University, that still amounted to eleven years before a young man could practice as a physician. Samuel Johnson advised Arthur Lee of Virginia to attend Oxford or Cambridge, with Edinburgh or Leyden as second choices, because, he said,

> the Scotch or foreign education is like a house built to last a man's life time only; the English is like a palace or fortress intended to last for many ages. The first build lightly, the last lay a very strong and firm foundation before they begin the work.[41]

Students who could not afford to build a palace had to look elsewhere for an MD, to Edinburgh, which required three years of study for most of the period, or to Glasgow, where 'the medical students were less able to support the expense of education than those of London or Edinburgh'.[42] Students who could not afford that would have to forego an MD, or apply for one from St Andrews, or Marischal College or King's College, Aberdeen. Surgical apprenticeship for entrance to a guild was also expensive unless the young man was a son or son-in-law of a guildmember.

To these, tangible restrictions must be added other, less tangible reasons for choosing one form of education over another. Students seem to have preferred, generally, to stay close to home, both for reasons of cost and out of preference for their own national institutions. Where they did travel, they frequently followed lines of family or business or confessional connections. American students at Edinburgh provide a good example of this. The largest group came from South Carolina, Virginia, and Maryland, the regions with the largest concentration of Scottish colonists.[43] Another large group came from Philadelphia, originally because of the connections between Philadelphia and British Quakers. Since Dissenters were excluded from Oxford and Cambridge, Quakers who wished to get an MD could not have followed Samuel Johnson's advice if they had wanted to, and frequently graduated from Edinburgh. With the founding of the University of Pennsylvania medical faculty in 1765, the lines of connection between Philadelphia and Edinburgh were more firmly drawn. Very few students from New England went to Edinburgh.[44] Since the patterns of practice were different in different colonies, the geographical and confessional differences corresponded to educational differences as well. Students from Maryland and South Carolina tended to come to Edinburgh right after their apprenticeship, without attending medical courses at an American university. They remained in Edinburgh for an average of two years, generally without taking a degree there, though some obtained an MD from Aberdeen or Glasgow. Students from New York and Pennsylvania, in contrast, were generally older and had attended medical courses before leaving home. Students from Maryland and South Carolina generally returned home from Scotland, but those from New York and Pennsylvania often combined study in London and Paris with graduation from Edinburgh.[45]Other factors contributed to differences in medical education. Students might feel that purely medical education carried more prestige, or else that surgical training might be more useful. Parents might prefer the discipline and structure of universities, or the practitioners who advised them might praise instead extensive clinical training at hospitals. Oxford, Cambridge and Edinburgh might attract students because they educated 'youth of the highest ranks of society',[46] or because, as Mary Hewson wrote to her son Thomas, 'Having studied in a University gives a man a name'.[47] London and Paris might attract students because they were London and Paris. In many cases the weight of family tradition allowed no real choice, since one aspect of education was the preservation of tradition. The young man from Norfolk whose father, uncles, and brothers all attended Cambridge would do so in turn, though he might defend his choice with reference to Sir Isaac Newton. His counterpart from Lanarkshire would attend Glasgow for similar reasons, though defending his choice by invoking Francis Hutchinson and Adam Smith. If a student's father or uncle or brother were a successful practitioner, that too might dictate his education, as might the expectations of the men among whom he expected to practice. Thomas Hewson was warned by his mother that if he did not follow his original plan of studying at Edinburgh University, she would

> be ashamed to tell any friend who inquires after you that you have again changed your determination . . . you are my son and I should try to think favourably of you; [but] those who love you less will form a judgment of your character from the consistency or inconsistency of your conduct . . .[48]

Thomas Parke, like Hewson unwilling to leave London for Edinburgh, finally did so because, he said, 'almost every physician in Philadelphia had been in Edinburgh, and this tho' seemingly an imaginary superiority, yet not the most trifling when we come to practice'.[49]

Parke's comment brings us back to my third assertion, that medical education was deliberately chosen to enable young men to set up practice. Medical practice, like medical education, was free from national regulation for most of the period, and so was also governed by a mixture of old and new ideas and institutions. Margaret Pelling has shown that from the sixteenth century at least there was great variety of English medical practitioners and practices.[50] Dorothy Porter and Roy Porter have recently argued that during the eighteenth century there was an increase in lay interest in medical knowledge, in the number and range of activities of regular practitioners, and in the number and range of 'irregulars'.[51] The variety of forms of practice meant that the older functional division of practitioners into physicians, who treated internal diseases, surgeons, who treated external conditions, and apothecaries, who compounded medications, was very hard to apply. Still, the social distinctions between them persisted, and in Georgian Britain the social and professional superiority of the physician to the surgeon seems to have been assumed at least as often as it was challenged. The rank of Physician to the Army continued to outrank the Surgeon, with even the newest Physician given seniority above an experienced Surgeon and twice the rate of pay, even though the two men might treat similar conditions.[52]

The more applicable functional divisions were succinctly described by James Parkinson as 'the practice of physic, or of surgery, alone' or the practice of 'both branches of the profession combined'.[53] Physic or surgery alone required a large number of wealthy patients who could afford to pay for what was in effect a form of specialization, which meant a large city. The majority of the practitioners in Britain therefore practiced 'both branches of the profession combined', simply treating whatever ailments afflicted their patients. By the 1840s these divisions had become the more modern hierarchy of consultants, called in for 'rare, difficult, and dangerous cases', and general practitioners 'to whom the great majority of society look in the first instance for assistance'.[54] The older images of physician, surgeon, and apothecary, though, were still the most familiar in the period covered by this book, and many writers tried, somehow, to accommodate the new division of professional activity with the social distinction embodied in the old. William Taplin used them as basic divisions in the professions in his satire on medical life, *The Aesculapian Labyrinth Explored: or, Medical Mystery Illustrated*, published in 1789.[55] Even Thomas Percival, trying to formulate rules for professional decorum under the new conditions of hospital practice, fell back on the traditional hierarchy to do so. His *Medical Ethics*, first published in 1803, prescribed that in cases involving physicians and surgeons, surgeons should give their opinion first in order of progressive seniority, then physicians in the same order. This meant that the most junior physician would give his opinion after the most senior surgeon, rather than all the junior members of the hospital staff speaking before their seniors. Percival's reliance on the physician's traditionally superior status is especially noteworthy since he clearly felt that there were many cases which 'may admit of elucidation by the reciprocal aid of the two professions'.[56]

Whatever practitioners' formal titles, their income could vary enormously. The most successful London physicians could earn £10,000 per year, an income surpassing many landed gentlemen, though of course it depended on the exertions of the physician, not on rents.[57] Professor William Cullen earned enough to acquire a landed property in Kirknewton, eight miles outside of Edinburgh, and took up agricultural improvement as a hobby.[58] Professor James Hamilton had a fine town house in Nicolson Square and a country house in 'a sweet and retired spot about three quarters

of a mile from Edinburgh'.[59] Erasmus Darwin's provincial practice gave
him an income of £1000 per year,[60] while Irvine Loudon has estimated
that surgeon-apothecaries, generally without an MD, earned about £400
per year.[61] This was a good income for the times; it probably would have
supported Lesassier in the 'business in a country place' he initially aspired
to.

Any young man setting up private practice had to expect several lean
years before he would attract enough patients to support himself. The
Aesculapian Labyrinth Explored quoted the proverbial expression, 'A physician never begins to get bread, till he has no teeth to eat it',[62] but any
practitioner might find himself in the same position. If he was fortunate,
he might purchase or inherit a practice, or enter into a partnership with
an older practitioner; if he had other means of subsistence, he might simply
wait.[63] If neither was possible, he might try to seek his fortune outside
Britain. In 1747 John Murray wrote to home from South Carolina that his
cousin Billy

> was well advised when he applied to Physick, it being absolutely the
> best travelling business in the world, and one that will soon gain him
> an estate if you are liberal enough with his education.[64]

It was as a travelling business that medicine appealed to many young men
who could not afford to set up practice at home. As *The London Tradesman*
wrote in 1797, 'An ingenious surgeon, let him be cast on any Corner of
the Earth, with but his case of Instruments in his pocket, he may live
where most other Professions would starve'.[65]

In the 1740s, when Murray wrote, the 'corner of the earth' most likely
to attract Edinburgh medical students was North America. After the
American War, however, the patterns of medical migration shifted to the
medical services of the East India Company, Army, and Navy. These three
services provided the main opportunities for medical men who preferred
or whose finances required them to practice outside the country. All three
required patronage of some sort, but assistant surgeoncies in the East India
Company were most highly prized of the appointments and thus hardest
to obtain. This may have been in part because the salary seems to have
been higher than in the other two branches, ranging from £80 to £175
per year, depending on where the practitioner was stationed.[66] Another
advantage of the East India Company was the opportunities for trade, and
a third was the possibility of establishing a private practice among the
British community in India.[67] Historians might be inclined to offset these
advantages with the high mortality rate among those who joined the East
India Company: C.J. Bryant estimates that one in four Scots who went
East died there, and few made fortunes.[68] The 'contempt of risk and the
presumptuous hope of success' which Adam Smith thought characteristic
of young men[69] may have kept young surgeons from making that kind of

calculation. Instead, their image of the East India Company was coloured by the example of men like Patrick Muschet, who went to Bengal 'where in the course of ten or twelve years he made a competence with which he returned to his native country'.[70]

If surgeoncies in the East India Company were out of reach, another possibility was a position in the Army or Navy, where the demand for physicians, surgeons, and surgeon's mates grew dramatically as a result of the wars with America and France. The salary of surgeons varied between £100 and £200 per year, and of surgeon's mates, between £60 and £120.[71] The army was considered the more respectable of the two. Lesassier, despite his failure at practice in Rochdale, felt the 'little profit to be gained and the poor plight one's character is in when one wishes to settle in the world', were good reasons for not becoming a navy surgeon.[72] Still, many young practitioners did enter the army and navy services, having no other opportunities to set up practice.

With this variation in income, prestige, and style of life among practitioners, many decisions about medical education must have become cost-benefit analyses, with location, cost, and prestige of study carefully weighed against expected return in location, income, and gentility of practice. It was, in fact, common for a young man to refer to education as an investment in time and money, which, Adam Smith said, 'is a capital fixed and realised as it were, in his person'.[73] Robert Dalrymple wrote to his brother in 1737 that 'I have nothing to depend upon, but my business. Whatever therefore I spend in the pursuit of it, I always will reckon well spent'.[74] Robert Hamilton, writing about the need for army surgeons to be better educated, complained that they had little incentive for extensive study, for 'who would give himself the trouble, and run into the expence necessary for such an education, for the poor pittance of three shillings a day?'[75]

Medical education could be regarded as an investment in a number of different ways. First, and most obviously, it would enable a young man to acquire knowledge and skills he needed to practice. That was certainly Dalrymple's meaning, and it is commonly found among medical writers advising students how to prepare for a career. The *Guide for Gentlemen Studying Medicine*, for example, said that three years of classes were necessary for 'every one who wishes to study upon a liberal plan'.[76] Thomas Alcock insisted that a full nine months of anatomical dissection for nine hours per day, five days per week was essential to practitioners.[77] This is the view of medical education's value most congenial to modern assumptions, and one reason why Edinburgh University and London hospital schools are often held to have provided the best medical education.

But medical education was an investment in other ways as well. Former students setting up practice in Georgian Britain could not rely on the knowledge acquired by study in the same way as modern medical students can. Practitioners and their patients lived in a world where medical knowledge could cure some ills and ameliorate others, but had nothing like its modern efficacy. Patients might consult a practitioner, but they also might challenge his ability, or refuse his treatment.[78] Not only could this prevent a young practitioner from collecting fees, but also it directly interfered with treatment: unless a practitioner could persuade his patient to follow his advice, any skill he had was useless. John Bard was not being cynical when he told his son Samuel that:

> a Gentleman will make his practice valuable in proportion to his merit and address – an easy, obliging and attentive manner with a proper degree of skill will insure you the best practice and the highest fees.[79]

The 'easy, obliging and attentive manner' were not superficial additions to diagnosis and treatment. They were instead essential components to clinical interaction that depended on patient compliance for success, as modern medicine does, but without modern medicine's long history of success. Formal medical training imparted more confidence to the young practitioner, and more authority in dealing with patients, than independent study. Porter's study of quackery confirms patient preference for formal credentials in an indirect way, for one of the techniques used by irregulars to attract patients was to claim degrees from universities and scientific societies.[80] If the formal credentials were considered to be especially prestigious, as study in Britain and the Continent was for American students, so much the better.

A third way in which medical education was an investment was that it could confer specific privileges. In France, medical corporations were eliminated in the Revolution, but Great Britain retained the privileges of its colleges of physicians and surgeons until the 1850s. As mentioned earlier, members of surgeons' guilds in London, Dublin, Edinburgh, and Glasgow had a monopoly of practice in those cities. The Royal Colleges of Physicians in London, Dublin, and Edinburgh, and physician members of the Faculty of Physicians and Surgeons in Glasgow had monopolies on the practice of 'physick' in those cities, and restricted membership to MDs.[81] In each College certain universities had the privilege of admission as Fellows without examination. For most of the period only Oxford and Cambridge graduates could become Fellows of the Royal College of Physicians of London, while all other MDs were admitted, after examination, as Licentiates. Similarly, all graduates with MDs from Scottish universities could become Fellows of the Royal College of Physicians of Edinburgh without examination. The London Colleges of Physicians and Surgeons also had licensing privileges for the military medical services.

Any student, or his family, had to weigh carefully all these aspects of education, and to do so without any guarantees of success, for investment in education, like all investments, carried with it some risk. A young man might be indolent or dull, or study too little to practice successfully. Or he might become too enamoured of study for its own sake, to the neglect of practical considerations, and find he had 'exhausted his stock' in paying for it like Peter Mackenzie, who had to seek an appointment in the East India Company.[82] Or he might set up practice, and find he could attract no patients, like Lesassier.[83] It was this risk that let Adam Smith to conclude that the attraction of the professions was due not only to the tangible benefits of success, but also to 'the natural confidence which every man has more or less, not only in his own abilities, but in his own good fortune'.[84]

From this perspective it is impossible to conclude that study at Edinburgh was always the best investment since, if it had been, no others would have flourished. I would like, therefore, to summarize by giving what information I have been able to find about student numbers for other choices, coupled with contemporary testimonials. Oxford and Cambridge together graduated approximately five MDs per year; medical students did not go there to attend classes without taking a degree.[85] In 1806 William Baillie advised the mother of a Glasgow student to send him to Oxford, even though he warned that 'his medical education will not be improved by this plan, for there are no lectures of reputation upon any branch of medicine given at Oxford'. There were other advantages, however:

> he will thereby become acquainted with the manners and the people of this country, may form some connections which may be of use to him in future life, and will more easily advance in his profession when settled in London.
>
> The people of England have a strong attachment to their two universities; the Fellows of the College of Physicians in London receive kindly all those who have been educated at Oxford or Cambridge; and there is a better chance of being chosen a physician to an hospital than if the medical education had taken place at a Scotch university.[86]

Susan Lawrence has found that Oxford and Cambridge men did indeed dominate, though they did not completely control, hospital practice;[87] they thus provide a good example of the way that the seemingly archaic privilege of Fellowship could be transformed into the progressive and extremely advantageous position of hospital consultant. For the small number of students who were eligible, then, graduation at an English University might have been the most secure investment of all.[88]

It is difficult to know how many students studied in London, but Lawrence has found that the number of pupils at the most important hospital schools went from between 100 to 150 per year between 1780 and

1798 to over 350 per year by 1815.[89] 'Indeed the opportunities of information here are so great,' wrote James Parkinson, 'as to authorise me to describe them, as constituting the first schools of practical medicine in the world.'[90]

Approximately forty students per year matriculated as medical students at Trinity College Dublin, with perhaps an additional 100 per year attending medical classes, but only an average of two per year graduated.[91] Those graduates were, however, granted all the privileges of Oxford and Cambridge graduates. In 1818 one writer admitted that 'the Dublin School has not yet obtained in other countries that celebrity which we shall see it entitled to receive'. Yet, he continued, 'from the increasing number of its students, and the activity manifesting itself among those high in the profession, . . . the period cannot be far distant when its merits shall no longer be concealed'.[92]

The University of Glasgow kept careful records from 1803, and the number of students enrolling in medical classes each year fluctuated between 300 and 500. Dow and Moss have estimated that the number may have risen to 1,000 by the late 1820s.[93] The number of graduates fluctuated between five and fifteen until 1820, and by the late 1820s had risen to an average of thirty.[94] In 1826 the Royal Commission noted that 'Glasgow has of late years risen into great eminence'.[95] Kings College granted ten to fifteen MDs per year,[96] Marischal College fifteen to twenty,[97] and St Andrews an average of twenty per year.[98] Contemporaries were not lavish with their published testimonials for any of these schools, but the large number of Fellows of the Royal College of Edinburgh who received their degrees might serve as living testimonials. Andrew Duncan senior, Professor of Medical Theory, received his degree from St Andrews in 1769, and James McGrigor, who became Director-General of the Army Medical Department, received his from Marischal College Aberdeen in 1804.[99]

At Edinburgh University, the number of medical students attending classes each year went from 300 in 1763 to between 900 and 1,000 from 1815 to 1825. The number of graduates went from 10 per year in 1763 to over 100 between 1815 and 1826.[100] John Morgan, in 1765, wrote that Edinburgh's reputation 'already rivals, if not surpasses, that of every other school of Physic in Europe'.[101] Professor Andrew Duncan junior called it 'the first medical school in the empire' in 1826.[102] The rest of the book will serve as additional testimonial.

2

Student life

The students here, denominated medical, may be referred to
three ranks or orders. 1st the Fine Gentleman [sic], or those
who give no application to study, but spend the Revenues of
Gentlemen of Independent Fortunes. 2ly. The Gentlemen, or
Students of Medicine strictly speaking, these live genteely and
at the same time apply themselves to study. 3ly. The vulgar,
or those who, if they are not indolent, are entirely devoid of
everything polite and agreeable. I believe you will not doubt
for a moment with which of these orders I ought to associate.

Walter Jones to his brother, 1776[1]

Medical students could arrive in Edinburgh by coach from England or
western Scotland, or by sea to the port of Leith. According to George
Logan in 1777, 'the first thing that attracts the attention of a stranger on
his arrival at this place, is the wretchedness of the Inns'.[2] A less waspish
account came from Lesassier, who had been so anxious for his first view of
the city that he sat up with the coachman. They arrived just before 3 am,
and he wrote that his vigilance had been rewarded, for

within about 2 miles of Edinburgh ye moon shone out with a most
vivid splendour So that ye night was as fine as any I had ever seen
The entrance to town here is beautiful just like going thro' a garden.
I was very happy when I felt ye rattling of our coach wheels on ye
street pavement.[3]

The greatest influx of students was from mid-October, in time for the
start of the medical lectures during the first week of November. By 1760
the academic calendar followed a regular rhythm. The Winter Session
lasted until the end of April, with an eight-day vacation for Christmas and
New Year's Day. Several professors complained about the bad effects of the
holidays. James Russell told the Royal Commission that 'young people get
habits of industry, and if they are broken in upon they do not always begin
to study again as they did before'.[4] On the other hand, when some
professors insisted on lecturing during the holiday, the students who had
left town for it were 'vexed', according to Professor John Thomson, 'that

the Professor should have gone over a subject, which they considered as of importance, in their absence'.[5] All medical courses except Botany were offered during the Winter Session. This was considered rigorous in 1760, when no other school offered as many courses of that length, but by 1826 six months had become the standard length for medical courses. Botany was offered only in the Summer Session, which lasted from the beginning of May through the end of July; additional courses in clinical lectures and midwifery were offered in the summer as well. Most students did not stay for the summer, though: by the beginning of May, Professor James Hamilton told Lesassier, 'great numbers of young men will be flocking to London for situations'.[6] Even those who stayed in town must have found it harder to concentrate, for John Thomson told the Commission 'Whenever good weather sets in, it is extremely difficult to keep up the numbers [of students in class]; there is no danger of the class being ill attended in bad weather'.[7]

Many students would have arrived with letters of introduction from fathers or family friends to professors or other Edinburgh connections. These were formal introductions serving in lieu of the personal introduction required in saluting people a student would not presume to address familiarly. Students simply met each other, but they 'waited on' professors or eminent professional men or father's friends. These letters also operated as a kind of currency, circulating through the networks of reciprocal obligations and 'interest' permeating Georgian Britain. Letters of introduction, however phrased, were always designed to present the bearer 'to a circle of connections who may be essentially serviceable' to him.[8] The way in which the recipient might be of service varied widely, from lending the young man credit to inviting him to dinner to welcoming him into the family. James Rush came to Edinburgh with a number of letters from his father, Benjamin, who had studied there forty years before. He was all but adopted by several of his father's friends, but he was disappointed and annoyed when his letter to Professor Andrew Duncan produced no more than a dinner invitation in return, especially since it also meant he had to attend Duncan's class. 'I can only regret having been placed under obligations to attend him,' James wrote to his father, 'he gave me a dinner, and I took his ticket.'[9] Thomas Ismay, in contrast, was very grateful for his letter of introduction from a Mr Sharp to Thomas Williamson, a Member of the Incorporation of Surgeons of Edinburgh. 'I shall always esteem Mr. Sharp, a particular Friend,' he wrote home, 'from whose Recommendation I have received so many civilities from Mr. Williamson.'[10]

Letters of introduction could also serve as mechanisms for parents to keep some control over students. Professor William Cullen, for example, had been waited on by a student who presented a letter of introduction from his father. Cullen wrote that he had been meaning to write back, but 'as I could not do that properly till I should know your son and observe his conduct, this put off my writing for some time . . . Now indeed when I have had a very particular and full opportunity of knowing your son I can no longer delay giving you my opinion of him', which was very favorable. [11] Cullen began by assuring his correspondent 'that from the time your son came here to this moment his morals have been perfectly correct, and his manners have been always polite and engaging'. He then went on to praise the young man's 'parts and genius . . . his close and unceasing application to study, and . . . his great and singular proficiency in medical knowledge'. We may assume that Cullen began with morals and manners because that would have been uppermost in his father's mind. Only by enlisting the help of a professor or other family friend could fathers find out what their sons were doing, since it was not usual for tutors to accompany students to Edinburgh. The desire of parents for some kind of supervision over students was strong enough for Professor James Russell to recommend to the Royal Commission the creation of a medical tutorial system. [12] During this period, though, the letters of introduction were the only mechanisms for parental control, and any student who presented a letter to his father's friend might expect his father to hear of his subsequent behaviour.

We cannot determine precisely students' backgrounds, but there were certainly real differences within the Edinburgh student population. There is no complete survey of the social origins of the medical profession in Britain in this period, nor can I offer one of the entire Edinburgh student population. The information we do have, though, is worth discussion. Of the 300 graduates between 1760 and 1805 whose fathers can be traced, the majority came from the middling ranks, gentry, medical practitioners, military men, ministers, and lawyers. The same holds for fathers of Edinburgh surgeons' apprentices between 1696 and 1730: Rosalie Stott found that they were medical men, gentry, Advocates and Writers to the Signet, ministers, and merchants and burgesses. [13] The few indentures which have survived for the period 1709 to 1811 confirms this pattern. [14] Medicine then, seems to have been primarily an occupation for genteel, though not aristocratic, families. Patricia Otto's study of daughters of the Scottish aristocracy found that physicians were seldom considered suitable husbands, and medicine therefore seems an unlikely occupation for younger sons. [15]

Nor were Edinburgh students likely to come from the opposite end of the social hierarchy, the labourers, village artisans, and tenant farmers. The ministry, not medicine, was the traditional route for the Scottish village 'lad of parts' who wished to improve his circumstances, for the good reason that bursaries were available for study. Any poor man who wished to study medicine would have had to overcome formidable obstacles. He would have first had to undergo preliminary schooling, and although Scotland was noted for its system of parish schools and high standard of literacy, a recent debate has suggested that for many people literacy extended only to reading the Bible and writing their name.[16] Even if the boy had the opportunity to learn to read and write, as well as acquire some Latin, the family would have had to be able to afford to support a non-wage-earning member, as well as the cost of school and preliminary apprenticeship. Robert Burns, an exceptionally talented child, still did not acquire the kind of education he would have needed to become a medical student.[17]

Yet in each group of medical students I have mentioned, there were also a few students from the other side of the great divide separating gentlemen from the lower orders. Among the graduates, for example, we find Andrew Marshall, son of a tenant farmer, who began his studies by obtaining a bursary to study theology at St Andrews. After receiving his MA degree, he acted as a tutor and was eventually able to finance medical education by taking private pupils, with the help and encouragement of his former employer.[18] John Brown, the author of the famous Brunonian system, was another such exception. The son of a village artisan, he first attended the parish school and was then apprenticed to a weaver. His exceptional abilities had attracted the attention of the parish schoolmaster and, with his encouragement, Brown was able to attend the grammar school at Duns, supporting himself by day labouring work. At twenty he, too, obtained a position as tutor, but after several months decided to go to Edinburgh to study divinity. Once again, his exceptional abilities, especially in classical scholarship, attracted attention, and when, after several years, he decided to study medicine, the medical faculty presented him with free tickets to their lectures. Brown supported himself by coaching medical students in Latin for their oral and written examinations, and by translating graduation theses into Latin.[19] An even greater success story was John Thomson, son of a silk weaver in Paisley. He was first apprenticed to his father, who then decided his son should become a minister, but John was so interested in medicine that he convinced his father to apprentice him to a physician in Paisley at the age of twenty. He spent the next seven years in study in Edinburgh and London, supporting himself by teaching. He was able to borrow money to enter the Edinburgh surgeon's guild, and ultimately became Professor of Military Surgery at Edinburgh University.[20] James Rush's later comment perhaps captures some of the effort required for the village lad to become a professor. 'John Thomson – a very worthy man,' Rush wrote, 'he seemed to work hard among learning . . . But he never seem'd to raise his own head above the chaos of books about him.'[21]

A few surgeon's apprentices, too, came from humbler origins. Three of the thirty-eight indentures in the records of the Royal College of Surgeons of Edinburgh were from guilds in Edinburgh: George Riddell, son of 'George Riddell, wright burger [sic] in Edinburgh', John Lizars, son of 'Daniel Lizars, engraver', and Alexander Morgan, son of 'Thomas Morgan, late Watchmaker'.[22]

These examples suggest that medicine provided some limited upward social mobility, precisely because access to it depended primarily on education, which, in Edinburgh at least, depended only on cost. That did not make it an egalitarian profession: Georgian Britain, like eighteenth-century Germany, recognized that poor students could be talented, but preferred that they be sons of impoverished gentlemen.[23] Artisans or farmers or tradesmen should spend their money on their sons' apprenticeship, according to contemporary prejudice, and not in trying to make them gentlemen. Tobias Smollett's Roderick Random was told by his examiners at Surgeon's Hall in London, 'that my friends would have done better if they had made me a weaver or shoemaker, but their pride would have me a gentleman . . . and their poverty could not afford the necessary education'.[24] Once their funds were spent on their education, however inadequate, poor students would have no reserve to set up practice, and few of the accomplishments required to attract paying patients. The gentry, especially, seems to have preferred their practitioners to have all the visible characteristics of gentlemen;[25] those characteristics might have helped practitioners establish authority for treatment with other ranks in society as well.[26] One reason for this preference is that patients seem to have been genuinely concerned about practitioners prescribing unnecessary treatment in order to make money.[27] Surely, they felt, a man who depended on their illness, not only for his income, but also for his rank in polite society, was less to be trusted than one who would be known as a gentleman whatever occupation he followed. According to contemporary opinion, a poor practitioner might be as intelligent as a wealthy one, but his poverty would inhibit his independence of judgement. 'A man that's pinch'd, let him be never so clever in his business,' wrote Adam Murray,

> must have a slow depress'd mind, think and act without freedom and
> courage, be little regarded by the people he lives among, and
> consequently be less employed and draw smaller fees.[28]

Young practitioners, like Murray, found they had to live in the style of gentlemen of fortune to reassure patients that they had no 'interest' in their illnesses. This was common enough for the author of the satirical 'Hints to Young Practitioners' to recommend claiming 'that you took your degree at a foreign university, rather for amusement than with a view to practise'.[29]

Another more concrete reason why medicine provided only partial upward social mobility was that family wealth translated into time and leisure for a more 'polite and agreeable' education, which in turn could translate into better preparation for the study of medicine. Coming from a well-to-do family could mean preliminary study at the Edinburgh High School rather than the parish school, enough facility in Latin to read and discuss Professor James Gregory's *Conspectus Medicinae Theoreticae*,[30] cultural sophistication to recognize David Hume's philosophy in Professor William Cullen's lectures on Medical Practice.[31] More family wealth also simply translated into more years of medical study, which was generally equated with better preparation for practice.

All these assumptions and prejudices were reflected by the writer from Trinity College, Dublin, who in a real-life echo of Smollett's fictional examiner, wrote that some Edinburgh students presented

> so much the appearance of rustic life, that every one must give their parents credit for the laudable ambition of making them gentlemen, however unfit they may be for such a station . . . The caution with which some of them go about to form a letter, seems to show that they had been but just emancipated from the rod of a country school-master.[32]

What this unpleasant remark also reflects, of course, is that such 'rustic' students did form part of the Edinburgh student body.

Young men carried their social and educational differences with them into their lives as medical students, for Edinburgh University was not a melting-pot. Edinburgh students did not wear gowns based on their rank, as at Oxford and Cambridge, but the differences among their background and styles of life must have been quite as obvious. Surgeon's apprentices generally lived with their masters, where they were regarded as an uneasy mixture of member of the family and servant.[33] Students also sometimes boarded with professors, where they were regarded as perhaps an equally uneasy mixture of family and guest. The majority of students lived in lodgings near the University. This was located at the present site of Old College, but in the mid-eighteenth century that was next to Potterrow port near the south city wall. Medical Edinburgh was concentrated by that south wall, with the Royal Infirmary directly to the west of the University and Surgeon's Hall to the west of that. South of the University were fields, except for the cluster of Potterrow suburbs; to the north, the 'Town' seemed very far away. When David Skene studied at Edinburgh in 1751 his father thought it 'preposterous' for him to pay seven pence to dine near the University between classes when he could dine for six pence on the High Street,[34] but to get there David would have had to walk downhill through one maze of wynds to the Cowgate, then uphill through another to Tollcross. By the 1780s, students would have found the walk much easier, for South Bridge had been built to connect Nicolson Street — extended between the University buildings and Infirmary — with the High Street. The combination of Nicolson Street and North and South Bridges had become a major transportation route linking the London Road in the south with the New Town, and the area south of the city had grown up accordingly. Medical Edinburgh had been extended to include the Public Dispensary on West Richmond Street, and most students lived in the cluster of streets bounded by the University, Surgeon's Hall, and the Dispensary: Richmond and Chapel Streets in the south, the old city wall in the north, Bristo to the east and Nicolson Street to the west.[35]

This system of students living in private lodgings, rather than in colleges controlled by the University, was extolled by Sir John Carr, in his *Caledonian Sketches*, as giving students 'power to visit among genteel families, and to temper the austerity of learning with the amenity of manners'.[36] It was severely criticized by a writer from Oxford who claimed that the 'Student of Medicine is placed under no restraints . . . even in the slippery period of early youth he is exposed to every temptation, and very often sinks to the lowest debauchery'.[37] Evidence from student diaries could be found to support both opinions. One incontrovertible result of the lodging system was that students' expenses at Edinburgh depended not on fixed costs, but, as George Bell told the Royal Commission, 'upon their rank in life'.[38] Professor Andrew Duncan junior, asked by the Commissioners to describe a typical medical student's expenses, replied, 'I have known instances of students getting through the winter on less than £10; I have known other medical students spend almost £500 or £600'.[39]

We have no records of actual students living on less than £10 for the winter, if by that Duncan meant the Winter Session, which was a period of six months. The cost of a room in Edinburgh seems to have included breakfast and supper, and the students' main choice was where to get dinner, the main meal of the day, usually eaten between 3 and 4 pm. In 1751 David Skene, whose father was a physician in Aberdeen, paid eighteen pence for 'a little, snug, Boxed Room (at ye top of a high house indeed)', just beyond the Potterrow port.[40] This would have amounted to £7 per quarter-year, or £14 for the Winter Session. He began by dining out at a cost of 6d, but later decided to save money by dining 'allways at home, but when invited abroad', and breakfasting upon pottage.[41] His younger brother, George, also began by trying to dine in town, but found that 'the lads in town join into clubs, and when they have a certain number, they make an agreement with the Landlord, to allow no more to come in but whom they please'. George could not find a club that would allow him to join, so that, he said, 'I must have wanted dinner every day, and I think two meals is but a scant allowance'. He therefore took a room for £9 per quarter which included 'fire and candles, four meals in the day . . . so that I have nothing to do with money but to buy paper and pens and washing'.[42]

Thomas Ismay, son of a Yorkshire vicar, paid £10 per quarter for room and board in 1771, which, he told his father, 'is the lowest one can get Boarded in a genteel manner'.[43] Ismay gave a description of what his board consisted of

> Tea twice a day if I chuse; have a Hot Dinner and Supper. The Dinner generally consists of a large *Tirene* of Soup, which I like extremely well, a Dish of Boiled Meat and another of Roast. There (sic) Mutton and Beef is very good. Veal, I have not seen any yet; Puddings, only one. Generally to Supper, Fish, Eggs, Beefstakes or what you please. Candles what you have occasion for, and a good Fire.

He went on to say that 'The greatest economists we have who take a Room, and live in a hansome manner but no ways extravagant, cannot live under £16 the half year and have everything to seek in'.[44]

The Skene brothers and Ismay show how the 'greatest economists' could live: £20 for room and board for the Winter Session, £40 if they stayed twelve months. Other expenses would include washing, clothes if necessary, paper, pens, books, and, of course, the classes themselves. Walter Jones, however, wrote home to his brother in Virginia that 'less than 100 pounds per ann. will not maintain a gentleman in Edinburgh'.[45] He came to Edinburgh intending to spend £90 per year, but ended spending £118 per year. His three-year stay nearly bankrupted his brother, who was paying for Jones' education.[46] Job Harrison, son of a yeoman in Chester, likewise spent over £100. He wrote home that though his expenses might seem high, still

> I can mention with certainty, there is not an English student has resided here during twelve months, for less, and very few within those bounds, nay there is not one in the house where I am an inhabitant that has lived for less than £150 p. annum.[47]

Of course, both Jones and Harrison were writing to justify their expenses. It presumably occurred to neither of them that costs could be cut back by as much as £50 per year, for to do so would be to jeopardize their 'genteel' style of life. Robert Whyte, son of Professor Robert Whyte, no doubt spent even more while a student, for his expenditures included one guinea per month pocket money, £3 per month for riding lessons, and twenty-five shillings for 'silk stockings and other necessaries'.[48] Sylas Neville, who had a small private income, also spent more on his household. In his second year he rented chambers with private kitchen and garden in order to accommodate his housekeeper, who was also his mistress; his costs included her pregnancies in addition to other expenses.[49]

Wealthy students, like Neville and many of the Americans, also spent time and money on the theatre, since it was one of the diversions polite Edinburgh offered. Students went to plays often enough for the Royal Medical Society to pass a rule that if a member missed a meeting, the president had the right to accuse him of attending a play. The member had to answer whether or not he had gone to a play, under penalty of paying half a crown.[50] A 'genteel' student could also attend the Assembly Hall, the focus of Edinburgh's social season. 'If you are known to be a Gentleman, you will meet with every civility and attention,' George Logan warned, '. . . otherwise you will find the young ladies very much on the reserve.'[51] American and English students made an especial point of travelling extensively, for experiencing foreign manners and customs was part of the point of studying abroad. Benjamin Rush sent his son James £200 as 'ample provision' for a trip to Liverpool, Bath, and Oxford, which, Benjamin told James, 'will contribute to your health, as well as improve you in knowledge, if not necessary, yet ornamental to a physician'.[52] Indeed, for wealthy students, these assorted activities were by no means frivolous: they ensured that the young physician received the same education as the young gentlemen among whom he hoped to practice. Still, James Rush's expenditures and his father's approval of them were in striking contrast to David Skene's account that he had not been 'at a Play, Concert, Assembly, or Tavern',[53] and his father's reproaches for David's spending seven pence for dinner, when he could dine for six.

Edinburgh medical students, then, found themselves thrown together with hundreds of other young men of very different social and educational backgrounds, all of whom claimed the status of student. They often reacted in shocked dismay. George Logan complained to his brother that

> Among such a number of students you will no doubt judge that we have plenty of companions but I do not think that a Man of your good sense & taste would be able to select 20 out of Monro's 300 with whom you would wish to associate.

Indeed, he said,

> On account of there being such a large proportion of the low class among the students, the others are not paid that respect which is due to them neither from the Citizens nor Professors considering that quantity of Money they annually spend among them and their genteel behaviour.[54]

Sylas Neville also complained that the townspeople did not have a high regard for students, 'on account of the riotous behaviour of some of the students, which they . . . unjustly impute to all.'[55]

Both Logan's and Neville's comments demonstrate their concern with being classed among the multitude of students. Logan's reaction, especially, reveals student concern with breeding, wealth, and taste as defining characteristics of their own circle of friends. A fourth defining characteristic, professional abilities, was implied by an earlier remark to his brother, 'As to myself', he wrote, 'I am happy in pursuing a subject to which I am particularly attracted and with which I am determined to get perfectly acquainted'.[56] Walter Jones combined all four characteristics when he

divided Edinburgh students into 'students of medicine strictly speaking',
who were gentlemen, but nonetheless seriously intent on their studies,
'fine gentlemen', who 'give no application to study, but spend the revenues
of gentlemen of independent fortunes' and the 'vulgar', who were, if not
indolent, 'entirely devoid of everything polite and agreeable'.[57]

Jones' distinctions did, as we have seen, point to real differences among
Edinburgh students. Yet it is more important for showing students' perceptions about their own social and professional rank. Modern sociologists
have found that people's images of occupational prestige are coloured by
the position of their own occupation on a prestige hierarchy, and that
'individuals engage in tactics of cognitive distortion (shifting the frames
of reference for evaluation and so forth) in a continuing effort to maximize
their individual prestige'.[58] Walter Jones' comments can be taken as an
eighteenth-century example of this. Polite Edinburgh society would surely
have ranked a 'gentleman of fortune' as higher than even an accomplished
physician. Jones effectively maximized his own perceived rank by contrasting the value of the industrious student of medicine with the uselessness
of the landed gentleman on the one hand, and drawing a sharp distinction
between his own gentlemanly status and the 'vulgar' who made up the
majority of Edinburgh students on the other. Sylas Neville adopted the
former criteria when he wrote that 'being at last tired of the insipid life of
a gentleman without employ, I had determined to study physic'.[59] He
adopted the latter in his many criticisms of the lack of gentility of
Edinburgh students.[60]

'Fine gentlemen', to Jones, might have included Robert Whyte junior,
or William Thornton, who spent his time at Edinburgh travelling,
attending learned societies, and cultivating his acquaintance with titled
gentlemen.[61] The 'vulgar' might have included students like Ismay or
David and George Skene. Yet they, too, defined themselves at students of
medicine strictly speaking, occupying a similar middle ground. Ismay
wrote to his father than £10 per quarter was the lowest one could get
boarded in a 'genteel manner', which implied that there were some ways
of boarding which were not genteel and therefore not acceptable. David
Skene wrote to his father than he supposed he 'should live as other
Gentlemen's Sons of a very moderate fortune did', which again carried
assumptions of his own genteel status.[62] 'Fine gentlemen', for Ismay and
the Skenes, might have included those who could afford the extravagance
of taverns, theater, concert, and Assembly Hall, all useless for the purpose
of conveying knowledge necessary for practice. For Ismay and students like
him also shifted the frame of reference to maximize their own positions in
the prestige hierarchy, away from breeding, wealth, and taste towards the
one characteristic they had in common with the most accomplished
physician, medical study itself. What his comments suggest is that Ismay,

too, regarded himself and his friends as students of medicine strictly speaking, occupying a middle ground between 'fine gentlemen' who lived extravagantly on the one hand, and the 'vulgar' who were not genteel on the other.

This fluid definition of 'student of medicine strictly speaking' was related to the fluid definition of a 'liberally-educated gentleman'.[63] Every student and indeed every writer on medical education seems to have defined a liberal education in a way to stress his own possession of it, so that it is impossible to define precisely a liberal course of study. Often the phrase 'liberal education' was used to mean classical studies, but medical writers used it to describe study which had nothing to do with classical Greek and Latin. One common usage was based on the sense of 'liberal' as 'generous' or 'bountiful',[64] so that a liberal education was a generous education, one where a father had not stinted to provide for his son's future. This was the sense in which John Murray used it, when he said medicine would gain his cousin an estate if William Murray was 'liberal enough with his education'. Another was that a liberal education was a literary education, and so always involved formal study from texts, though a wide range of authors could be recommended as 'liberal.'[65] The reason for the lack of precise definition in terms of subjects was that the operative definition at Edinburgh was the one given by Johnson's *Dictionary*, 'Not mean . . . Becoming a gentleman',[66] a definition echoed a hundred years later by William Whewell, who wrote 'the education of the upper classes is termed *Liberal Education*'.[67] The purpose of even classical studies was to make gentlemen, not scholars,[68] and as Sheldon Rothblatt has said, 'The proof of a liberal education lay in behaviour, expressed as style, taste, fashion, or manners'.[69]

Any Edinburgh student who considered himself a gentleman, and I have found none who did not, considered his own education to be liberal. The problem he faced was redefining a concept designed originally for a landed gentleman into a useful characteristic for medical education. For a medical practitioner could not rely simply on manners; he required what John Bard had called the 'proper degree of skill' as well. Presumably the more skill he had, the more successful his eventual practice would be, and the more like a gentleman he would be able to behave. The question was what, given those assumptions, would be the most liberal form of education. Obviously classical studies alone were not enough.

The most sophisticated way of adapting the concept of liberal education to medicine was to take the pedagogical assumptions underlying a gentleman's classical studies and modify them for medical subjects. We can get some idea of how this was done from a letter of advice written by Sir John Clerk of Penicuik to his son John, on the latter's indenture to Adam Drummond and John Campbell, surgeons in Edinburgh. Sir John's

letter both shows what Lowland gentry expected in their medical practitioners and is an unusually shrewd piece of advice. Unlike medical writers,
he made no distinction between different branches of medicine; instead,
John was to prepare for as extended a practice as possible, whether as
'physician chyrurgeon or druggist', rather than surgeon alone. His preliminary education had been classical, and his father urged him to continue
his studies, for 'Physick', according to Sir John,

> can never be understood or studied as it ought without a perfect
> knowledge of the Latine. Therefore I advise you every day in your life
> to glance over these books you have been learning, that something
> may be rather added to your stock than diminished, by laziness or
> supine negligence.

Sir John especially advised 'Virgil, Ovid, Horace, and Lucretius amongst
the poets', Livy and Salust 'among the prose'. These were the standard
authors among eighteenth-century schoolboys. To them young John Clerk
was to add Celsus, for 'most of the medicinal words and phrases that can
be of any use to a physician at this day'. Celsus was, again, a standard
author, so much so that abridgements and translations of his *De re medica,
Of Medicine* went through many editions.[70]

This advice allows us to glimpse some of the assumptions behind the
frequent assertion that Latin was necessary to a physician. Horace, Ovid
and other, general authors had already given John, not only a knowledge
of Latin language and literature, but also a stock of literary allusions and
images that he had in common with other young gentlemen. Celsus was
intended as a medical version of the same shared culture, providing not so
much the literal 'medicinal words and phrases' – appended, in some
editions, in a glossary at the back of the book – but rather a vocabulary
of medical ideas and images, which would allow him to communicate with
other, similarly educated medical men.[71]

This is seen most clearly in Sir John's recommendation of Greek,
'because much of all the terms used in physick and anatomy are originally
Greek. Hippocrates therefore is an author which every physician ought to
study and understand'. Again, he had in mind the mastery of a body of
classical literature, not merely vocabulary in the narrow sense, for he also
recommended 'dayly use of Homer and Xenophon's works', and carrying
'to church a Greek Bible or New Testament'. 'I own,' he said, 'that a man
may be a great physician without the knowledge of the Greek language
but yet he will never have the honour of being reputed a scholar, without
it.'[72]

Sir John recommended other subjects in addition to Latin and Greek,
including Mathematics and Experimental Philosophy, penmanship and
bookkeeping. Yet it is not the subjects themselves that make the education
'liberal', but rather their expected outcome. Mastering them, learning the

language of medicine as he had learned the language, broadly defined, of Horace, would allow young John to enter the world of the learned physician, and of course become eminent and successful in his business. This is a view of medical knowledge as a common literary heritage shared by physicians similar to the classical literary heritage shared by gentlemen. Its impact can be seen in the clinical lectures of Professor John Rutherford, who assimilated the vocabulary of Hippocrates so thoroughly that it seemed entirely natural to him to present his careful clinical descriptions in the language of Hippocratic cases.[73]

By the second half of the century, however, there were many successful professional men who had not had John Clerk's classical education, and therefore could not see its utility, or saw only its prestige and not its pedagogical purpose. At Edinburgh and elsewhere, lecturers presented courses and wrote textbooks that assumed no knowledge of the classics, based on eighteenth-century medical concepts, observations, and vocabulary. The division between ancient and modern was not absolute: as we will see, both Hippocrates and Celsus could be adapted to eighteenth- and early nineteenth-century medical ideas. But instead of being the foundation of medical study, they became stylistic ornaments, recommended, not required, reading. 'I allow we derive much knowledge from the Ancients,' Professor William Cullen told his students,

> but they have many deficiencies from their Ignorance of Anatomy, Chemistry, and natural knowledge. They therefore cannot give us much instruction. The confusion also that prevailes in their writings is such that I cannot set them up as Models in our studies.[74]

In 1826, when the Royal Commission, unwittingly echoing Sir John Clerk, said that all medical graduates should know Greek because 'many of the medical terms [are] Greek words', Professor William Pulteney Alison found the recommendation pointless. 'A great proportion of them are diverted from their original meaning in Greek . . .' he said, 'we should rather deceive ourselves than derive any benefit from a knowledge of their precise meaning in that language.'[75] Obviously he was thinking literally of the etymology of medical words, which is not what Sir John meant at all. Alison, born in 1790, could have used Chemistry as an illustration of a branch of medicine where the vocabulary marked a complete break with the classics. In 1785, a student who knew Greek might have realized that the new chemical term oxygen meant 'begetter of acids', and therefore might have found it easier to understand that part of Antoine-Laurent Lavoisier's chemical theory. He would not have found 'oxygen' in Hippocrates, however, and by the 1820s, the new chemistry had lost even that limited connection to Greek.[76]

By the second half of the eighteenth century, then, medical education had lost the direct link to classical studies assumed by Sir John. The subjects he recommended continued to be a kind of list of course requirements for a liberal education as defined by medical writers for the following eighty years, largely because gentlemen like Sir John and the Royal Commissioners, expected practitioners to have them.[77] Classical languages were expected of the highest ranks of medical practitioners: Neville wrote that he was 'at a loss to know how a man can be a Physician and Professor without classical learning'.[78] Mathematics and experimental philosophy were considered part of a liberal education by the Royal College of Surgeons of Edinburgh.[79] John Bard told his son Samuel to pay careful attention to penmanship.[80] Only bookkeeping, which Sir John thought necessary 'in all stations in life' found no other adherents.

The opposite of a liberal education was apprenticeship, the training of an artisan, or 'mechanick' in the eighteenth-century sense.[81] At Edinburgh University the image of the apothecary's apprentice was of a social and intellectual inferior, always ready to mock his betters. 'A gentleman can declaim on the causes of diseases,' warned Professor John Gregory, '. . . but [if] he was never conversant with the sick, he is embarrassed with his erudition, and perplexed in cases, in which an apothecary's apprentice would find no difficulty.'[82] The *Guide for Gentlemen Studying Medicine* gave as a reason for the student taking Materia Medica to make sure he was never exposed to the embarrassment of being 'obliged to confess his ignorance [of drugs] to apothecary's apprentices'.[83] This distaste for servile apprenticeship, like the value placed on a liberal education, was prevalent in Georgian Britain, but it too posed a particular problem for medical students, since apprenticeship remained a common form of medical education; we will discuss some responses to it in Chapter Six.

Students' accounts of their friends show little crossing of social boundaries. David Skene roomed next to Willie Gordon, who had come with him from Aberdeen. Ismay's 'principal acquaintance' was Matthieu Cadoux, apprenticed to Thomas Williamson, the surgeon to whom Ismay had been given a letter of introduction.[84] Cadoux was Dutch but may have had some English connections, for Ismay wrote that his mother was staying at Newcastle, and that Cadoux spoke English very well. 'He generally comes and writes with me every evening till 12 O'Clock,' Ismay said, adding for good measure 'He is a very hansome and genteel young Gentleman and worthy of any person's acquaintance.'[85]

Neville's friends were more varied and less consistently studious. They could afford to be, since they, like Neville, intended to graduate, and so had the luxury of spreading their study over three years. Moreover, the concept of liberal education discouraged 'pedantry', and taverns, excursions, and membership in the Royal Medical Society were part of the required sociability.[86] Nationality played some role in determining friendships, for Ismay wrote that the students were 'Scotch, English, French,

Dutch, Irish, and from almost every Kingdom in Europe; besides a great many from America'.[87] James Rush missed having his countrymen to speak to, for he wrote at one point, 'It is so pleasant to meet an American that I must record it'.[88] Irish students may have been even more pleased to meet one another, for there was a good deal of anti-Irish feeling in Edinburgh: Sylas Neville wrote 'The Irish have an exceeding bad character here & in general they deserve it'.[89] Job Harrison's remark about expenses of English students reflects his own national bias, as does his comment that the people in Edinburgh 'are extremely civil, but speak very bad English'.[90] Most likely he had few Scots friends. Differences in religion were mentioned less frequently in student letters than differences of nationality, but Quaker students formed their own 'chain of friendship',[91] and the three Roman Catholic students who boarded in the same house as Harrison may have done the same.[92]

All these differences among students make it difficult to speak of the typical student experience. Charles Camic has argued that students at Edinburgh University received 'lessons in universalism' despite the heterogeneity of the student body, that the process of going from class to class with a mixture of other young men meant they acquired a sense of uniform standards, universally applied.[93] I have been more struck, however, with the way each student assumed his own personal experience was the standard by which others should be measured, and the pains each took to find criteria to define an 'us', consisting of his circle of friends, against a 'them'. These differences in social background and friendship were reinforced by different courses of study, as we will see.

There were at least some points of intersection among groups of students. If David Skene really never went to a tavern he was probably in the minority, and students from as varied backgrounds as Neville, Rush and Lesassier visited the Castle and Holyrood Palace, the New Town and Arthur's Seat.[94] Students also appeared to have had similar patterns of intensity and instability in friendships. 'How fickle are the friendships of young men,' Alexander Lesassier wrote after a quarrel with a man who had been one of his closest friends.[95] 'Both he and I were very proud and tenacious of our own opinions – towards the close of our friendship we each suspected the other of great duplicity. Thence, many trifles were thought of in a serious manner'.[96] Neville's principal acquaintance for his first two years at Edinburgh was Thomas Baker; Neville confided to his diary that Baker 'was not sublime', but nonetheless considered him 'a very honest, good-natured man'.[97] Yet by the time both were ready to graduate, Neville was calling Baker 'a fool & a coward',[98] told him that his conduct 'was a mixture of meanness and duplicity', and accused him of having bought his thesis.[99] Lesassier concluded that the perfect friend could only be found in a diary, and his definition explains why:

> One in whom we can confide our inmost thoughts, whilst we remain
> assured that they will never be revealed – One who is impartial and
> uninterested [and] can listen to our anxieties & misfortunes [and]
> afford us consolation & in our perplexities direct us in that line of
> conduct the most eligible – One who may serve as a memorial of
> where we formerly have erred; by reviewing which, ourselves, or
> others may, in similar circumstances avoid those breakers on which
> we foundered . . .[100]

Lesassier's definition is, we might say, typically adolescent in its intensity;
it is also extremely sentimental, and serves as a reminder that the student's
age of improvement was also his age of sentiment.[101]

Women, too, were objects of sentiment. Most students were in no
position to marry, since they could not support a wife, and young ladies
of independent fortune were not likely to wish to marry them. Thomas
Knowles, mentioned by Neville, though married, had left his wife with
her family during his year of study.[102] Sex was available in brothels,
frequently mentioned in student diaries, though not in letters to their
fathers.[103] There were other 'irregular' connections as well. Neville and his
housekeeper were one example, and he mentioned an American student
who apparently abducted a young lady from London.[104] It is hard to say
how frequent such connections were. It does not seem to have been easy
to keep them private. Neville heard about the American student from his
mother, so presumably there had been some talk about it in town. Neville
had a hard time maintaining the pretence to his landlady that his
housekeeper was only his housekeeper, and not his mistress, writing 'I hate
such prying Devils. The chambers are all so close together that what we
say or do is liable to be overheard'.[105] Neville's landlady did not actually
interfere, but clearly such arrangements could not be openly acknowledged.

Young ladies – or one particular young lady – were usually considered
off-limits for sexual intercourse, and were frequently regarded with
intense, but temporary, affection. 'I did not say love, I am sure; or if I
did, I did not mean it;' James Rush wrote, thinking of Miss Ferguson,
with whom he had spent several days taking long walks through Edinburgh; '*or* if I meant it, I did not say there was any danger of my falling
into it; or if there was, I did not say, that I had not an iron curb of reason
strong enough to back me out of it'.[106] Alexander Lesassier expressed
the same feelings, though without using the word, when he described
parting from his 'dear Laura' at the end of his first year in Edinburgh, when
he left to become an assistant surgeon in the army. He described his last
walk with her on a fine Thursday evening, when

> everything conspired to render this the most delightful walk I ever
> had . . . Our conversation turned chiefly on my approaching journey

> – But oftener we walked in silence responsively sighing – that thus we
> should be torn from each other – never perhaps to meet again . . .
> alas how blessed I should be with such a girl as she is . . . When we
> had nearly half finished our walk home . . . I chanced to touch a
> tender key – & my poor Laura burst into tears – In the height of
> enthusiasm she vowed never again to go to Arthur's Seat . . . so long
> as she lived unless in my company. [107]

If this was love, it led to neither marriage nor sexual consummation, and
there is no sign that any of those involved expected it to. Rush sternly
told 'thou little wicked god, who with thy smooth wings so often contrived
to slip between us and our duty . . . draw near . . . and read this, '*This
day commenced my attendance on lectures that is to continue for six months*'. [108]
Miss Ferguson left town, and any pangs Rush felt were gone within a
week. Lesassier wrote in his diary, 'Adieu dear Laura & may you be blest
with as good a partner for life as you deserve', but did not arrange his life
to be that partner. Even Laura, despite her tears, may have taken it for
granted that her involvement with Lesassier was temporary: she agreed
readily that she should not come to the post to see him off, and of course
never offered to accompany him. [109] Information from student diaries is
inevitably one-sided, but it may be that young ladies, too, regarded their
student admirers with intense, but temporary affection; the long walks in
Edinburgh and even the inevitable parting may have served as pleasurable
diversions from the serious business of preparing for adult life.

The most important feature of Edinburgh life shared by all students was
the study of medicine itself. More than pens and paper were needed to
prepare for lectures, for medical studies were especially known to be an
unpleasant business. Sylas Neville found it difficult to watch the dissection
of a woman in Professor Monro *secundus'* anatomy class. He wrote in his
diary,

> We had a recent subject at Monro's Theatre today for the first time.
> It is the body of a woman. The melancholy nature of my present
> studies increases the lowness of my spirits. [110]

Neville had no medical experience prior to his arrival in Edinburgh, and
his reaction was probably similar to that of many of the students confronted
with the realities of dissections and operations. Neville did get used to
such subject matter: within a week he could write, 'The dissection of the
recent body I daily see makes me think what poor corruptible creatures we
are but does not affect my spirits so much as I feared'. [111] Even after several
years of medical study, though, James Rush could not sit through one
operation for breast cancer. 'The mamma was taken off very expeditiously
indeed,' he wrote,

> and I was about to give credit to the hand of the operator – But just
> as the ligatures had all been applied, and the dressings were about to

be put on – It was discovered that the diseased part had not been entirely extracted . . . the barbarous handling and even *punching* of wounded flesh . . . which followed – was too shocking to look at.[112] Nor was he the only one so affected, for 'let me add' he wrote, 'of some medical students whose rough exterior, scarcely justified a suspicion that there was any feeling within – that a number of them left the room'.[113] Medical studies were known to induce melancholy in students, and Dr Manning, who had recommended to Neville that he study in Edinburgh, wrote and inquired after Neville's state of mind, saying 'Physic was not the most proper study for one that had not good spirits'.[114]

There was much in the content of medical studies to depress the spirits. The phenomenon of students fearing that they were suffering from diseases they read about apparently occurred in the eighteenth century as it does today. Alexander Monro *secundus* told the story of a student who was afraid that he had dropsy, the cure for which could have been paracentesis, an operation which involved cutting into the abdomen and applying pressure to make the fluid run out.[115] Monro had mentioned in a lecture that one symptom of dropsy in the pleura was the sound caused by the fluid which collected in that part of the body; the practitioner could, he said, hear the noise of the fluid 'as we hear the dashing of water in a bottle half full'.[116] One student, hearing this, 'took a fancy he had a dropsy and wrote as much to his friends'. Monro went to see him,

> and was surprised to find a fat well coloured fellow dying of a dropsy, but he told me it was beyond all doubt, for not merely a motion was felt, but it could be heard, and I heard it most distinctly.[117]

Presumably after a little gentle inquiry, Monro found the reason for the noise: before diagnosing himself, the student 'had drunk pretty freely', and Monro thought 'he had done so on purpose, for his idea was that the stomach needed to be distended before it could press against the water in the pleura'.[118] No doubt the student was genuinely frightened, and Monro may have told the story as much to reassure students concerning their own fears of diseases as to illustrate the necessity for careful attention to symptoms in dropsical patients.

Monro's student's illness proved to be imaginary, but medical students were known to suffer from genuine illnesses. Neville complained after two months in Edinburgh, 'Have a most disagreeable cold in my head. Have had more colds since I came here that I had had for 3 or 4 years.'[119] Professor John Gregory warned students of a particular form of fever, which 'several young gentlemen of our own profession here, are liable to'.[120] This fever, he said, was 'more commonly owing to their living rather under what they were accustomed to at home; from their giving too great application to their studies, and from too great anxiety of mind'.[121] The remedy for the fever was strict attention to regimen: students should restrict themselves to a vegetable diet, should abstain from alcohol, should take exercise, either on horseback or in a carriage, and take, Gregory advised, 'a total cessation from business'.[122]

Medical students, because of the nature of their subject matter, were even more vulnerable to illness than students generally. There is a special poignancy in Ismay's writing to his father, 'When I consider the Money that it will cost me during my stay at this place, it makes me confine myself too close to my study; more so than is conducive to my health',[123] for Ismay died at the end of his year of study at Edinburgh. A note attached to his letter said that he 'died in the Bloom of Life, much regretted by his Friends and Acquaintances and was interred in Grey Friars' church yard . . . The Pall was supported by ye Medical Professors'.[124] Charles Darwin, a particularly promising student, fell ill and died as a result of performing a dissection.[125] Professor Andrew Duncan senior had Darwin interred in his own family's burial plot, as he did for several other students who died while in Edinburgh. There are five or six who surround Duncan's own grave in the family mausoleum in Buccleuch churchyard.

Yet disease was a part of the profession which had brought all these young gentlemen to Edinburgh. Having arrived, presented letters, found lodgings, and made acquaintances, they were ready to choose courses. How they went about it is the subject of the next chapter.

3

The courses:
a guide for gentlemen studying medicine

> I waited upon Dr Rutherford who received me very kindly,
> and desired I would give his Service to you, when I wrote you.
> I told him: if he would be at the trouble to give me his advice
> as to what Colleges I should attend, you had desired I should
> follow it. He replied he would willingly assist me in anything
> he could as to the Classes. He thought the students commonly
> erred in attending too few, as their time would admit of more
> and these were opportunities that are not to be often had.
>
> David Skene to his father, Dr. Andrew Skene[1]

The first step in understanding patterns of medical education at Edinburgh
University is to look at the available courses. Formal matriculation took
place in November at the beginning of the Winter Term, when students
convened in the university library to sign the Matriculation Album.
Thomas Parke, who matriculated in 1771, wrote that the process was
accompanied with some ceremony: the Principal, William Robertson,
attended in full academic dress, and each student was called in turn to pay
his fee of half a crown to the library, and sign the Album.[2] From 1762,
medical students were listed separately because, as the statute explained,

> That as the Library at present is not properly stocked with medical
> books, the sum arising from the contributions of the students of
> Medicine shall be entirely appropriated to purchase such books as
> shall be thought most usefull to them.[3]

At the time of matriculation students also wrote down, or told the clerk,
what courses they intended to take that year. The Matriculation Albums
are thus our main source for student course attendance, and seem to have
been taken seriously by the University as a way of keeping track of
students, for additional information was inserted into the lists at certain
points, to make sure they were accurate. One such note stated that 'Dr
Monro attested that the above James Young attended the Anat in 1754',[4]
another that 'NB John Moffat studied this year Bot, Anat & Chir, Med
Pract'.[5] The University may have wished to keep a record for administrative purposes, for on March 31, 1763, just after the enactment of the

regulation concerning the Matriculation Albums, a University meeting established

> that all students of the University who desired to have a certificate of their attendance upon the different classes should hereafter have a certificate from the Secretary of the University upon their paying five shillings ster[ling] for the same . . .[6]

Matriculation, though, was not absolutely necessary to attend classes. What was absolutely necessary was paying the professor a class fee for each course and receiving a ticket, for the janitor in each lecture hall had orders to admit only students with tickets. A comparison of professors' class lists and matriculation records reveals that many students between 1760 and 1811 attended classes without matriculating.[7] Their reasons for not matriculating varied. There seems to have been some unwritten rule that students who had graduated the previous spring could attend classes in the fall without matriculating, for many did so.[8] Some students may have taken literally the idea that matriculation gave access to the library, and decided it was unnecessary. The library was open four days per week, from 10 am to 1 pm, according to Peter Mark Roget, who did matriculate. 'I borrowed a few [books],' he wrote, 'but as I have no time to read at present, shall defer it to the summer.'[9] Other students may also have assumed they would not have time to read books, and thus did not matriculate. Some may have arrived in town after matriculation, and so never bothered to sign. Some may simply have wished to save half a crown. Even the desire to obtain a certificate from the University was not necessarily a reason to matriculate, for class tickets could be used to correct the Album. One note in the Album recorded, 'It appears from his tickets that James Malcom was this year a student of Anat & Chir, Chem, Med Pract'.[10]

Despite the ways of getting around it, matriculation appears to have been taken seriously by the majority of medical students from 1762 on. It became even more formal after 1811, when the increasing size of the student body made it impossible to convene everyone in the library at once. Instead, students would come to the library over a period of several days in November and give their name, county, and whether they were enrolling in the faculties of law, medicine, theology or arts. Professor Andrew Duncan junior, as University Librarian, passed a resolution in 1812 that raised the matriculation fee to ten shillings, extended the hours of the library, and warned students that matriculation was 'the only legal record of their attendance in the University'.[11] The University sub-librarian, Nicholas Bain, put their names in rough alphabetical order and issued each a ticket with a unique matriculation number. Bain then collected all professor's class lists, and checked each student listed against his matriculation records. Next he compiled a complete list of medical students, in rough alphabetical order, with the courses they had actually paid to attend. This immense effort worked to decrease the number of non-matriculating students, though not to eliminate them entirely, since it was still possible to attend classes without matriculating. Many students, as we will see, did not need a legal record of having attended a University.[12]

The Edinburgh University matriculation albums kept unusually careful, detailed records of course attendance.[13] Some of the reason for it is obvious: professors were paid by their students, and so had an obvious incentive to keep careful lists of attendance. Similarly, medical matriculation paid for medical books, and every fee collected by the clerk or librarian presumably had to be accounted for. Still, the University had no obvious financial incentive for recording which courses students attended, or, after 1811, what county they came from. One reason for doing so seems to have been a general concern for careful records found in many Edinburgh medical institutions such as the Royal Infirmary and the Royal Colleges of Physicians and Surgeons.[14] Another was that all disputes among faculty, between faculty and the Town Council, the University patrons, or between faculty and students were apt to end either in court or in print. Careful records of the University activities, including student course attendance, could provide useful evidence if the University's authority or actions were ever questioned.

The main reason was probably that Edinburgh University, to a greater degree than most educational institutions in the period, relied on its students, not just for professor's fees, but also for its reputation. What students did there was not incidental to the successful functioning of the University, but vital; Edinburgh could not afford to have students merely matriculate, and leave their education to tutors, like Oxford and Cambridge. Medical students came to take medical lectures, and the large numbers of students who came provided the criterion for measuring the success of the lectures, and indeed all of University medical education. Nearly all professors who wrote any pamphlet proclaiming the value of their courses referred to the large number of students they attracted;[15] Andrew Duncan senior made a similar point for the medical faculty as a whole when he proudly published the numbers of 'students of physic' in *Annals of Medicine* in 1799.[16] What made these claims different from those of professors at other Universities is that at Edinburgh, from 1762 on, those figures could be verified. It was essential for Edinburgh's reputation that they had to be verifiable.

In this chapter we will examine each of the medical lectures in order of student attendance, though we might wish to reserve judgement as to whether their value should be gauged by their attendance alone. Each course was offered every year, and each was scheduled at a separate hour, and, wrote Ismay, 'The Colledge [sic] Bell generally rings to every class'[17] so that it would have been possible for a student to attend them all in a single year, though few did.[18] All classes except those that made use of the Royal Infirmary met five days per week. This was the most extensive selection of medical lectures available at any university in Britain, a source of pride to the faculty and convenience to the students. Mary Hewson exhorted her son Thomas at great length to go to Edinburgh, for, she said,

> It is very likely that more practical knowledge in medicine may be acquired in London or even in Paris, but the question is, will a young man apply as much in either of these cities, as he will in a University where every branch of science is regularly taught, and drawn together so compactly from one to the other?[19]

No, was her reply, leaving no room for Thomas Hewson to disagree. Professor John Rutherford told David Skene to take as many courses as possible, since 'these were opportunities that are not to be often had'.[20]

To understand these opportunities, we must examine just what 'every branch of science' consisted of. Let us assume, then, that it is the first week of the Winter Session, when professors gave introductory lectures for free to aid students in choosing courses. We have no strict instructions from parents or teachers, and since the cost of each course is the same, three guineas, we can consider each course on its own merit.[21] To make up for our lack of letters of introduction to professors who might advise us as to courses, we can take with us J. Johnson's *Guide for Gentlemen Studying Medicine at the University of Edinburgh*, price 1s 6d, which described the content of each course, and gave the author's own opinions on their importance. The occasionally polemical comments of the *Guide* led Alexander and James Hamilton, Professors of Midwifery, to be accused of writing it, but as students we would be unaware of that.[22] To balance the remarks of the *Guide*, and for further assistance, we can turn to the opinions of eminent medical authors, and to reports of students who have been to Edinburgh before, and can tell us what they found.[23]

The best-attended course was Anatomy and Surgery, attracting an average of 65 per cent of the students in each cohort. Anatomy, according to the *Guide*, was 'very properly considered to be the foundation of all medical studies', since a knowledge of the structure of the body in its healthy state was necessary to anyone who wanted to treat its diseases.[24] Anatomy was taught in this period by the Alexander Monros, *secundus* and *tertius*. Monro *secundus* had taken over the course from his father, Alexander Monro *primus*, in 1754. He has usually been considered the ablest of the three Monros, a distinguished anatomist as well as an eminent lecturer.[25] Under Monro *secundus*, an average of 88 per cent of the students per cohort attended Anatomy and Surgery. The course had originally been called, simply, Anatomy, but in 1777 Monro *secundus* had the name of the chair changed to Anatomy and Surgery. This was a direct response to a petition of the College of Surgeons to the Crown requesting a new Professorship of Surgery, with the appointment of one of their Members to the new position. Monro claimed that he had originally been appointed Professor of Anatomy and Surgery, and he requested that the Town Council consolidate his position by giving him a new commission 'expressly authorizing him to be professor of medicine and particularly of anatomy and surgery'.[26] The Town Council supported Monro against the College, perhaps because of the numbers of students he succeeded in attracting to his course each year. The Town Council may have seen no reason to quarrel with a professor who had such a proven record of success.

The lectures of Monro *secundus* were highly commended by the *Guide*, for in addition to discussing the structure of each part of the body, he considered 'the different diseases which may be occasioned by the derangement or accidental injury of any of the organs'.[27] This was usually covered in the first half of the course; in the second, Monro discussed the different surgical operations, 'and performed them on a dead body to impress the rules'.[28] He ended the course with a general discussion of physiology and comparative anatomy.

Not everyone was as impressed with Monro *secundus* as the *Guide*. George Logan complained that Monro was

> too great a Philosopher to enter so minutely into his subject as the demonstrative part of it requires, on which account Students may attend him three or four years without gaining a proper knowledge of this kind.

But, he added, 'in his Physiology, perhaps no person is equal to him for perspicuity and strength of argument'.[29] Logan had in fact picked up one of Monro's main points, though without being aware of it. Monro's course was an ongoing argument for the value of the philosophical anatomist, who used his understanding of anatomy to devise new surgical procedures. When he referred to 'surgeons' he usually meant only a competent operator, and he was not, in fact, very interested in merely demonstrating existing operations.[30] Not even Logan thought of skipping the course entirely, though, for since Monro lectured 'on Anatomy and Surgery it is necessary for persons in every department of Medicine to attend him'.[31] Students who attended the lectures were getting an introduction to essential aspects of medicine, anatomy, physiology, and surgical operations. This was enough to make even those critical of Monro's style or ideas attend his course.

The subject matter of the Anatomy and Surgery course was so important that not even Alexander Monro *tertius*, a notoriously bad lecturer, could drive students away entirely. When Monro *tertius* took over the course from his father in 1798 the percentage of students who attended the course did drop, from an average of 88 per cent of the students in each cohort to an average of about 70 per cent; after 1810, the percentage fell to only 38 per cent of the students per cohort. Not all of this was Monro *tertius'* fault. From 1800, he faced more competition than his father, from private lecturers like John Barclay and John Bell,[32] from London lecturers like Sir Charles Bell or the hospital schools, or from Professor James Jeffray's Anatomy lectures at the University of Glasgow[33] and James Macartney's at the College of Surgeons in Dublin.[34] Even more competition came from the fact that anatomical dissection increasingly became essential for medical study, and cadavers were hard to obtain in Edinburgh. Monro *tertius* may not have seen any reason to be concerned about this, since the number of students increased so much over the period that the number actually enrolled in his class each year stayed about the same, fluctuating between 150 and 200 from 1800 to 1826. He may have assumed he was carrying on his father's tradition, since the same number of students took his class as had attended his father's.[35] Anatomy and Surgery was offered from 1 pm to 3 pm, 'because', the Royal Commissioners were informed, 'for many anatomical demonstrations, the best possible light is required, and the dissections for these must immediately precede the lecture'.[36] Monro *tertius* also offered a practical anatomy class at 4 pm, in addition to his lectures, which enrolled twenty-three students in 1815.[37]

If the percentage of students in Anatomy in each cohort declined by the end of the period, the percentage of students in Chemistry increased. An average of 76 per cent of the students per cohort attended Chemistry from 1763–1826. William Cullen taught the Chemistry course from 1755 to 1766, when his student, Joseph Black, took over.[38] Black was not a very inspiring lecturer, 'good Language & very instructive', wrote Thomas Parke in 1773, 'but I blush for his delivery'.[39] Even so, he managed to attract an average of 58 per cent of the students in each cohort through the 1770s. John Gregory set out the reasons for Chemistry's importance to medical students in his *Observations on the Duties and Offices of a Physician; and on the Method of Prosecuting Enquiries in Philosophy*. A knowledge of natural philosophy, he said, would help students understand the mechanical principles of the body, but they also needed to understand the chemical principles, by which 'various changes are induced upon the fluids'. It is, he said,

> therefore necessary to be acquainted with the chemical history of the animal fluids, with the chemical history of whatever is taken into the human body as food or physic, and in general, of all the substances which can, in any degree, influence it.[40]

Anatomy and physiology would teach students about the mechanical changes in the human body; chemistry would teach them about the chemical changes.

From the early 1780s, the percentage of students in each cohort who attended Chemistry began to rise, reaching an average of 81 per cent in each cohort after 1798, when Thomas Charles Hope took over the course. Many of these students, such as Lord Cochrane and Josiah Wedgewood, came expressly for the purpose of hearing about the 'New Chemistry' expounded by the celebrated Dr Black, rather than for general medical instruction. Black seems, in fact, to have directed his course at that audience, rather than the more pragmatic medical students. According to the *Guide*, he divided his course into two parts. In the first, he discussed the effects of heat, including his own research into latent heat; in the second, he gave a general account of mixture. The lectures were, the *Guide* explained,

> admirably well adapted for the ordinary run of his pupils, for they are calculated to exhibit general views of chemistry; nothing more is necessary either for gentlemen, or for the greatest numbers of practitioners of the healing art.[41]

No doubt Wedgewood and others like him were pleased, but at least some students were not. George Logan said that Black's lectures, like Monro's, 'were more calculated for the physician as philosopher than as a practitioner',[42] and Sylas Neville was annoyed that Black cut short the section of the course that dealt with pharmacy.[43]

Students in Black's chemistry course, then, might have the satisfaction of knowing they were attending the lectures of a great philosopher, but they would not learn how to compound medicaments. This tradition was continued when Thomas Charles Hope taught the course. He turned it into a series of colourful and dramatic demonstrations, in order to play to a fashionable audience as well as attract students; John Leslie, Professor of Natural Philosophy, referred to Hope as the 'Showman in the other corner'.[44] Chemistry was offered at 10 am.

The course in Medical Practice was not, despite its name, a course where students actually got practical experience with patients, but instead an explanation of pathology, the various diseases with their causes, symptoms, cure, and prognosis. It attracted an average of 61 per cent of the student per cohort. The *Guide* called it 'the important object of medical students', but did not explain its contents, obviously assuming that all his readers would be familiar with it.[45] As one such student, J. T. Ford, explained, pathology followed naturally after the study of Anatomy and Physiology, which discussed those powers in the human body which preserve health, because it dealt with 'when those powers are counteracted or their effects diminished or obviated or their actions irritated'.[46]

Robert Whytt taught the course from 1747 to 1765. According to David Skene in 1751,

> Dr Whyte is reckoned a very clever fellow, and the book he has just now published very well esteem'd: But few people recommend his

lectures; and as far as I can hear, I would be giving him 3 Guineas for reading over Haller; which may be cheaper done at home.[47]

It was probably for similar reasons that only an average of 34 per cent of the students in each cohort attended Whytt's lectures between 1763 and 1765; in 1766, when John Gregory began teaching the course, the enrollment jumped to 60 per cent of the students in that cohort.

Some students were not pleased by Gregory's appointment to the chair, and would have preferred William Cullen. Cullen was one of the most popular professors in Edinburgh, and in his position as Professor of Chemistry, he had built up a student following, which lasted throughout his life. 'The inimitable Dr Cullen', Thomas Parke called him;[48] to other students he was 'the Scotch Hippocrates', 'that shining oracle of physic', 'the great the unrivalled Dr. Cullen'.[49] He was appointed to the chair of Medical Theory at the same time that Gregory became Professor of Medical Practice, and some students petitioned the Town Council to reverse the appointments, making Cullen Professor of Medical Practice, and Gregory, of Medical Theory.[50] The Town Council refused to make the change, but in 1769 Cullen and Gregory agreed to alternate teaching the two courses, so that one year Cullen taught Medical Theory and Gregory taught Medical Practice, and the following year the men switched. This continued until 1772, when Gregory died, and Cullen was appointed Professor of Medical Practice.

Cullen did draw more students than Gregory between 1769 and 1771, even when he taught Medical Theory, which usually attracted far fewer students than Medical Practice.[51] However, not even Cullen teaching Medical Practice could attract as many students as Monro *secundus* in Anatomy and Surgery: 184 in 1769, 193 in 1770, and 211 in 1771.[52] A popular lecturer, then, could certainly attract more students to his course, but he could not alter basic patterns of course attendance.

Thomas Ismay illustrates the point that students did not choose courses merely on the basis of the professor. He studied in Edinburgh in 1771, when Cullen was teaching Medical Practice. Ismay would have preferred to hear Gregory, for, he said, Cullen

is accounted very clever, but generally deals too much upon Theory. Dr Gregory is liked by some persons much better, as he only regards theory as far as is requisite for practice.[53]

Ismay, evidently, had come to Edinburgh to learn about rheumatism, apoplexy, and so on, not Cullen's theory of disease causation. Yet he did not consider paying an extra three guineas to hear Gregory in Medical Theory, or returning another year to take Gregory's Medical Practice. His main object was to learn about diseases and their treatment; he would do that in Medical Practice no matter who was teaching it. Of course, Ismay had only attended Cullen's class for two weeks at that point, and had never attended Gregory's; presumably his information came from other students.

Cullen arranged his lectures on Medical Practice according to the principles of his Nosology.[54] Nosology literally means the study of disease, but in the eighteenth century the word referred to the classification of diseases into classes, order, and genera according to their symptoms. Learned opinion varied as to whether the classification reflected real differences in the cause of disease, or was simply a convenient way of arranging diseases. Linnaeus, whose 'passion for order and classification extended to his medical work',[55] may well have believed that his nosological system described different species of disease. It is hard to tell if Cullen did. His lectures stressed the utility of classification as a learning aid for students, for 'you cannot too soon begin to learn the general characters of diseases', Cullen told his classes.[56] James Ford may have reflected this pragmatic approach to nosology when he wrote that 'too much dependance cannot be placed upon this kind of knowledge . . . as must appear from the multitude of cases which act upon the human body, and which are therefore incapable of being particularized in a scheme of nosology'. However, he concluded, such a scheme was 'a good introduction to the knowledge of diseases – and observation alone can supply its defects'.[57] Nosology continued to be used as a pedagogical tool: James Gregory followed Cullen's system when he took over the course in Medical Practice in 1790, despite his misgivings over the value of nosologies in actual treatment.[58] An average of approximately 60 per cent of the students in each cohort attended the class under Cullen and the number rose slightly to an average of 70 per cent under James Gregory. After Gregory died in 1821, James Home took over the professorship, and the students per cohort declined to an average of 42 per cent. Medical Practice was offered at 9 am.

Medical Theory, or Institutions of Medicine, was not as well attended as Medical Practice, going from an average of 36 per cent of the students in each cohort to 50 per cent after 1811. It was certainly not a prerequisite to Medical Practice, as the name seems to imply, since it attracted far fewer students. In 1773, when Cullen began teaching Medical Practice, Alexander Monro Drummond was appointed Professor, 'the most learned, most ingenious, and most ornate Physician ever bred at this University', Neville reported Cullen as saying.[59] However Drummond, who had been in Italy when appointed, never returned to Edinburgh to teach, preferring to remain in Naples.[60] Francis Home taught the course for two sessions, and Andrew Duncan senior was given a temporary position as lecturer in the course for another two, until 1778, when James Gregory began teaching. Probably the chair had been kept vacant deliberately for James Gregory, to give him time to get his MD in 1774 and study abroad, for Gregory was the son of John Gregory, and the Edinburgh professorate looked after its own.[61] Gregory taught Medical Theory until 1790, when he took over the position of Professor of Medical Practice on Cullen's death. Andrew Duncan senior was then appointed Professor of Medical Theory.

In the nineteenth century, Medical Theory became the Physiology course, but in the eighteenth century its subject matter was not that well defined. Its object, according to the *Guide*, was 'to explain the principles on which the practice of physic is founded'.[62] William Cullen divided his course into three parts:

> The first treats of life and health. The second delivers the general doctrines of diseases. The third delivers the general doctrine concerning the means of preventing and curing disease.[63]

Andrew Duncan, according to the *Guide*, also divided his subject matter into three parts, but differed from Cullen's arrangement. The first covered the 'nature, properties, and diseases', of the human body, the second, therapeutics, or the use and operation of medication, and the third, medical jurisprudence. The second and third parts reflected Duncan's own interests, and so were presumably his own additions to the course.[64]

The content of the course explains its comparatively low attendance, for much of the material in it was presented in other classes as well. The material on the nature and properties of the human body in health, as the *Guide* pointed out, was covered in the Anatomy lectures; though he went on to say that the Medical Theory course would give a 'connected view of the whole', students may have found this unnecessary. Diseases were discussed in detail in the Medical Practice class, and medications, in Materia Medica, for those students who had not learned about them during apprenticeship. Medical jurisprudence, the third part of Duncan's course, would have been entirely new to most students, but most students would not have found the material useful for practice. When, in 1807, Medical Jurisprudence became a separate course, comparatively few students attended.[65] The course on Medical Theory, then, was a grab-bag of topics covered elsewhere. The low course attendance cannot be blamed solely on Duncan, either, for James Gregory, who later attracted 70 per cent of the students in each cohort in Medical Practice, attracted an average of only 35 per cent when he taught Medical Theory. Medical Practice was taught at 11 am.[66]

Clinical Lectures were given twice a week at the Royal Infirmary of Edinburgh, three months by one professor and three months by another. It attracted an average of 33 per cent of the students per cohort. The course had been started by John Rutherford in 1748, but from the 1750s were given by whichever two professors wished to do so.[67] Two wards of the Infirmary, one men's and one women's, were set aside for the patients whose cases were discussed in the lectures. According to the *Guide*, 'their cases were explained, and the reasons for the various remedies which have been employed clearly pointed out'.[68] Clinical Lectures were one of the few places where medical students could actually see patients, and few other universities provided similar opportunities.[69] It is all the more surprising, then, to find that only an average of 33 per cent of the students in each cohort attended the Clinical Lectures. More students may have made use of the Infirmary, for tickets for admission to walk the wards were sold separately from those for Clinical Lectures. The Infirmary was open for this purpose between 12 noon and 1 pm. The cost was one guinea for apprentices of Fellows of the Royal College of Surgeons, and two guineas for the rest of the students.[70] We have no way of knowing how many students purchased tickets and visited the Infirmary patients on their own. Still, one would have expected more students to take advantage of the opportunity to hear lectures.

One reason why more students did not attend may have been the overcrowding in the course, which seems to have afflicted the class very soon after its inception in 1748. By 1751, David Skene was already complaining that during the Clinical Lectures

> there is always such a crowd of students about the physician and surgeon, that there is nothing either to be seen or heard, nor even a great deal of benefit if both were to be had. A few superficial questions are asked and some medicines prescribed without saying why.[71]

Josef Frank, in 1804, gave a vivid picture of the overcrowding in the Clinical Lectures, where only those near the patient could follow what was going on, and students in the back pushed and jostled, or else chattered among themselves.[72]

An even more important reason for the comparatively low attendance is that the Clinical Lectures co-existed with other forms of patient contact for the novice practitioner, such as apprenticeship or walking the wards of a hospital. Even students eager to see patients might have decided to save their three guineas, and perhaps find a surgeon who would allow them to accompany him in his practice.[73] Or they might simply have gone to London, the 'Metropolis of the whole World for practical Medicine', or Paris, where there were many more opportunities for clinical experience.[74]

Students may also simply have felt, like twentieth-century students, that they would learn more from studying texts than from the routine practice they would see on the wards.[75] Silas Neville, after Professor John Gregory's death, arranged to get a copy of his Clinical Lectures, saying 'they are the best cases and reports I ever read';[76] apparently he saw nothing incongruous in reading cases which began with an exhortation for students to learn clinical medicine from patients, not from books.[77] Samuel Lewis, sixty years later, refused an offer to be a dresser in the Infirmary, because, he said,

> If I had become a dresser I should have been obliged to spend at least

an hour and a half daily in the Hospital, and that would have been so much time lost in making myself fit for my approaching examination. There is little to learn as a dresser, all that you are allowed to do is to bandage ulcers etc. and one must be a very stupid fellow who can't learn all the mystery of bandaging in three months.[78]

Hospital practice was still primarily limited to charity patients as well, which meant that students would acquire experience with diseases of the poor, generally not a group they wished to treat as practitioners. Edinburgh medical students, then, may have been even less willing than modern ones to forego studying medicine from texts for attending clinical lectures. Clinical Lectures were held on Tuesdays and Fridays at 4 pm.

The Midwifery course also provided an opportunity for students to have contact with patients, and it attracted an average of 27 per cent of the students in each cohort. The course was taught by Thomas Young from 1756 to 1780, when he was joined by Alexander Hamilton; in 1800, Hamilton's son James took over the professorship.

Thomas Young seems to have given two courses each year in Midwifery. The first cost each student three guineas, and, according to Ismay, the second another two and a half guineas. There was substantial inducement to taking the second course, for, Ismay wrote, 'If I attend [Young's] second course, I shall then deliver myself, but now I am only present at them'.[79] The *Guide* describes the Hamiltons as also using the inducement of patient contact to increase their fees. For the three guinea fee, students received a series of lectures on the care of pregnant women, the management of labour, the care of women immediately after childbirth and the diseases of early infancy. If a student took the course a second time, he paid two guineas, and three times, one guinea. For an additional 11s 6d he could watch and assist at deliveries in the Lying-In Ward of the Royal Infirmary, which was under Alexander Hamilton's direction. Or for ten guineas, he could become an Annual Pupil, and visit Hamilton's own private patients, have charge of his own cases, and attend the lectures and Lying-In Ward without extra charge.[80] After 1793, students could also attend James Hamilton's Lying-In Hospital, established 'for the purpose of affording relief to the wives of indigent tradesmen'.[81]

The Midwifery professors might use the carrot of seeing patients to attract students, but they could not use the stick of graduation requirements, for Midwifery was the only course taught by a member of the medical faculty which was not required for graduation. The *Guide* posed the question of whether this was due to 'the jealousy of other professors, the negligence of the professor of midwifery, or the ignorance of the patrons of the university?'[82] The *Guide*'s concern over the status of the Midwifery course was one reason why Alexander and James Hamilton were each accused of writing it. Midwifery was offered at 3 pm.

Materia Medica attracted an average of 38 per cent of the students per cohort from 1763–1826. Francis Home taught Materia Medica from 1768 until 1798, and only succeeded in attracting an average of 25 per cent of the students in each cohort to the course, 'as it is a thing not very necessary to a Person, that has been acquainted with Medicine before', according to Thomas Ismay.[83] Home was succeeded by his son James, who taught until 1821. Under James Home, the percentage of students increased, to 50 per cent per cohort. Perhaps Home can be given credit for this, but more likely other changes in medicine contributed to the increase, as we will see in Chapter Eight.

The *Guide* described Materia Medica as essentially a course in pharmacy. In the first part, Francis Home discussed the 'history, qualities, doses, etc, of all the animal vegetable and mineral substances' used in medication. In the second part, he explained how to compound them. Since, according to the *Guide*, most of the medication in common use were easily learned, 'it has become fashionable for the young gentlemen studying at Edinburgh, to despise or neglect Dr Home's class'.[84] Indeed, according to Neville, it was not only Home's class, but also his knowledge, that was 'despised by the generality of the students'.[85] The *Guide* could not come up with many reasons why Materia Medica was essential; its main argument was that the practitioner should take the course to make sure he was never exposed to the embarrassment of being 'obliged to confess his ignorance [of drugs] to apothecary's apprentices'.[86] Materia Medica was offered at 8 am.

Botany only attracted an average of 25 per cent of the students in each cohort. It was taught by John Hope from 1761 to 1785, who behaved, according to Neville, 'with much good nature to his pupils, doing every thing in his power to instruct them . . . '.[87] Daniel Rutherford, son of John Rutherford, taught the course from 1786 to 1820. The attendance at Botany may have been under-reported in the Matriculation Albums because it was given only in the Summer, not during the Winter term. It may also have attracted few students simply because it was given in the summer. They may have reasoned that there was no point in staying on in town, and paying rent and an additional three guineas, just to look at plants 'which may be cheaper done at home', to borrow David Skene's phrase. Job Harrison was certainly not pleased to be in Edinburgh in July. He wrote that

> Edinburgh is now more filthy and disagreeable than in winter, particularly at night after eleven o clock, when the inhabitants discharge their daily excrement thro' the windows, and in the morning before the scavengers have cleaned the streets. I am obliged to go quite thro the town every morning to the Botanical Garden, and whenever the morning is hot, and at the same time free from wind, the stench is intolerable.[88]

Botany hardly seemed worth the effort. The *Guide* did not speak favourably

of Daniel Rutherford's course, and mentioned that most vegetable preparations could be obtained in shops and were described in Materia Medica
treatises. The author still recommended that students take Botany,
however, for reasons similar to those for attending Materia Medica: it
would keep the practitioner's abilities from 'being called in question by
his ignorance of the principles of a science which is vulgarly believed to
be necessary'.[89]

These were the courses given by the medical faculty throughout the
period 1760–1826. On the basis of attendance, they fall into two groups.
The first consists of the three best-attended courses, Anatomy and Surgery,
Chemistry, and Medical Practice, which attracted an average of 65 per
cent, 76 per cent and 61 per cent respectively of the students per cohort.
The second group consists of the rest of the courses, Medical Theory,
Clinical Lectures, Midwifery, Materia Medica and Botany, which averaged
between 20 per cent and 40 per cent of the students in each cohort. See
Table 3.1.

In addition to those courses which were offered throughout the period,
there were several which were only offered for part of the time. Cullen
gave a course in Nosology, beginning in 1770 and continuing until his

Table 3.1 Average course attendance, total student body, 1763–1826

Anatomy and Surgery:	65%	Medical Theory:	37%
Chemistry:	76%	Clinical Lectures:	33%
Medical Practice:	61%	Midwifery:	27%
		Materia Medica:	38%
		Botany:	25%

death in 1789. The course is listed in the Matriculation Albums after that date, but it is not clear who taught it.[90] According to the Album, twenty to thirty students took the course each year, most of them older students, interested in hearing more of Cullen's ideas from the great Professor himself. Cullen also gave private lectures for students who were attending his courses for the second time. Samuel Bard attended them in 1764, when Cullen lectured on chemical pathology, but the topic mattered less to him than the informal contact with his revered professor. 'What I greatly admire is the manner in which [Cullen] gives these lectures,' Bard wrote,

> we convene at his own house once or twice a week, where after lecturing for one hour, we spend another in an easy conversation upon the subject of the last evenings lecture, & every one is encouraged to make his remarks or objections with the greatest freedom & ease – I can not help comparing him upon these occasions to *Socrates* or some other of the ancient philosophers surrounded by his admiring pupils.[91]

These informal conversations go a long way towards explaining why students – the select group of students who attended these private lectures – regarded Cullen with such affection, and listened to him 'with the greatest pleasure and attention', according to Bard. They also suggest that professors, too, had their own ways of defining 'students of medicine strictly speaking', and that however important Cullen's courses in Chemistry and Medical Practice were in maintaining his genteel style of life, it was his smaller classes which, as Bard thought, 'must certainly make him very happy'.[92]

Other courses which appear in the matriculation records were instituted between 1800 and 1826: Clinical Surgery, taught by James Russell, in 1803, Military Surgery, taught by John Thomson, in 1806, and in 1807, Medical Jurisprudence, taught in succession by Andrew Duncan junior, William Pulteney Alison, and Robert Christison. These courses will be discussed in more detail in later chapters.

Students could also attend courses given by extra-academical lecturers, that is, teachers unaffiliated with the university, who lectured on medical subjects. Sylas Neville, together with five other students, attended a 'private course of Anatomy' given by John Innes, Monro's demonstrator.[93] Since Monro's course was so large, students had little opportunity to actually see dissections close at hand, and there was no provision for students to dissect as part of the course. In Innes' class, students could observe much more, and according to Neville, 'As so small a number were admitted and we had so good an opportunity of attending to every demonstration, I received much benefit from it'.[94] When Andrew Fyfe became demonstrator, he too offered private classes.[95] Neville in 1771 also took a course in Therapeutics, taught by Andrew Duncan senior, who was at that point 'a private Lecturer and thought clever'.[96] Duncan was, as mentioned earlier, appointed temporary university lecturer in Medical Theory. When the permanent appointment was given to James Gregory, he went back to extra-academical teaching. In 1776 he set up his own clinic, which became the Public Dispensary, in order to attract students.[97]

Since many students, like Neville, were anxious for further instruction, extra-academical lectureships could be quite lucrative, and were a common employment for young men who had just completed their studies, especially those who aspired to university positions. James Russell and John Thomson started out as extra-academical lecturers, as did Duncan. Other lecturers were never appointed to university posts, but became prominent teachers in their own right, such as John Barclay and Charles Bell, both lecturers in anatomy. Extra-academical classes were offered in practical chemistry from 1800 and, like practical anatomy, provided opportunities for students to learn manual techniques which were only demonstrated in University lectures.[98] No class lists are available for any of the extra-academical courses, but since some of them continued for many years, they must have been successful in attracting students. Andrew Duncan claimed that his lectures in the Dispensary attracted over 100 students in the first session in 1776, an impressive figure considering that only twenty-six students signed the Matriculation Album as attending Clinical Lectures that year.[99] Duncan's claim may well have been exaggerated, but the Dispensary did become a well-established teaching institution, suggesting that extra-academical lectureships could indeed be very successful.[100]

University classes did not admit women, but extra-academical courses sometimes did. James Hamilton, professor of Midwifery, offered a class for 'female practitioners' on completion of which they each received a certificate 'of her being qualified to practice midwifery'.[101] Hamilton taught this course in question-and-answer form, rather than through lectures, so that he could satisfy himself that his pupils really were well qualified. It is noteworthy that he was more concerned about testing the qualifications of his female than of his male students; presumably it was because his female practitioners were certified only through his personal authority, rather than through the University. University certification to practice was not required for female midwives any more than for their male counterparts, but they, too, may have found it useful in attracting patients.[102]

With all these courses available, how did students actually choose which ones to take? They relied a good deal on information from other students, but, as James Rush found, 'every set of men have their favourites and their prejudices'.[103] He intended, he said, 'to choose for himself', but few students were allowed that freedom. The most common procedure seems to have been for students to come with strict instructions from parents, or seek advice from medical professors or other practitioners in Edinburgh. David Skene's father, Dr Andrew Skene, had told him to follow John Rutherford's advice as to classes, but nonetheless kept questioning his expenses, much to David's annoyance. 'You say I can attend Dr Rutherford's lectures on the Royal Infirmary Patients without paying to the Infirmary', David complained,

> The Dr himself was my authority to the contrary. Nor is there any such thing as seeing an Operation for 6 pence; tho I have been often told I could before I left Aberdeen. [104]

Obviously Dr Andrew intended to keep strict control over David's studies. David kept similar control when it was his turn to pay for his younger brother George's studies. [105] Once a young man was in Edinburgh, though, there was little his father could do short of cutting off funds, and David in fact relied heavily on Rutherford's advice.

Sylas Neville also had a letter of introduction, in his case to the geologist James Hutton, who introduced him to Joseph Black and Alexander Monro *secundus*, both of whom advised him on his course of study. [106] Thomas Ismay 'advised with' the surgeon Thomas Williamson about courses as about other things; Williamson also took Ismay to see Monro, whose opinion may have been especially valued on this issue. [107] The advice given to each student was tailored to their different circumstances. Neville, who had no previous medical education, and intended to graduate, was told to take Anatomy and Chemistry his first year, and postpone taking clinical lectures until he had more experience of medicine; the faculty consistently gave this advice to students who expected to spend more than one year at Edinburgh. [108] Ismay, who expected to study only one year, did not have time to postpone classes. He was therefore advised to take the 'most material' courses, 'Anatomy, Medical Practice, Midwifery, and Clinical Lectures'. [109] These were rigorous schedules. Ismay wrote to his father that he rose

> about 7, read till 9, then go to Dr. Cullen's Class, come back at 10, then breakfast and transcribe the Notes which I have taken at his Lecture. From 12 to 1 walk in Infirmary, from 1 to 3 attend Dr Monro. Then come and dine, and as you may suppose I am very hungry. From 4 to 5 attend Dr Young, from 5 to 6 transcribe the notes I have taken of Dr Young or Dr Monro's Lectures; from 6 to 7 attend Dr Innis [sic] Private Demonstrations, from 7 to 9 transcribe the Lectures I have borrowed and at 9 get Supper; from 10–12 write Lectures besides every Tuesday and Thursday from 5 to 6 o'clock I attend the Clinical Lectures. [110]

Though presumably not all students were this conscientious, their surviving letters and diaries indicate that hard study was expected at Edinburgh, in contrast to the English or many French Universities. [111] Benjamin Rush wrote that there was 'such a spirit of emulation reigning among the students here that a man must forego all hopes of making a figure unless he is always employed'. [112] Neville's diaries contain many references to how hard he worked. [113] Lesassier's diaries present indirect evidence that he, too, was working hard: he did not write very often in his diary while at Edinburgh, because, he said, 'My present mode of life tho' a very busy one, yet is extremely dull nothing but running from Class to Class all day long'. [114] By the end of the session the number of hours spent in lectures often increased, for when professors began to run out of time needed to finish their courses, they sometimes lectured twice a day during the week or on Saturdays. [115] The latter was too much for a group of seventy-nine graduates who protested to the Royal Commission about this 'deprivation of our only holiday', which required them 'to appropriate, either to recreation or study that day [Sunday] which we feel should be devoted to far different purposes'. [116]

Some students must have chosen courses based on their own interest or the professors' reputations, but as the enrollment patterns discussed in this chapter shows, these factors alone cannot account for course attendance. David Skene, again, illustrates the limitations of intellectual interest. He wanted to attend Andrew Plummer's lectures on Chemistry, as he believed he 'should have liked them more than any of the rest as he performs all the experiments before his students'. Despite his interest, he chose to take other, more useful courses. [117] Intellectual curiosity, then, was not the sole or even the most important factor in a student's choice of courses. Professors' reputations, too, though clearly influential in attracting students to Edinburgh in the first place, could not change basic patterns of attendance. The bad reputation of Alexander Monro *tertius* did not drive students away from Anatomy and Surgery entirely, and the excellent reputation of William Cullen could not attract a majority of students to Medical Theory.

More generally, it is misleading to associate particular course material only with particular professors. Students often referred to Monro's Anatomy or Black's Chemistry, but the real significance of Edinburgh's medical lectures was that there were always lectures in Anatomy and Chemistry whether or not there were Monro or Black. 'In a University', Mary Hewson wrote in response to her son's objection that Edinburgh professors were getting 'old and infirm', 'a young man who is attentive will acquire science tho' the professors are not in full vigour of mind, for what they have taught a great number of years they continue to teach with the same method'. [118] It was the collective task of the medical faculty to regularly teach medicine in all its branches so attentive students might learn. The students' responses will be the subject of the following chapters.

4

Gentlemen physicians

[We] received the reward of all our labours – the Degree of
Doctor of Medicine, which was conferred by the Principal in
the name & by the authority of the University. I thank God
for thus carrying me through this important business with the
approbation of all the Professors & much satisfaction & credit
to myself. I hope He will enable me by the Profession I have
now authority to practise to be of use to my fellow-creatures.
  Immediately after the ceremony the Principal & Professors
gave us their hands as brethren.

Silas Neville, Diary[1]

The students who graduated *'Doctoratûs in Arte Medica'*,[2] Doctor of
Medicine, were the official product of the Medical Faculty and the
University of Edinburgh. The distinguishing feature of their education was
their required conformity to regulations prescribing a set course of study,
a Latin thesis, and oral and written examinations for graduation. These
students constituted an elite within the Edinburgh student body, and
indeed a deliberately-constructed one, for by formulating strict requirements that applied to the graduates and no one else, the University
implicitly divided the students into those who graduated and those who
did not. The requirements were restrictive enough, both because of the
cost of study and the preliminary education they assumed, that graduates
at no time amounted to more than 20 per cent of the student body. The
dignity and honour claimed by physicians gave graduates an impact out
of proportion to their numbers, however; these were the students who gave
the Medical Faculty its reputation and set the standard for University
medical study throughout Britain.

Edinburgh University formally began to award medical degrees in 1726,
when the medical faculty was instituted by an act of the Town Council.
The minutes of the Town Council said nothing about any educational
requirements for the degree, stating simply that the then four Professors of
Medicine had full power

> to profess and teach Medicine in all its branches . . . as fully & freely

as the said science is taught in any University or Colledge in this or any other country: . . . [and] to examine candidates, and to do every other thing requisite and necessary to the graduation of Doctors of Medicine as amply and fully and with all the solemnities that the same is practiced by the Professor of Medicine in any Colledge or University whatsoever.[3]

Though this statute empowered faculty to both teach and examine, it did not explicitly require students to have attended courses before being examined for a degree. A student could simply present himself as a candidate for a degree, be examined by faculty, and receive the MD. This was the procedure in many universities throughout Great Britain and the Continent.

From the first, though, most students seem to have studied at Edinburgh prior to being examined by the faculty, even though a regulation specifically requiring 'a course of study in all the branches of Medical teaching in this or some other University'[4] was only passed in 1767. It was certainly the most efficient way for students to combine learning about medicine and being examined on their knowledge; I have only found ten of the graduates after 1762 who did not sign the matriculation album at all. In 1777, the University statute was modified to clarify what 'all branches of Medical teaching' meant. It stated that no student would be admitted as a candidate unless he had attended courses in Anatomy and Surgery, Chemistry, Botany, Materia Medica and Pharmacy, Medical Theory and Practice, and had attended the Clinical Lectures in the Royal Infirmary.[5] These were all the subjects taught by Professors of Medicine whose appointment stipulated that they could examine candidates for degrees. These were the men who technically made up the Medical Faculty. The Professor of Midwifery, whose appointment had not so stipulated, was formally not a member of the faculty, could not examine for degrees, and could not require his course for graduation. In 1783, the regulations were clarified still further to require a set period of study, stating that

No person shall be received as a candidate for a degree in Medicine until he has applied, during three complete years, to the study of Medicine in this or in some other University. It is expected of candidates to attend the University of Edinburgh at least one of these years, that the Professors may be acquainted with their character, conduct, and diligence in prosecuting their studies.[6]

These regulations were probably prompted by the scandal surrounding the credentials of Samuel Leeds, who graduated in 1766. Professor John Thomson, in his biography of Professor William Cullen, quoted the description of Leeds as 'an illiterate person, who had been brought up to the trade of a brush-maker'[7]; on setting up practice in London, his competence was questioned by Dr John Fothergill, and the resulting lawsuit led to Fellows of the Royal College of Physicians of London casting aspersions on the value of Edinburgh degrees. Thomson implied that Leeds had been awarded a degree without attending classes, and that the scandal prompted Cullen to work to prevent degrees from being awarded in Scottish Universities without proper study.[8]

Thomson's biography was begun in the 1820s at a time when he was deeply concerned with the reform of the medical graduation requirements proposed by the Royal Commission. That may have coloured his account, for whatever Leeds' origins – he may well have been, like Thomson, originally intended for trade – Leeds had in fact signed the matriculation records in 1764 and 1765, and is listed as attending Anatomy and Surgery, Chemistry, Materia Medica, Medical Theory, and Medical Practice.[9] This was nearly all the classes offered by medical professors: only Botany was missing, and students who took it in the summer frequently omitted to record it when they matriculated in the fall. There is of course no guarantee that Leeds went to classes, but there is equally no reason to assume he did not. According to the matriculation records, at least, Leeds had fulfilled all the requirements later published in statute.

It is much more likely that the series of statutes issued from 1767 to 1783 were intended to publicize existing policy rather than establish new requirements. Prior to 1767, students arriving in Edinburgh could wait on a professor to find out what they needed to do in order to graduate. The requirement of three years' study was not formally published until 1783, but students must have known of it, because Samuel Bard wrote home to his father in 1764 that 'by the Laws of the University I can not Graduate in less than three years from the time I began',[10] and George Logan wrote in 1778 that 'You cannot graduate here without having studied medicine at this or some other University for three years'.[11] Moreover, graduates who matriculated before the 1777 statute requiring specific courses attended substantially the same lectures as those matriculating after.[12] The informal advising system apparently worked almost as well as later published requirements to enforce behavior.

The problem with unpublished 'Laws of the University' was not only that other practitioners could dispute the value of an Edinburgh degree, as in Leeds' case. It also led to conflict between faculty and students. The medical faculty, like other faculties at other Universities, occasionally made exceptions to their requirements for study in the case of older or experienced practitioners. When Richard Pulteney, for example, came to Edinburgh to graduate in 1764, he was already an established practitioner, 'a man of eminence in the Literary World and a Fellow of the Royal Society', according to Samuel Bard.[13] His graduation without attending classes, though, led to a protest signed by twenty-nine students, Bard

among them, since, they said, 'we are unanimous in thinking that the
Superior Honour and Importance of Medical Degrees in the University of
Edinburgh, over those from other Scotch Universities, depend wholly upon
their being bestowed agreeably to proper Regulations'.[14] Most, including
Bard, later backed down, but they were right on principle: the value and
distinction of Edinburgh degrees did depend upon conformity to
regulations.[15]

Whatever inclination the medical faculty may have had to keep the
regulations vague in order to make exceptions disappeared after 1770,
when William Black, 'student of medicine', applied to Professor William
Cullen for permission to graduate in the spring. He had not yet attended
Botany, but, he assured Cullen, he intended to do so in the summer.
According to Black, Cullen initially told him that 'he would use his
interest with the Professors to attain my request; telling me, that he did
not imagine they would refuse me'.[16] After Cullen consulted with other
professors, though, according to Black, 'Dr. Cullen has (it seems) forgot,
and contradicted almost every circumstance that passed between him and
me relative to this affair'.[17] Black was especially angry not only, he said,
that other students had been allowed to graduate without fully completing
all the courses, but also because his request 'was agreeable to the then
established rules of the University; and . . . the refusal of it was equally
repugnant to these rules, as to reason and practice'.[18] He refused to apply
for graduation at Edinburgh.

Black's difficulty demonstrated the problem with vague regulations, and
with students' interpreting them according to their own perceptions of
'reason and practice'. The specificity of the 1777 regulations, followed by
their publication in 1783 by Principal William Robertson 'at the request
of the Senate Academicus, in order to show the practice of the University
and do justice to its graduates',[19] may well have come from the desire to
avoid similar misunderstandings. Known as the *Statuta Solennia*, the 1783
requirements remained in effect until 1825, and I have found no instances
of students graduating without signing the matriculation records after they
were published.

The reality, then, is not that Leeds, and other students prior to 1767,
were sliding by without attending classes, but that the faculty faced the
much more complicated problem of ensuring that they only granted
degrees to students who would become good physicians. This is of course
a problem faced by modern medical schools as well, and indeed most
degree-granting institutions have had to wrestle with some form of it. The
difficulties were succinctly put by Adam Smith, who wrote in a letter to
Cullen that

> A degree can pretend to give security for nothing but the science of
> the graduate; and even for that it can give but a very slender security.

For his good sense and discretion, qualities not discoverable by an academical examination, it can give no security at all.[20]

For Cullen or other medical professors to have agreed with this whole-heartedly would have meant denying the value of University study and examination, something few faculty members have ever been prepared to do. What they did instead was adopt a solution they had seen to be effective in enhancing the prestige of medical degrees at Leyden University, requiring lectures in subject matter deemed relevant to a physician, and testing knowledge of that subject matter prior to awarding a degree. This solution may seem obvious to modern observers, because it is commonly adopted by modern educational institutions. It was not at all common in the 1760s. Nor did it always work, any more than it does today: Adam Smith was correct to note that the medical faculty could not give security that all of their Doctors of Medicine would be good physicians. But even Smith would have agreed with Cullen's later statement, that 'the title of Doctor acquired here, more certainly than in several other Universities, proves its possessor to be both learned and skilfull'.[21]

Having set course requirements for graduation, the medical faculty then had the responsibility of enforcing them. Students had to present either class tickets or a certificate of completion from their lectures in Edinburgh or elsewhere in order to be admitted a candidate for graduation.[22] Joseph Black explained at some length, in answer to a query concerning requirements for graduation, that

> every course of medical chemical or botanical lectures which has been attended in any other university and of the attendance on which proper certificates are brought by a student of medicine coming to us is admitted as a part of the qualification entitling him to sit for a degree — We require that a student who begins and finished his medical studys here should employ three years at least in these studys (the greater number employ more) . . . But if he sh[oul]d have begun his studys in another University . . . we do not require of him to study here over again those branches . . . and far less do we require that he should fee the professors of those branches here altho he should not attend them.[23]

By the end of this letter, Black's interlocutor could have no excuse for not understanding the regulations: students could attend courses at another university and graduate at Edinburgh only if they could present proof that they had attended those classes. The Dean of the Faculty appears to have been quite strict in requiring proof, since Caspar Wistar was not allowed to graduate in two years, because he did not have formal proof of attendance from the University of Pennsylvania Medical College.[24]

The enforcement of regulations produced formal compliance with the requirements, as Table 4.1 shows.

Table 4.1 Graduates' course attendance, 1763–1826

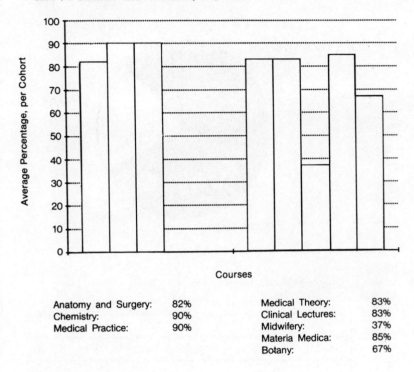

Courses

Anatomy and Surgery:	82%	Medical Theory:	83%
Chemistry:	90%	Clinical Lectures:	83%
Medical Practice:	90%	Midwifery:	37%
		Materia Medica:	85%
		Botany:	67%

Edinburgh graduates did indeed take the required courses, though at no point was course attendance 100 per cent, either because some students took courses elsewhere or because some managed to evade the requirements. This level of course attendance was much higher than that of any other group of students, as we will see in subsequent chapters. The majority of graduates also attended courses for three years, though there was more variation, see Table 4.2.

The largest single group of graduates, 42 per cent, studied for three years; the next largest group, 25 per cent studied for four or more years. Although Joseph Black was thus wrong to say that the 'greater number' of graduates studied for more than three years, at least a large number did. Of course his information would have come from the students who asked him for advice, the majority of whom may well have studied for four years if he recommended it. Only 12 per cent studied for one. Their course attendance suggests that they did study elsewhere, as the regulations required, since only 48 per cent attended Anatomy and Surgery. It is hard to imagine any student being allowed to apply for graduation or being

Table 4.2 Graduates' period of study, 1763–1826

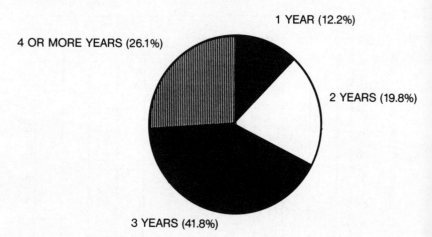

1 YEAR (12.2%)

4 OR MORE YEARS (26.1%)

2 YEARS (19.8%)

3 YEARS (41.8%)

Table 4.3 One-year graduates' course attendance, 1763–1826

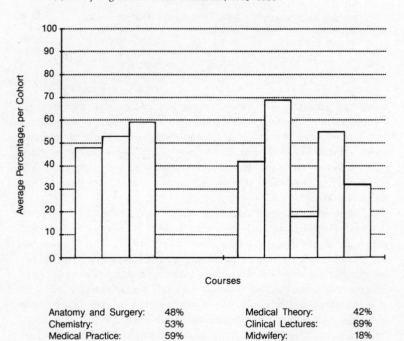

Courses

Anatomy and Surgery:	48%	Medical Theory:	42%
Chemistry:	53%	Clinical Lectures:	69%
Medical Practice:	59%	Midwifery:	18%
		Materia Medica:	55%
		Botany:	32%

Table 4.4 Three-year graduates, by year of study, 1763–1826

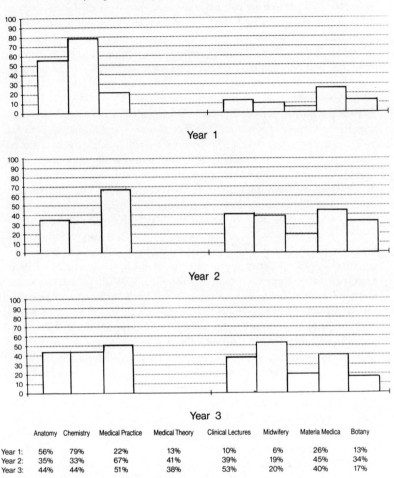

	Anatomy	Chemistry	Medical Practice	Medical Theory	Clinical Lectures	Midwifery	Materia Medica	Botany
Year 1:	56%	79%	22%	13%	10%	6%	26%	13%
Year 2:	35%	33%	67%	41%	39%	19%	45%	34%
Year 3:	44%	44%	51%	38%	53%	20%	40%	17%

able to pass the examination without having studied anatomy and physiology.[25] (See Table 4.3.)

The graduates who studied for three years have the course of study most usually associated with Edinburgh medicine, beginning with the basic sciences of Anatomy and Chemistry followed by courses in more strictly medical subjects and Clinical Lectures.[26] See Table 4.4.

Three-year graduates attended, in their first year, Anatomy and Surgery, and Chemistry, 56 per cent and 79 per cent respectively. Their attendance at Anatomy followed the same pattern as the student body generally: prior to 1805, an average of 88 per cent took it in their first year, while only

35 per cent of the graduates took it in their first year after that date. This is an especially interesting pattern among the three-year graduates, because it is likely that many of them, like Neville, came with little prior experience, and the faculty probably continued to give them the same advice he had received, to take Anatomy and Chemistry the first year. If they followed that advice, they must have studied with private teachers, not Monro *tertius*.

Sixty-seven per cent of the three-year graduates took Medical Practice in their second year. Medical Theory, Materia Medica and Clinical Lectures also attracted more students in their second year, 41 per cent, 39 per cent and 45 per cent respectively. These three courses would have introduced students to the central aspects of the study of medicine: they would have learned the basis of physiology, pathology, and medication, illustrated by examples drawn from the cases at the Royal Infirmary. Thirteen per cent remained in Edinburgh during the summer after their first year to attend Botany – Samuel Bard hoped he had by this, 'so far mastered it, as to be able to lay it aside now, until I can pursue it with less disadvantage to my other studys'.[27] If they did not, they would have had to take it the next summer, as did 34 per cent, in order to graduate in the spring of their third year and not face the problem confronted by William Black. During the third year, many students – 44 per cent – attended Anatomy, probably for the second time, and 44 per cent attended Chemistry, many of whom were no doubt also repeaters. Fifty-one per cent attended Medical Practice, and 53 per cent Clinical Lectures. Third year students were in the best position to appreciate those courses, and they may have been the most attentive, knowing that their knowledge would soon be tested in their examination for graduation, and in their practice.

It is naturally too much to expect that all students were able to relate their courses in this way. Indeed, it is almost certain that they did not. 'It has long been a matter of regret', Professor Robert Christison wrote in a letter to the Senatus Academicus in 1824,

> that, so far as regards the fundamental sciences of anatomy, chemistry, physiology, and materia medica, the attention of the student to them is almost confined to the period during which he attends each class. One science drives out the last, just as he passes from one classroom to another.[28]

The process of dividing medicine up into 'branches' and teaching each branch as a separate course had created this pedagogical problem which many modern medical professors would recognize, for there, too, medicine is divided up into separate subjects, each extensive enough to monopolize the attention of students on its own.[29] Each course offered by the Edinburgh medical faculty had its own body of material, not obviously related to the others. In order to master Chemistry, students had to learn about elective affinities as well as the composition of the blood; to master Medical Practice, they had to learn about diseases they would never see in the Royal Infirmary. Perhaps they, like twentieth-century students, adjusted to the demands on their time by concentrating their attention on whatever course, or classroom, they were currently in.[30]

What the regulations left out was as important as what they put in. Christison raised this issue as well when he wrote that the Medical Faculty

> are probably not aware how much their Regulations influence the students in their medical pursuits. These Regulations, it is presumed, are intended, by their framers, only to enforce such studies as are absolutely indispensable for graduation – not to point out what course of study is desireable to form a thorough physician.

At the time he wrote this, Christison had graduated only five years previously, and, he said,

> From a very recent, extensive, and intimate acquaintance with the students, especially of the better class, I have some reason to assure you with confidence . . . that, besides following what you prescribe, they are too apt to stick to the strict letter of your statute, by not following what you do not prescribe.[31]

Christison illustrated his point by referring to his own subject, Medical Jurisprudence, but the same case can be made even more forcefully using Midwifery lectures. Midwifery occupied an ambiguous place in eighteenth- and early nineteenth-century medicine. It was of acknowledged utility, since many practitioners could expect to have to deliver babies at some point, and the Midwifery class at Edinburgh was one of the few courses where students would actually see patients.[32] However, Midwifery was not part of the traditional academic curriculum, and though the man-midwife was gaining respectability, the character of Dr Slop, the man-midwife in Lawrence Sterne's *Tristram Shandy*, suggests he still had a long way to go. The candidate for graduation was required to attend the courses given by the other professors, but, according to George Logan, 'his attendance on Midwifery is also expected but this they cannot insist on'.[33] According to Table 4.1, 37 per cent of the graduates did attend Midwifery, a higher percentage than those students who did not graduate, but still much less than in the required courses. Professors' recommendations, and presumably practical considerations, therefore, had some weight with graduates, but not as much as the actual requirements.

The requirements also left out any form of contact with patients other than one course of Clinical Lectures. Some graduates may have served an apprenticeship. Richard Dennison, who graduated in 1775, had been apprenticed to 'Mr. Donne, the first Surgeon in Norwich', according to Neville.[34] David MacLagan was apprenticed to Andrew Wood, Fellow of the Royal College of Surgeons of Edinburgh, and dedicated his thesis to him.[35] James Vernon dedicated his to Thomas Nasmyth, MD, who first taught him the elements of medicine,[36] and James Chew dedicated his to John Hill, MD, Blackburn Lancaster, '*Praeceptori*'.[37] There was nothing in the university regulations that required apprenticeship though, and as we shall see, some medical professors discouraged it. This meant that a student could arrive in Edinburgh with no knowledge or experience of medicine, and leave with a degree three years later, having fulfilled the course requirements, written a thesis and passed the examinations, but never having seen a patient other than from the far end of a crowded ward during the clinical lectures.

Sylas Neville was in this position: he went to Edinburgh to study largely because he had spent his inheritance, tried studying law but gave it up after a year, and could not afford to support himself as a country squire. From his diary, his only contact with patients during his Edinburgh stay, aside from Clinical Lectures, appears to have been bloodletting his own servants, a skill he had acquired from one of his fellow-boarders, rather than from courses. 'I did it', he said, '. . . with success, for which I thank God . . . if I had made a mistake, it might have given the lower people here a mean opinion of my abilities in my profession'.[38] The 'lower people' might have been justified in their opinion, for Neville had less clinical experience than the much-despised apothecary's apprentice. He had, however, attended enough courses to allow him to present himself as candidate for a medical degree.

Graduates' education differed from other students' not only in the number of courses attended but also in that their knowledge was tested at the end of their studies. The first step for this was for the student to go to the Dean of the Faculty[39] with certificates of attendance from his classes, three months before the date he wished to graduate. The cost of graduation was £10, which was split among the six professors who had the privilege of examination. Until 1814, graduation was held in June and September, so the student had to notify the Dean in either March or June. After 1814, as the number of graduates rose, the date of graduation was changed to 1st August, to give faculty time to complete the examinations after their classes had ended.[40] Sylas Neville took the precaution of calling on Monro *secundus*, before he spoke to the Dean, since he was concerned that he might not be fully prepared for the examination, 'not from want of industry, but from an indifferent state of health', he was careful to add in his diary.[41] Neville almost always complained of his health when he was nervous,[42] and Monro, perhaps recognizing the symptoms, encouraged Neville 'by saying [he] had been more industrious than many others, and that they do not ask difficult questions, but only such as may put Gentlemen in a proper way of prosecuting their studies'.[43]

The graduation exercises were a mixture of traditional academic forms and modern eighteenth-century medical content. Tradition was maintained by requiring that all parts of the examination be in Latin, the language of scholarship and of gentlemen. Neville wrote that he was 'at a loss to know how a man can be a Physician and Professor without classical learning',[44] something he was in fact proficient in. One purpose of the first private examination was to see whether a student's Latin would allow him to fulfill all the graduation requirements, and Neville found 'that if the questions do not require very long answers, I can speak the language with tolerable fluency and correctness'.[45]

Other students had more difficulty. Most of them would have learned Latin in school, but probably quickly forgot it afterwards. By the second half of the century, Latin was no longer the language of the Scottish universities, even in the medical faculty;[46] it was certainly no longer the language of medical practitioners, whether surgeon-apothecaries or physicians. Moreover, students had to discuss in Latin material that they had heard lectures on in English. '[The faculty] cannot but acknowledge that it is extremely unreasonable', George Jardine, Professor of Philosophy at Glasgow, complained in 1825,

> to discourse to the young men three or four years in English, without asking a single question in any other language; and then all at once to mount upon their Latin stilts, and to come forward with all the learning of a Celsus . . .[47]

The result was that those who had difficulty with their Latin or other subjects, and wished to pass the examinations, had recourse to coaches, called 'grinders', who would question them, in Latin, on subjects they would be expected to know for their examination. The number of students resorting to grinders appears to have increased over the period. Robert Christison, who graduated in 1819, said he went to be 'polished by a grinder' before his examination, not because he needed it, but 'because everyone did it'.[48] By that time the grinders had become established private teachers, meeting with classes of eight to ten students for three months in the winter before their expected graduation. The faculty did not necessarily disapprove of this, because it was a useful form of auxiliary education to the lectures. Professor William Pulteney Alison told the Royal Commission 'there are some very respectable men who devote themselves to that kind of instruction', and was in favor of giving grinders some sort of official status as tutors.[49]

One indirect indication that more graduates were resorting to private teachers for review comes from the changes in course attendance among three-year graduates. Table 4.4 gives the averages from 1763 to 1826. If we divide up the period, though, we find that prior to 1805, an average of 62 per cent attended Anatomy and Surgery in their third year, 66 per cent attended Medical Practice, and 71 per cent attended Clinical Lectures.

This suggests that graduates were attending these courses for a second time in order to prepare for examination. From 1805 to 1826, though, only 31 per cent attended Anatomy and Surgery in their third year, 45 per cent attended Medical Practice, and 47 per cent attended Clinical Lectures. Perhaps students were supplementing University lectures with private lectures or grinders to prepare for graduation.

Archibald Robertson, who graduated in 1813, was probably one of these private teachers, for he published a series of books designed to help students through their examinations: *Colloquia Anatomica, Physiologica atque Chemica, Quaestionibus et Responsis, Colloquia de Morbis Practice*, and *Colloquia de Rebus Praecipuis Chemiae, Pharmaceutices, atque Botanices*.[50] These were serious study guides, not mere cribs of possible examination questions. A memory of the basic grammar, a good coach, and books like Robertson's and Professor William Cullen's *Nosologia*[51] might have done wonders for the student whose feeling for his classical heritage was a little shaky. The use of Latin during the examinations was maintained at least until the 1820s, for Professor William Pulteney Alison told the Universities Commission in 1826 that permission to conduct the examinations in English if the candidate had trouble with Latin had only 'lately' been granted.[52]

The written examination consisted of commentaries on Hippocrates' aphorisms and on case histories, which were part of a long-standing academic tradition for medical degrees.[53] The founders of the Royal College of Physicians of Edinburgh had imported these exercises from Leyden, in 1682, to use as tests for admission into the College.[54] When the Medical Faculty was founded in 1726, it incorporated the exercises into its own degree requirements. The public defense of a written thesis, performed before the entire faculty, was another aspect of long-standing academic tradition.

The Edinburgh medical faculty took these traditional forms and transformed them into a thorough test of eighteenth-century medical knowledge. The questions were not especially difficult for anyone who had attended lectures, as Monro assured Sylas Neville, but that was of course the point: graduation at Edinburgh was deliberately tied to mastery, and public presentation, of material taught in classes in Edinburgh. The first part of the graduation exercises was a private oral examination, held in the home of one of the professors shortly after a candidate notified the Dean that he wished to graduate. In this examination the faculty took turns asking the student questions on medical subjects, to see whether he was in fact well enough prepared to apply for a degree. The Dean recorded the name of student, the faculty member who presided, the date of the examination and the outcome.[55] If a student's answers were acceptable, he would be allowed to continue with the rest of the examinations; if they were not, he could apply again, usually after another year of study.[56] Not more than one or two students per year were rejected outright; another two or three were often allowed another oral examination a few weeks later.

The Faculty's records of the subjects covered in the first oral examination tend to be sketchy lists of topics. The most common question was for students to discuss the circulation of the blood. This was hardly an advanced topic, but its frequent use suggests that faculty regarded it as a touchstone by which to gauge a candidate's knowledge of anatomy and physiology. If his answer was acceptable, they could move on to other topics; if not, they could question him more fully.[57]

Students gave a more detailed account. According to both Samuel Bard and Sylas Neville, the graduation exercises began innocently enough with the first, private examination at the home of one of the professors. The Faculty seem to have gone to some length to put the candidates at ease; as Bard wrote to his father, 'altho' they kept up the strickness of Professors, they never lost sight of the politeness of Gentlemen'.[58] The examination was held in the evening. Bard, not knowing what to expect, 'went in trembling'; probably realizing this, 'Dr Cullen, after desiring me to sit down, began my examination, by asking me some general Definitions, as Quid est medicina? and so on'.[59] This would certainly have reassured Bard. To the question '*Quid est Medicina*', What is medicine, he might have responded, from Celsus, '*ut alimenta sanis corporibus agricultura, sic sanitatem aegris medicina promittit*',[60] 'As agriculture promises food to the healthy, so medicine promises health to the sick'.[61] Or he might have said, from Cullen's lectures, it was 'the art of preserving health and of curing disease'.[62] Either way, he would no doubt have been calmed and encouraged by his ability to respond. Neville was pleased that Cullen, who was the second Professor to question him, 'began by telling me that he was so well satisfied with the answers he had heard from me, that he did not think it necessary to ask me any further, but as it was the custom . . .'[63]

The medical faculty were not always so kind. When Robert Jones had his first oral examination on 4 May 1781, the Dean carefully wrote out every question he was asked, taking pains with handwriting and using full sentences. Jones was an outspoken follower of John Brown and had publicly clashed with Professor Andrew Duncan over the treatment of a fellow student.[64] In his case, the faculty may have assumed the justice of their decision would be questioned, and we may assume that his examination was more adversarial than Neville's. Jones was allowed a second examination five days later, but was ultimately rejected.[65]

The preliminaries over, the professors went on to ask more specific questions. After questioning Bard on general definitions, Cullen went on to ask him some questions upon the structure of the stomach and alimentary canal, thence made a digression to the diseases, examined me upon the colic, Illius [sic], the Diagnosis and method of cure; then Doct[o]r Monro junior [*secundus*] asked me the distinction between Illius and Inflammation, some physiological questions upon the Pulse in inflammation; the causes of Intussusceptio in the Intestines, and the method of cure in both these diseases.[66]

This description is especially interesting, because the repetition of words beginning with 'I' — ileus, inflammation, intussusceptio, intestines — suggests that Bard was being tested for his knowledge of Latin as well.

Neville's examination was similar, as he described it in his diary:

Dr Home examined me on the circulation and the diseases of the skin. Old Cullen took me next upon the insensible secretion or halitus from the lungs, catarrh, measles, and the peripneumony, which is often the companion of that disease . . . Dr Black, who with Dr. Monro came in after the examination was begun, asked me concerning the influence of the excretion by perspiration and urine. Dr Hope then asked me the definition and symptoms of Diabetes. Dr Monro asked me some questions concerning the cure of the same disease.[67]

All these questions were on subjects that came from lectures. Monro's lectures on Anatomy and Surgery, and Cullen's and Gregory's on Medical Theory and Practice, would have provided answers to the questions concerning the structure of the stomach and alimentary canal, as well as other physiological questions. The definition of Diabetes, and other diseases was also in Cullen's *Nosologia*.[68] The first examination lasted about forty-five minutes.[69]

Students who had passed the oral examination might have passed on to others the questions they were asked. Thomas Ruston mentioned having met Bard shortly before Bard's graduation,[70] and in Ruston's papers are a list of Latin questions and subjects, beginning with '*Quid est medicina? Quid est sanitas? Quid est morbus?*' and including questions on the function and diseases of the stomach and intestines, and on the circulation of the blood.[71] Perhaps Bard described the examination to him as well as to his father. The list does not include answers, so probably Ruston used the list as study questions to prepare for his own graduation.

This private examination was the main test of whether a student was to be allowed to graduate. It may have been the medical faculty's way of fulfilling their obligation to be familiar with the candidate's 'character, conduct, and diligence in prosecuting his studies', required by statute of the University. The next requirement for graduation was to write and publicly defend a thesis, a copy of which had to be given to the medical faculty six weeks before graduation. The thesis, like the rest of the graduation requirements, was a traditional academic form adapted to

eighteenth-century medical scholarship. It was generally considered to be
a literary exercise, which marked the candidate's entry into the academic
profession. Unlike theses for some Continental universities, these were not
propositions put forth by a professor, which a student was required to
defend. Edinburgh theses were, instead, much closer to a modern term
paper: a student chose a topic, read up on it, and composed it. The amount
of work students did varies, but generally theses did require substantial
research into the available literature on a subject, and graduates were
expected to cite the pertinent works on their chosen topics. Christison gave
the example of William Stroude, who read every work on Gout in the
University Library, and had to put his analysis in one section of the thesis,
and the references in another.[72]

Professors might have recommended topics for some students, or at least
offered suggestions, since Sylas Neville consulted with Cullen as to the
topic of his 'Inaugural Dissertation', as the theses were officially called.
'After telling him that I had been anticipated in one subject, the *Diaeta
Aquia*', Neville said,

> which I had chosen on account of my reading Italian, by which I
> thought some authors of the country where this practice chiefly
> prevails would have been open to me, I informed him that I intended
> to study the Ancients and therefore had thoughts of writing some-
> thing on the Prognostic, in which they particularly excelled, and that
> I meant to confine myself to the Prognostic in Fevers.[73]

Neville's second choice of topic had also been prompted by his linguistic
skills, since he was reasonably fluent in classical languages; it might also
have been prompted by the desire to please Cullen, who was especially
interested in fevers. But Cullen obviously had not dictated the topic of
Neville's thesis, and certainly did not write it for him.

As Neville's choice of topic indicates, the thesis could be a commentary
on an aspect of classical medicine. However, it could also be on topics of
current interest, including experimental science. Professor Joseph Black
provided the shining example of a student who used the thesis requirement
to carry out independent research. His own experience was exceptional,
however: he came to Edinburgh an already proficient chemist, trained by
Professor William Cullen while at Glasgow University, and was able to
discern in a dispute between two professors a chemical question which
could be answered by experiment. He was also exceptional in his access to
apparatus, since there were no courses in practical chemistry at Edinburgh
University until the 1820s,[74] and students therefore had to rely on being
taken under the wing of sympathetic faculty. His dissertation, *On Magnesia
Alba*[75] attracted much more attention than was usual for MD theses: it
received the commendation of several of the Edinburgh professors, as well
as Baron de Montesquieu and the Academy of Sciences of Bordeaux, to

whom it was shown by Black's father.[76] The essay which came out of his dissertation, 'Experiments on *Magnesia Alba*, Quicklime, and some other Alcaline Substances', was presented to the Edinburgh Philosophical Society, and published a year after Black's graduation in a collection of essays written primarily by professors. It is considered by historians as one of the major works of eighteenth-century chemistry. This was not the ordinary response to 'the great majority of Theses', which, Professor William Pulteney Alison told the Royal Commission, 'cannot be expected to contain any thing worthy of being published'.[77] However, Joseph Black's case does show the possibility that the scholarly research required for a thesis could become experimental research.[78] Daniel Rutherford's MD thesis, *On Fixed, or Mephitic Air*, is the first analysis of nitrogen, carried out under Joseph Black's guidance.[79] William Meade performed chemical analyses of the water from St Bernard's Well, on the Waters of Leith, for his thesis,[80] which presumably stood him in good stead during his later analysis of mineral waters in New York State.[81]

Several students carried out physiological experiments. In order to examine the effects of digestion on food in the stomach, Benjamin Rush made himself and a friend experimental subjects, by eating and then taking Tartar Emetic to vomit, a procedure that had the merit of requiring no apparatus beyond willing friends and a strong stomach.[82] George Kellie carried out experiments on Animal Electricity;[83] Alexander Philip Wilson experimented on Opium for his thesis on Dyspepsia.[84] Even students who did not actually perform experiments often chose experimental subjects for their theses.[85]

The majority of the theses, though, were on well-established medical topics, well-represented in the literature. Most of them fit perfectly into the categories of either 'Case Histories' or 'Questions on Medical Subjects' that the faculty might have proposed to the graduates in their examinations. Certain diseases were especially popular: Apoplexy, Dysentery, Dyspepsia, Fever, Hysteria, Jaundice, Pneumonia, Rheumatism, Typhus, and Smallpox. These were all standard diseases, and students might well have seen examples of them in the Royal Infirmary. At least one student did, in fact, cite a case he had seen there.[86] The number of books that existed on any topic might have been an equally compelling reason for a student choosing it: Stroude, after all, chose to read every book on Gout in the library, rather than examine every case in Edinburgh.

The amount of time and effort spent on a thesis varied with the student. Stroude spent two years preparing his, but Neville, in contrast, first discussed his topic with Cullen on June 18, only six weeks before a draft had to be completed and shown to Cullen, before the final version was given to the Dean. Cullen warned him he had started very late, which made Neville, '. . . not a little uneasy as I am afraid it is almost impossible to produce any thing tolerable on a subject of so much nicety in so short a time'.[87] He managed to complete it only just in time, giving a copy of the plan to Cullen on July 4, and receiving 'his approbation in very genteel and candid terms'.[88] Some students intending originally to graduate in June found they could not complete the thesis in time, and ended up graduating in September.[89]

Neville himself almost did not make the deadline, for he continued to procrastinate, even though he was so pressed for time, and even though the unfinished thesis weighed heavily on his mind: as he said, after one day trip, he 'should have enjoyed the excursion very much if my Thesis had been done'.[90] On July 31, one day before the final copy had to be delivered to the Dean, Neville called on Cullen again, to say the thesis was done, but he had not yet made a presentable copy. This time Cullen was not so pleasant, pointing out that he had given Neville 'more indulgence than any body else, tho' some other Gentlemen had applied for more time'.[91] Finally he told Neville that he would sign the thesis, as he was required to do before it could be delivered to the Dean, if it was delivered to him before 10 pm on August 1. Neville made the necessary heroic effort, familiar to most who have been students, of staying up nearly all night in order to finish the thesis. Even this was not quite enough, and he had to call on a scribe to help him transcribe it. He did in fact manage to get a copy to Cullen the next day, and to the Dean by August 2. Graduates must have been allowed a little leeway, for the Dean, having seen the thesis, permitted Neville to take it home for a day or two to make a few minor changes. On August 3 the completed and corrected thesis was finally out of Neville's hands. 'Sent the thing again to Dr. Cullen before dinner', was his only comment − he was no doubt pleased to be rid of it for the time being.[92]

Theses may have been expected to be a student's own work, but there were apparently ways of getting around this. Just as a student whose Latin was poor could hire a grinder to practice for his oral examination, and perhaps also for his written, he could also hire a translator to translate his thesis into Latin. A thesis could be twenty to fifty pages long, and many students would have had difficulty writing that much grammatical Latin, especially if they, like Neville, waited until the last minute to begin work. According to Thomas Beddoes, most students wrote their theses first in English, and translating them was an 'occupation from which a good scholar may derive emolument in Edinburgh'.[93]

It also seems to have been possible to hire someone to actually write the theses. Again according to Beddoes, 'the ordinary gratuity for a translation was five, and for an original composition, where that is required, ten guineas', though his account is somewhat suspect.[94] Neville was certainly concerned about faked theses. He wrote in his diary,

As I took some pains in the composition of my Thesis, I thought I had the right to take notice of the mean and dishonorable conduct of those who publish the compositions of other men as their own. I have therefore done it in my conclusion . . .[95]

He decided he had better check the paragraph with Cullen, however, who apparently approved of it.[96] There seems to have never been an official inquiry into the subject, and so it is hard to know how widespread the practice was.

A different kind of problem was actually produced by the fact that the thesis was expected to be the student's own work. Some students clearly hoped their thesis would become the same route to fame and fortune as Black's on magnesia alba. 'You know how necessary it is for a young man to begin the world with some degree of character', James Jeffray wrote to William Hamilton, Professor of Anatomy at Glasgow, when describing his theory on the circulation in the placenta '. . . You will smile I know at me — but the little eclat my industry & attention can now gain me, is all my fortune'.[97] The way for a student to obtain 'some degree of character' was, as Samuel Allvey put it, 'to contribute those observations which he has made, and the opinions, which he has formed; rather than to collect the facts and opinions of others'.[98]

Students clearly believed this was required of them even if the 'others' happened to be the medical faculty. The fact that the faculty made no restrictions as to choice of topics, and generally seem to have exercised little control over the theses, sent a clear message to graduates that they were free to develop their own ideas. Neville was cautious enough to check a doubtful paragraph with Professor William Cullen, but some students felt that professorial authority was a form of censorship. According to Robert Jones' account, in 1781 John Wainman was told by Professor Alexander Monro *secundus* to remove quotations from John Brown's *Elements of Medicine* from his thesis *On Epilepsy*.[99] Wainman protested, because he said '1st . . . I am prevented from saying what *I really believe*, to the manifest injury of my Dissertation. 2dly, . . . I am deprived of the liberty other candidates have always enjoyed, in making quotations from any author'.[100] Monro did not challenge Wainman's point that a thesis should say what the author really believed, for to do that would undermine the value of writing theses. He did, however, assert his authority by responding that 'As to the liberty you say "candidates have always enjoyed" . . . I never heard of it before; and *am determined* to give it *no quarter* neither now nor hereafter'.[101] As was frequently the case in faculty-student disputes, Monro had University policy on his side: the faculty had to formally approve each thesis before the University gave 'sanction to its publication'[102] and therefore they did have the power to refuse it. Wainman was probably not convinced, though, and Robert Jones concluded that the faculty's purpose was 'by downright outrage, to carry their point of quashing this doctrine'.[103] James Jeffray resented the faculty even more, believing they opposed his ideas in public only to steal them in private. 'I do think they do not use me well', he wrote, 'if it be nonsense let the laugh come against me alone & if there be any thing in it why should these people whose careers are already established filch it from me.'[104]

Since the thesis was due six weeks before graduation, the remaining period was devoted to the rest of the graduation examinations. The second oral examination took place in the University Library. All candidates met on the same day, but were examined separately on medical subjects by two of the professors, 'particularly with respect to points not touched upon in [the] former examination'.[105] Neville was examined by Professors Hope and Cullen, on Erysepalis, but said only that he had 'passed my 2nd examination before the Faculty for my degree'.[106] Student rumour said that the first oral examination was the only true test, and that, as George Logan reported, 'there is hardly an instance of a Gentleman being degraded after passing his first'.[107] Unfortunately for James Mosely, though, student rumour was not always accurate: he did not pass his Library examination the first time around, and had to undergo a second examination in the presence of the full faculty two days later.[108]

The next requirement was to write commentaries on an aphorism of Hippocrates, a general medical question, and two case histories. Daniel Rutherford, Professor of Botany from 1786 to 1820, kept some of the essays written in response to questions he proposed to candidates.[109] His records consist primarily of essays written in response to aphorisms and questions, but include two case histories, written between 1787 and 1790, and gives an indication of the kind of essays candidates were expected to write. The examinations were intended to be written at home, with the aid of whatever books or notes the student might have available. According to Christison, students sometimes simply turned their commentaries over to their grinders to write, but we have no way of knowing how many did so.[110]

Despite the traditional form of the commentary on Hippocrates' aphorisms, graduates were clearly expected to draw on current medical concepts and information, and paid more attention to eighteenth-century authors than classical ones. Samuel Allvey, for example, in his essay on '1. We ought to consider whom it may be convenient to feed once or twice a day, more or less, and by little and little. 2. We must attribute something also to custom, season, country and age',[111] cited at length from James Gregory's *Conspectus Medicinae Theoreticae*.[112] The essay was only seven pages long; the citation thus made up a substantial portion of it. Allvey also cited Celsus, as did George Harries, in his commentary on

'1. In the beginning of diseases, 2. if there appears to be a cause for moving of any thing, move it. 3. But when they are advanced, it is much better to let it alone'. [113] But Cullen also cited from Celsus, and there is no reason to assume that either student was very familiar with classical authors: eighteenth-century editions of Hippocrates' and Celsus' works often came with subject indexes for rapid reference to a specific topic. [114]

Most of the aphorisms came from Book 2, and dealt with general topics that the students would certainly have covered in Medical Practice, or Clinical Lectures, such as 'When a delirium or raving is appeased by sleep, it is a good sign', [115] or 'In any diseases, if the mind is sound, and those meats which are offered are willingly accepted of, it is a good, but if otherwise, a bad sign'. [116] Henry Stanistreet, in 1787, and George Kittsom, a year later, were both asked to comment on Book 2, Aphorism 13, 'To such as expect a crisis, the night before the paroxysm is very tedious, but the night following is commonly more easy'. [117] Stanistreet used the essay to discuss several different aspects of crises in fevers, most probably as many as he could think of. He contrasted the crises in fevers where the diseases came on gradually and left gradually, with those more serious cases where the crises were accompanied by delirium and convulsions. [118] He discussed possible explanations for crises, mentioned that Hippocrates was right to say that the night preceding a crisis was more uncomfortable, since fevers tended to get worse at night, and concluded that it was not surprising that the night following a crisis would be better. [119] The phenomena and possible causes of crises in fevers was one of Cullen's favorite themes, and the first part of his *First Lines of the Practice of Medicine*[120] was devoted to it. Stanistreet probably took much of his discussion of the different sorts of crises, and their causes, from Cullen, and may even have referred to his notes while writing, since his comments on the hypothesis that crises were the result of the efforts of the *vis medicatrix naturae*, the healing power of nature, to expel morbific matter from the body follow Cullen's closely. [121] It is easy to picture him receiving his aphorism, going back to his lodging, and taking down his copy of Cullen's *First Lines* to read up on the subject before starting to write.

Stanistreet's essay shows more preparation than George Kittsom's: Kittsom appeared generally familiar with the concepts, but fuzzy as to details. He, too, felt that the truth of the Aphorism could not be doubted, but he spent only a page and a half discussing it, concentrating mainly on the action of the *vires Naturae Medicatrices*, the healing powers of nature, in expelling the disease. [122] Kittsom probably did not refer either to his notes from Cullen's course, assuming he had them, or *First Lines*, since Cullen spoke only of one healing power of nature, rather than several. Both students must have convinced the faculty that they knew the subject well enough, though, since both did graduate.

The questions on medical topics also dealt with specific topics covered by Edinburgh professors in class. Rutherford appears to have been especially interested in various aspects of medical chemistry. He asked several questions on medication, such as 'What are the powers of digitalis in the human body? In which diseases is it made use of? In what form? And in what doses?'[123] and 'What evils spring from the imprudent administration of Mercury? How is it possible to help in such cases?'[124] Other questions concerned physiological processes: 'What changes occur in blood through the circulation through the lungs? Is something lost, or gained? What?'[125] or 'What changes occur in food in the stomach and intestines?'[126] Rutherford also repeated certain subjects, such as the composition of human urine, and where its salt content came from, asked of both Patrick Baron Seton in 1787, and John Benjamin Jachmann in 1789, or whether calculi could be dissolved within the body by ingesting solvents, asked of Charles Ker in 1785, and Andrew Ker in 1790.

The commentaries on the case histories, though again a traditional form, were similarly answered with reference to eighteenth-century texts. Thomas Trotter was given the case of an elderly woman, overweight, who suffered from bad headaches, accompanied by ringing in the ears and frequent numbness, which was succeeded by a slight fever or heat, weakness, quick pulse, and perspiration.[127] The headache, ringing in ears, and numbness were a sign that this was what Cullen had classed as a Neurosis, or a disease which affected sense and motion. If Trotter had taken down his copy of Cullen's *Nosologia*, and looked under Neuroses, he would have found that the first order in the class was Comata, which involved the disruption of voluntary motion, and the first genus in that class was Apoplexia. Trotter might have remembered that apoplexy was most likely to affect older, overweight men and women, or he might have looked it up in Cullen's *First Lines*. In either case he would have decided, as indeed he did, that his case was one of apoplexy, and his account of it began with the definition taken from Cullen's *Nosologia*, 'Motus voluntarii fere omnes imminuti, cum sopore, plus minus profundo, superstite motu cordis et arteriarum',[128] or 'The whole of the voluntary motions in some degree abolished; with sleep, more or less profound; the action of the heart and arteries continuing'.[129]

Trotter then went on to discuss the disease. He first gave the History, or general description of the illness as it was likely to appear in a patient. Next he turned to the Causes, which were the Predisposing and Exciting causes. Predisposing causes were those having to do with the usual habit and temperament of the patient, such as old age, obesity, or frequent inebriation. The exciting causes were those which were responsible for bringing on the disease at a specific time, such as vigorous exercise or drinking to excess. These two types of causes were intended to explain why this particular patient was likely to be subject to this particular disease, and why it would come on at this particular time. Trotter obviously took much of his commentary from Cullen's *First Lines*, since his description, though of course in Latin, follows Cullen's closely. [130] For example, he stated that the proximate cause of the disease was whatever compressed the brain, or else interfered with the mobility of the nervous power from the brain to different parts of the body. [131] This came straight from *First Lines*, where Cullen suggested that the disease was caused by 'either some compression of the origin of the nerves, or by something destroying the mobility of the nervous power'. [132]

What all these examinations rewarded was serious medical study, rather than experience with medical practice, though that would not necessarily hurt. Even case histories were tests of the student's knowledge of diseases as they appeared in lectures and textbooks rather than actual consultations with specific patients. Once his diagnosis was complete, Trotter made no further attempt to refer to the specific elderly woman who had prompted his account of Apoplexy. This, again, confirms the accuracy of Adam Smith's observation, that examinations for degrees could give security only for the 'science of the candidate'; they could not guarantee his ability to practice medicine.

Once the examinations were finished, the only remaining formality was defence of the thesis at graduation itself. Neville was to graduate on September 12, and the day before took the precaution of calling on Dr Hope, who was to examine him, and 'telling him that I was glad I had fallen into such good hands'. [133] He also spent the few days before graduation by 'considering the doctrine of my thesis, [and] finished my preparation . . . by reading over the Thesis itself'. [134] On the day of graduation, all the candidates met in the Public Hall of the university, and heard the oath they were to subscribe to. [135] The candidates were then questioned on their dissertations in turn. Hope seems to have been very kind to Neville, who wrote that he

> paid me many high compliments and then made only two observa-
> tions, to which it pleased God to strengthen me to give proper
> answers, even in public. He then concluded with further praise of my
> dissertation, saying that it was *bene eleganter et erudite scripta.* [136]

Hope's compliment translates literally to 'well-, elegantly-, and learnedly-written'. We should not make too much of this fragment of faculty evaluation, but it seems worthwhile to point out that these were all comments on Neville's literary style, rather than medical content. If professors frequently made these kinds of comments it would help explain student preoccupation with their own style. [137]

Once the examination was over, the candidates left the room, while the Principal asked the Faculty if they wished him to confer the Degree of

Doctor on the candidates, 'to which they assented'. The candidates had in the meantime put on black Doctor's gowns; they re-entered the Hall, subscribed the Oath, and 'received the reward of all our labours', said Neville, 'the Degree of Doctor of Medicine, which was conferred by the Principal in the name and by the authority of the University'.[138]

That was the way in which Edinburgh students became Doctors of Medicine. They must have spent that night celebrating, and the next few days preparing to leave town. Many would have had their theses elegantly bound, perhaps, like Neville, in 'green morocco and gilt'[139] to present to family, teachers, and patrons. Then they would have left, again perhaps like Neville, hoping to bring credit to 'the Profession I have now authority to practice . . .'[140]

5

Industrious apprentices

It was formerly, I believe, customary for apprentices to be employed in many duties which we now consider as menial and servile. Under this regime a good deal of their time must have been misapplied, and it cannot be doubted that their sense of self-respect must have been lowered to an injurious degree. But these days are past . . . An apprentice receives the same education which another student does, he attends the same classes, he embraces the same opportunities, and besides these, he receives additional advantages from the general inspection of his master, from the frequent examination on professional subjects which he undergoes . . . and from those real clinical lectures, though not dignified by the name, which are so much the more useful, that they are occasional, private, and frequent.

William Brown, FRCSE[1]

Besides the graduates, the other group of young men who formed a natural pool of Edinburgh students were the apprentices of the surgeons' guild in Edinburgh, known as the Incorporation of Surgeons until 1778, when members received a royal charter to become the Royal College of Surgeons of Edinburgh. The change of name was part of the ongoing effort of Edinburgh surgeons to raise their status while retaining the legal privileges of a guild. Central to their effort was the change in the image of surgical apprenticeship, from a 'menial and servile' form of education to a liberal one. The 5 per cent of the student population who were apprentices therefore acquired an importance out of proportion to their numbers.[2]

The Edinburgh surgeons were not unique either in their attempts to improve their status, or in their concentration on education as the way to do it. The status of surgeons, as individuals and as an occupation, improved throughout Europe in this period. Oswei Temkin's original analysis is still the most useful summary: he pointed to the improvements in technique, the limiting of major operations, like trepan and amputation, in favour of more conservative methods, and more careful attention to the impact of disease and the constitution of the patient in considering surgical procedures.[3] Temkin attributed these improvements primarily to the advance of anatomy and experimental physiology, but he also mentioned as a factor a higher educational standard for surgeons.[4]

Edinburgh surgeons were unusual, however, in their heavy reliance on existing University medical lectures. Elsewhere in Europe, surgeons were excluded from the universities, and developed separate educational institutions to train their students and apprentices.[5] Edinburgh apprentices, welcome like all other students to attend University lectures, 'embraced the same opportunities', to borrow William Brown's phrase, for social mobility through University education. Whether this was good or bad depends on one's point of view, for historians of medicine have noted that Edinburgh surgeons did not develop the distinctive surgical view of disease that led to the intensive study of pathological anatomy among surgeons in Paris, and ultimately to modern pathology.[6] For the individual surgeon's apprentice, it was undoubtedly good, for it increased his own respectability and that of his associates. 'If gentlemen studied it, it must be a fit subject for gentlemen,' was a familiar tautology in Georgian education, and it eventually came to dignify even the messy, bloody and painful business of surgery before asepsis and anaesthesia.

The 'Calling', as the Incorporation of Surgeons of Edinburgh was often referred to, was first granted a charter to form a guild and elect a Deacon by the Town Council in 1505. Members had the exclusive right to practice surgery within the 'liberties' of the city, extending from the High Street to the city walls, and excluding the suburbs of the Canongate, Potterrow and Leith. In 1657 the Incorporation formed an alliance with the apothecaries' guild, and Members thereafter practiced as surgeon-apothecaries, with a monopoly over the largest part of medical practice within the town. In 1695, the Incorporation was granted the privilege of licensing country surgeons in the three Lothians, Fife, Peebles, Selkirk, Roxburgh and Berwick. In theory only men who had received a certificate from the Incorporation were entitled to practice surgery and pharmacy in those areas.[7] In practice this privilege was not actively enforced, but had important consequences, as we will see in Chapter Eight.

Edinburgh surgeons, called Members of the Incorporation before 1778 and Fellows of the Royal College thereafter, had political influence as well as professional authority. Edinburgh craft guilds had six permanent seats on the Town Council, and the Deacon of the Incorporation, called the President of the Royal College after 1778, was always appointed to one of them. He was also frequently chosen as a representative to the Scottish Parliament prior to 1707.[8] The surgeons seem to have made a reasonably smooth transition to Scottish political realities after the Union as well, for the minute books of the later eighteenth century indicate good relations

with Henry Dundas, 1st Viscount Melville, Scotland's political manager
during the late eighteenth century.[9]

Nor did Edinburgh surgeons have any difficulty attracting apprentices,
either those intending to enter the guild themselves, known as 'apprentices for the Freedom', or others simply looking for surgical training.
Apprentices were usually indentured at the age of fifteen or sixteen.
Apprentices for the freedom were bound for five years, at a cost of between
£50 and £60 during the period.[10] There was also a booking fee, set at £5
in 1782.[11] Room and board was ordinarily included in apprenticeship, but
not clothing. In order to join the guild, a former apprentice had to undergo
an examination and pay an additional fee. This was set at £8/6/8 for sons
of members, £16/13/4 for sons-in-law, and £43/6/8 for apprentices who
were neither of these, but had 'served for the freedom'. Surgeons wishing
to join the guild and obtain the privileges of the monopoly who had not
served an apprenticeship for the freedom had to pay £166/13/4.[12] This was
a substantial sum, but then membership in the guild conferred substantial
privileges. It is possible that members who bought their way into the guild
without apprenticeship continued to be treated as outsiders, however. John
Bell, for example, entered in 1786 after 'nine years hard toil in the
University of Edinburgh',[13] and a period as army surgeon, but without
having served an apprenticeship for the freedom. In his subsequent quarrel
with Professor James Gregory over 'younger surgeons' being denied access
to the surgical wards of the Royal Infirmary, he became convinced that
Gregory was acting in concert with a network of established Edinburgh
surgeons, trained by apprenticeship, who conspired against innovators like
himself. This was all the more unfair, Bell wrote, because by paying entry-
money the surgeon was doing more than just buying a share in a monopoly;
instead, 'the sum of two hundred pounds . . . puts him on a rank with
any profession in this city, and proves that he has had opportunities of a
respectable education'.[14] Bell ultimately left Edinburgh, but not until he
had booked a number of apprentices of his own, probably including his
more famous younger brother, Charles Bell, who entered the College in
1799. Charles Bell is not listed in the records as being indentured, but
that was fairly common for relatives of Fellows who later became Fellows
themselves. It is possible, but unlikely, that Bell was never indentured
and paid the £166 entry fee; it is more likely that John and Charles Bell
simply evaded the £5 booking fee. John Bell's investment of 'two hundred
pounds' was thus an excellent family investment.

Apprentices who did not intend to become Fellows, but were simply
looking for surgical training, were usually bound for three years, at a cost
of from £30 to £50, with a booking fee of only one guinea.[15] These
apprentices were referred to in the minutes as servants, originally to get
around the rule that no master could have more than one apprentice every

three years.[16] The cost even of a three-year apprenticeship was high, no doubt reflecting the fact that the monopoly over surgery and pharmacy in Edinburgh was valuable, and parents were willing to pay for it. Even apprentices not booked for the freedom would benefit from the professional success of their masters. As we have seen, apprenticeship was considered a reasonable form of education for sons of men of middling ranks, and Sir John Clerk of Penicuik's letter to his son John, when the latter was bound for the freedom to Adam Drummond and John Campbell, shows it attracted even sons of baronets.

Sir John's letter also shows that some apprentices, at least, had received the education of gentlemen. Generally, though, it was very hard to fit apprenticeship itself into any model of liberal education. For most of the eighteenth century, the guild's minutes used the term 'servant' to refer to apprentices not bound for the freedom, one sign of the status of apprentices. Throughout the period the apprentice pledged himself to a master surgeon for a set period of years, 'during which space the said apprentice [binds] and obliges himself to serve . . . faithfully and honestly by day and night, holiday and work day'.[17] Though not a schoolboy, he nonetheless lacked independence, the essential characteristic of a liberal gentleman; the apprentice, literally, was not his own master.

Unlike students, whose progress in medical education depended primarily on their own efforts, apprentices depended very much on their masters'. Practitioners took apprentices partly for the fees paid for the indenture, and partly because they were a convenient form of cheap labour. Apprentices took over much of the drudgery of keeping a shop: they swept floors, compounded medicines, cleaned bandages, and made up bills. An apprentice could also take messages or run errands, thus ensuring that a busy practitioner did not lose patients when he was himself out of the shop. As the apprentice grew more competent, he could act as an assistant when calling on patients, an especially important function for surgeons, for many operations required two men. In return, the master was supposed to teach the young man his business. According to John Bell, the apprentice 'accompanies [his master] on visits to persons of a certain class; and of the lower people he takes a more particular charge'.[18] The time allotted for instruction, however, as well as the type of instruction, was left entirely to the discretion of the master.[19]

There were many opportunities in this system for masters to exploit apprentices, but as long as it was the main form of medical education a young man could console himself with the thought that his reward would come when he set up his own practice. As long as it was common for most young men to serve a master at some point, there was no special hardship in being a surgeon's servant or apprentice. As long as apprenticeship alone guaranteed entrance to the lucrative monopoly over surgery in Edinburgh, or constituted sufficient credentials for country practice, it continued to be highly valued. As the availability of more 'genteel' forms of medical education grew, however, and apprentices competed with practitioners trained at Edinburgh University or London hospitals, the image of apprenticeship was tarnished. 'Now, on full conviction, I assert,' James Parkinson wrote, 'that of all the modes which could be devised for a medical and chirurgical education, this is the most absurd.'[20] Even James Lucas and William Chamberlaine, who wrote handbooks addressed to apprentices and masters, gave so many examples of unpleasantness on both sides that it is a wonder anyone ever took an apprentice. Young men were idle, or spoiled by their mothers and sisters, or expected to be treated as if they were at home. They seduced maidservants, forgot to take messages, or compounded medication incorrectly, thus ruining their master's business. Or they actually stole money or their master's patients.

These tensions between master and apprentice really existed, as Alexander Lesassier's brief period of apprenticeship to Mr Collier in Manchester shows. Collier gave Lesassier little formal instruction, and seems to have regarded him as an assistant in the shop, rather than a student. The only 'medical improvement' Lesassier mentioned was 'Finding that dissection in Mr C's house was not only inconvenient, but also dangerous', which raises the question of where he would have obtained a cadaver, and where in the house he had been planning to put it.[21] He did not steal, though Collier accused him of taking food from the house to share with his friends,[22] but he did sleep with a maidservant, subsequently making the unpleasant discovery that if he had been caught he could have been compelled to pay for his own board.[23] He was reasonably diligent, but he considered himself a young gentleman, not a servant: when Collier accused him of 'impertinence' during a quarrel Lesassier 'resolved not to humble myself at all'.[24] Indeed, though Lesassier initially was pleased to gain Collier's approval, he strongly resented any treatment which suggested he was not Collier's equal.

That was of course the main problem with apprenticeship. Young men, however much they might want the legal or professional advantages of apprenticeship, never wanted to be treated as servants. If they had friends or associates who were not bound, the problem became more acute. This was especially difficult in Edinburgh, when apprentices could see all around them young men learning medicine without having to serve a master. The College of Surgeons confronted this problem in 1770, when members complained that

> the greatest part of those who are intended for this branch, seem
> rather inclined to attend a shop for some little time as students, than
> to be put under an indenture for a limited space.[25]

This caused many difficulties,

these gentlemen students being under no sort of restraint, they take
liberties, which give the very worst example to the prentices. [26]
In the next meeting, therefore, the College passed a regulation forbidding
masters to take into their shops any students who were not properly bound,
being

> unanimously of opinion that such a plan of education is of the worst
> consequences, to the students themselves as it makes it almost
> impossible for them to lay a proper foundation, or to acquire practical
> knowledge: that their being under no sort of restraint or any
> obligation to attend business is hurtful to their morals as well as their
> improvement in knowledge: that their example has universally been
> hurtful to the prentices, and at the same time has been accompanied
> with many inconveniences to the masters. [27]

Of course this was 'hurtful to the prentices'. They were presented with the
example of young gentlemen learning in three months, entirely at their
own convenience, the practical knowledge they had to serve at least three
years to acquire. A 'gentlemen student' would not have to sweep the shop,
or perform other menial tasks; instead, he paid the master surgeon for
instruction in the same way as he paid the professor of medicine for
lectures. If surgical knowledge could be acquired so easily, in a period of
a few months, why should a young man bother to be bound at all? [28]

Why indeed, asked Professor Andrew Duncan junior, who had been
apprenticed to Alexander Wood, an Edinburgh surgeon, in 1789. [29] He
knew, he said,

> from personal knowledge, that apprentices must spend a great deal
> more time on mere manual operations than is required for mastering
> them; that their leisure hours for study are cut up and frittered away
> by frequent calls for their occasional service; . . . that a single idle
> lad taints the whole shop. [30]

So far from this early introduction to medicine giving them any advantage,
Duncan felt, former apprentices, 'could not stand comparison' with other
medical students, 'who had studied . . . from the beginning under proper
conductors'. The most important reason for the superiority of those
students was

> that, besides having their time entirely at their own or their
> conductor's disposal, they very seldom begin their strict professional
> studies till later in life, and thus spend one, two, or three years more
> in the invaluable pursuit of general knowledge. [31]

It was that general knowledge that gave the practitioner his liberal cast
of mind, contemporaries would have agreed, and Duncan was thus entirely
correct in assuming they would serve a young man better than apprenticeship. But of course most young men could not afford one, two, or three
additional years of study required to obtain a Master of Arts, as Duncan

had;[32] nor were schools or private teachers more accessible for most.[33] A young man might be able to stay at home and study, but the rapid connection of ideas in Lesassier's diary gives a good illustration of why that, too, was difficult. 'Sep 12 1803,' he began,

> My birthday This day through' the ill usage of my Father I resolved on leaving him: but am not yet certain what part of the world to move to I think of *Edinburgh* . . . Since writing the above I believe I shall be able to get a situation in Town at a Mr. Collier Surgeon Bridge St.[34]

The next day he wrote

> It is nearly settled that I shall go to Mr Collier for 5 years. He is a Quaker and a respectable man By which step I shall not only be out of my Father's reach but also save myself a world of trouble! for what would have become of me had I persisted in going to Edinburgh God only knows.[35]

Apprenticeship, for Lesassier, was a welcome alternative to running away from home, and the prospect of being 'out of my Father's reach' might have attracted many young men and presumably their fathers. Fathers could, of course, have allowed their sons to begin taking medical lectures early, as Parkinson suggested. But even he said that many 'who may read this passage, will exclaim – what! attend a course of lectures on anatomy at fifteen years of age',[36] and the hypothetical father to whom his advice was addressed, 'actuated by no small regard to old customs',[37] did apprentice his son.

If apprenticeship was unavoidable, then, the question was how to make it more genteel. One way was to insist that the young man was not a servant at all, but rather a member of the family. The author of the letter 'From a young apprentice to his father', included in *The Complete Letter Writer*, described the members of his new household in terms of that ideal. 'My master is an honest, worthy man;' the young apprentice wrote,

> every body speaks well of him . . . My mistress is a chearful [sic], sweet-tempered woman . . . And the children, after such examples, behave to us all like one's own brothers and sisters. Who can but love such a family?[38]

And how could apprenticeship, under such conditions, be described as servile? Such familial relationships could occur between Edinburgh apprentices and their masters, for they come through in letters from Alexander Wemyss, surgeon in Edinburgh, and his wife Katherine about their apprentice Bethune Lindsay. Bethune, son of George Lindsay of Wormiston, was briefly apprenticed to Wemyss before leaving to take up a commission in the army. His father wrote apparently apologizing for the inconvenience and asking what he owed. Nothing, Wemyss replied, 'you were extremely right in accepting the commission for your son . . . He is a very fine genteel lad & I heartily wish and expect he will do very well in the Army.

As for the short time he has been with us, you & he are extremely welcome'.[39] Katherine's letter to Lady Wormiston was equally affectionate. 'I rec'd yours with a piece of very pretty cloth', she wrote, 'for which the Doctor and I return you many thanks, you should not have done it, for we never intended to have taken any thing for the short time your son was with us . . .'[40]

It would be pleasant to think that apprentices were always accepted as part of the family in this charming domestic way. Even if they were, though, tensions could arise; that too, after all, was part of family life. Lesassier, for example, seems to have transferred to his master some of his feelings towards his father, with the result that his apprenticeship was not the escape from unwanted authority he had hoped. His diary also suggests that introducing a young man into the household could be disruptive in other ways. Collier was furious when he found out that Lesassier had taken long walks in the countryside with his thirteen-year-old daughter: it was the cause of the first major battle between master and 'prentice.[41] Probably Lesassier did not intend a seduction: taking long romantic walks with young ladies was one of his favourite occupations. Equally probably Miss Collier and Mr Lesassier did not regard each other 'like one's own brother and sister'.

Another, more successful way to make apprenticeship genteel was to insist on the gentility of the masters. In Edinburgh, the surgeons' guild occupied an ambiguous status. On the one hand, Edinburgh surgeons were prominent local practitioners. On the other, as the fame of the University spread, it was increasingly the Professors of the Faculty of Medicine who set professional and educational standards. Rosalie Stott has rightly stressed the connection between the educational activities of the Incorporation and the founding of the medical faculty in 1726: John Monro, who worked to found the faculty, was a member of the Incorporation, as was his son, Alexander Monro *primus*. Yet Stott's account also shows the tensions in the alliance between surgeons and professors. Only professors who were Fellows of the Royal College of Physicians could examine candidates for a degree, and only they could be specifically designated as part of the Faculty of Medicine.[42] The regulations of the College of Physicians prohibited Fellows from being Fellows of the College of Surgeons at the same time. Edinburgh surgeons were thus prohibited from becoming full examining members of the medical faculty as long as they remained Members of the Incorporation. Individual social mobility, in other words, could only be achieved by leaving the privileges of the guild behind.

Professor Alexander Monro *primus* for most of his life was a Member of the Incorporation, and thus not a Fellow of the College of Physicians. He resigned from the Incorporation in 1757 in order to become a Fellow.[43] His son, Professor Alexander Monro *secundus*, had also been a Member of the Incorporation. When he began lecturing, however, he resigned from the Incorporation to join the Royal College of Physicians of Edinburgh, saying he had entered into a business 'which was thought incompetent [sic] with the exercise of surgery and pharmacy'.[44] Thomas Young, Professor of Midwifery, likewise originally a member of the Incorporation, also resigned to join the College of Physicians in 1762.[45]

It is not clear whether the rest of the Incorporation resented the Monros' and Young's attempts to distance themselves from their guild origins, though they certainly resented Monro's monopoly over the teaching of surgery.[46] What is clear is that from the 1770s, the Incorporation took vigorous and largely successful steps to raise their status as a corporate body. The first of these involved changing their name to the Royal College of Surgeons, clearly inspired by the prestige of the Royal College of Physicians of Edinburgh. The new name appeared first in the minutes in 1770, in the diploma for country surgeons, where the candidate was described as appearing before the 'College of Surgeons of Edinburgh'.[47] In 1778 the Edinburgh surgeons petitioned for, and received, a royal charter to call themselves the Royal College of Surgeons of Edinburgh. The Members of the former Incorporation were now to be known as Fellows; the former Deacon became the new President. Surgeons could now claim equal legal status with the Royal College of Physicians of Edinburgh, since they had an equivalent charter. In addition, by changing the name of their society they could distance themselves from their long history as one of the Town's guilds. Upon receiving the royal charter, the College decided 'that as it was found from experience that their connection with city politicks had been a source of much dissention in the society', it was resolved that 'members of the Royal College of Surgeons of Edinburgh ought to be disengaged as much as possible from city politicks, with which as a corporation the surgeons of Edinburgh have hitherto been connected'.[48] Squabbling over city politics was hardly a suitable occupation for professional gentlemen; besides, the stakes were not as high as they had been 100 years earlier. The Fellows went so far as to submit a memorial to legal counsel, as to whether they could legally separate from city government. 'The plan of education which the memorialists now pursue' they wrote,

> places them on a very different point of view from that in which they stood two centuries ago and entitles them to be considered as a literary society and not in the line of mere mechanicks.[49]

Since their education was now liberal, not servile, the Memorial went on,
> They have long viewed their connection with city politicks as an interruption to the due prosecution of the various branches of their profession, and as prejudicial to their true interests, being thereby

led into disputes and altercations which tend often to destroy the
peace and harmony of the Society.[50]

It was the opinion of counsel, however, that the Royal College could not
disassociate itself from city politics without sacrificing their privileges, and
so the idea was dropped. This is an important point: the Royal College of
Surgeons saw no incompatibility between corporate privilege and a liberal
profession. Neither, of course, did the Royal College of Physicians of
Edinburgh, which also retained its privileges throughout the period.

Instead, the Deacon's council proposed 'that it might be for the honour
and advantage of the College to institute literary meetings and to elect a
President annually to preside on these occasions'.[51] The purpose of the
proposal was obvious: if the College could not entirely disassociate itself
from its 'mere mechanick' origins, it could at least behave like a society
of learned gentlemen. This proposal was never acted upon, any more than
Dr John Aitken's proposal of 1784, that the Royal College

> should assume . . . a proper connection and correspondence with
> similar associations and with respectable medical characters and . . .
> collect memoirs and essays belonging to our object without altering
> in any degree . . . our new limited corporate and burghal capacity.[52]

John Bell satirized the pretensions of the College as 'the busy bustling
awkwardness of such a society; their awkward ungainly attempts at literary
reputation; the inconsistency betwixt their trade of Apothecary-Surgeons,
and their assumed functions of playing the part, forsooth, of physician'.[53]
The description is apt, for the College, by any name, was an organization
of busy practitioners, not a philosophical society.

Yet if the College was not successful in becoming a literary society, it
was strikingly successful in becoming an educational institution. The
memorial to counsel had made it clear that it was by virtue of the 'plan of
education which the memorialists now pursue' that they were entitled to
be considered as gentlemen, and not 'mere mechanicks'. That was the most
effective strategy medical writers employed to make apprenticeship genteel: insisting that it was a form a professional study, which gave every
opportunity for professional improvement. In Edinburgh, professional
improvement for apprentices, as well as other young men, was always tied
to lectures. Apprentices routinely attended Professor Alexander Monro's
anatomy course, for, as Sir John Clerk had said, 'The foundation and
perfection of Chyrurgery is to understand the structure of the human body.
And for that end', he told his son, 'neglect no opportunity of studying
anatomy with the best masters'.[54] John Bell later echoed this advice when
he wrote that

> naming parts first, then describing, then dissecting them; dissecting
> them again and again in different directions, and in a variety of

subjects; dissecting, till names and parts are rightly associated in his mind, till he recollects, and can represent with ease . . . all their relations to each other . . . till, placing his finger on any point of the body, he can name the parts which lie within, will, indeed, make a man a surgeon.[55]

We do not know how many apprentices could have followed this advice, for we do not have class lists for private anatomy classes. The difficulty of obtaining cadavers in Edinburgh makes it likely that apprentices found it easier to follow the second part of Sir John Clerk's advice on professional studies, to 'study physick in all its parts'. Between 1770 and 1780, 77 per cent of the apprentices signed the matriculation album, meaning, of course, that 23 per cent did not.[56] After 1780, virtually all apprentices did. As Table 5.1 shows, they also attended a wide range of courses over the period.

Table 5.1 Apprentices' course attendance, 1763–1826

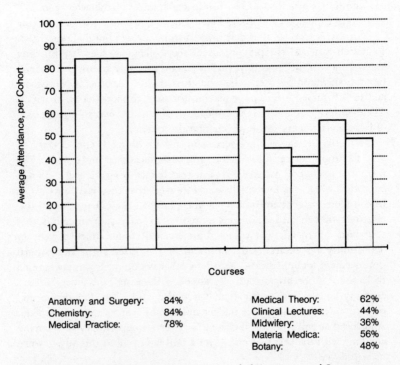

Courses

Anatomy and Surgery:	84%	Medical Theory:	62%
Chemistry:	84%	Clinical Lectures:	44%
Medical Practice:	78%	Midwifery:	36%
		Materia Medica:	56%
		Botany:	48%

Eighty-four per cent of the apprentices attended Anatomy and Surgery over the period. This shows that apprentices did follow advice like Sir John's of 'neglecting no opportunity for studying anatomy'. This pattern of attendance was consistent over the period, suggesting that however inadequate Monro *tertius'* course might have been for more advanced students, for young apprentices there was no substitute for a solid series of lectures on anatomy, physiology and surgery.[57] Attendance at other courses was lower than the graduates', but higher than other groups of students, as we will see. Less than half the apprentices − 44 per cent − attended Clinical Lectures, no doubt because they had opportunities to attend what William Brown called 'those real clinical lectures, though not dignified by the name', which came from attending their master's patients. Table 5.2 shows that 42 per cent attended courses over the period of their apprenticeship. It was thus the 'greater number' of apprentices who employed more than three years attending lectures, rather than graduates, as Professor Joseph Black had assumed.

Indeed, some apprenticeships at Edinburgh clearly came to be dominated by the presence of the university. An apprentice elsewhere was usually the only young man in the shop, with at most one older or younger associate. In Edinburgh, too, most masters took only five or six apprentices over their career; a small number had perhaps ten or twelve over a thirty year period. Benjamin Bell, Andrew Wardrop, and James Russell, however, consistently booked many more from the time they became Fellows in the 1770s, and in the 1790s the three men formed a partnership, whose main purpose seems to have been training apprentices.[58] One hundred and fifty-four apprentices were booked either to the three men individually or to 'Bell, Wardrop Russell & Co', 36 per cent of the total booked between 1780 and 1815.[59] That meant that the

Table 5.2 Apprentices' period of study, 1763–1826

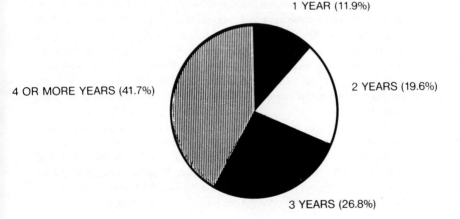

partnership trained five or six young men at any one time. Once Russell became Professor of Clinical Surgery,[60] his apprentices must have reaped the added benefits of frequent contact with surgical operations. John Bell accused the 'copartnery', as he called it, of being behind the expulsion of other surgeons from the Royal Infirmary; if he was right, it may well have been in order to limit control of surgical cases as far as possible to members of the partnership, and access to their own numerous apprentices.[61]

Apprenticeship under these circumstances must have been more like being in a small class than Lesassier's experience of serving a master. Certainly that was how William Brown described it in 1826. His father had been a Fellow of the Royal College, and William himself became one in 1817; he therefore grew up imbued with the principles of the new, liberally-educated Edinburgh surgeon. Writing in response to Andrew Duncan junior's derogatory comments about apprenticeship, mentioned earlier, Brown acted as spokesperson for the new image of the apprentice as student. 'It was formerly', he wrote

> . . . customary for apprentices to be employed in many duties which we now consider as menial and servile. Under this regime a good deal of their time must have been misapplied, and it cannot be doubted that their sense of self-respect must have been lowered to an injurious degree.[62]

By the 1820s, Brown wrote, those days were long past. Everyone agreed that attendance at medical lectures was important, and no master would prevent a worthy apprentice from attending them, at least not in Edinburgh. 'I never heard of a master hinder his apprentice from attending the classes', Brown wrote. 'Were he selfish enough to entertain the proposal, the number of classes, and the variety of lectures on all branches, make it, in general, an easy matter for the apprentice to carry on his course of study without interruption.'[63] Brown's purpose was obviously to put apprenticeship in its best possible light, but this may have been the simple truth. Edinburgh masters would not hinder apprentices from attending classes, because that was an important reason why they were so successful at attracting them. Moreover, given the number of apprentices the most popular surgeon-masters like 'Bell, Wardrop, Russell and Co', could have at any one time, allowing some to attend classes would have been no hardship: when the older ones went to class, the younger ones could look after the shop.

Yet if the benefit of becoming an apprentice in Edinburgh came from attending classes, why not follow Parkinson's advice and simply enroll the young man in lectures? Because, Brown might have answered, he would then be subject to all the temptations that Parkinson's anxious father feared. Far better to indenture him to a master, who would make it his business to monitor the young man's educational progress and moral conduct. 'A professor with 200 or 300 pupils, cannot inspect, with satisfaction to himself, their general progress and conduct . . .' Brown said,

> But a master, with half a dozen apprentices, possesses every advantage for instructing them in the most perfect way. He knows their dispositions, and can accommodate his mode of instructions to these; he knows their mental progress, and can deal out to them the kind and degree of instruction which they require.[64]

By the 1820s there was widespread concern about large lectures as a form of medical instruction, so much so that professors recommended making grinders University tutors, as we have seen.[65] Brown clearly was addressing that concern. But again, he was also describing an important feature of Edinburgh apprenticeship: some masters did have 'half a dozen apprentices', and made tuition, not sweeping the shop, the basis of apprenticeship. If, like James Russell or John Thomson or John William Turner, the master was also a lecturer, the apprentice would move easily from shop to lecture to private class.[66]

To Duncan's objection that 'an idle lad taints the entire shop', Brown replied that though it was true that not all apprentices were equally industrious, at least apprenticeship provided a much more protected environment than mere attendance at lectures. An apprentice, Brown said, will

> be exposed equally . . . to the contagion of surrounding vice . . . but he has (what every other student has not) in his master, a friend on the spot; a director qualified to advise and assist him, and whose duty it is to inspect his moral conduct as well as his professional improvement.'[67]

When Brown wrote this he was thirty years old, and had already booked five apprentices, the first when he was only twenty-three. It seems to have been common for young surgeons to book apprentices soon after becoming Fellows, no doubt because they had not built up lucrative practices and needed the income from apprentice fees. It did mean, though, that they had more time to direct their apprentices' studies. The fact that the master had only recently finished his own studies may have led his apprentices to agree that he was 'qualified to advise and assist' them, in the way that twentieth-century medical students look to residents for advice on getting through.[68] It is also possible that they would have been more likely to consider him a friend, though it is equally possible that they might not have accepted his authority: James Rush in Philadelphia faced both situations when he took private pupils soon after finishing his own studies.[69]

Brown's account of apprenticeship, then, answered all possible objections. Apprentices were not servants, but students, with the added advantages of a built-in tutor and moral guardian. 'An apprentice receives the same education which another student does', Brown wrote,

> he attends the same classes, he embraces the same opportunities, and besides these, he receives additional advantages from the general inspection of his master, from the frequent examination on professional subjects which he undergoes . . . and from those real clinical lectures, though not dignified by the name, which are so much the more useful, that they are occasional, private, and frequent.[70]

Apprenticeship, then, was simply another kind of tutorial system for medical students. Andrew Duncan junior acknowledged the force of Brown's arguments when he wrote that 'Mr Brown's animadversions . . . puts our readers in possession of the leading arguments on each side of an important question', though without, presumably, altering his own opinion.[71]

Apprentices, to the Fellows, were like students who attended classes to the Faculty, young men seeking medical improvement whom they had no ultimate obligation to certify. Like professors, the surgeons chose one particular group of men to test on their knowledge, the ones who wished to become Fellows of the Royal College. The examinations for membership underwent the same shift from guild practice to academic institution as the College itself. In 1712, the Incorporation of Surgeons had decreed that all prospective Masters undergo four 'lessons', as the examinations were traditionally called, in order to be admitted. The first lesson required the 'intrant', as the candidate was called, to make 'a speech . . . on any chirurgicall case, operation or surgery in general as he pleases. And to answer all practical questions that shall be enquired in any case or operation in chirurgerie'. The second was 'anatomicall' the subject was chosen by the Incorporation, and the candidate notified in advance. The third and fourth lessons were to be 'operations of chirurgery', and those were also determined by the Members.[72]

The formal statutes were not changed until 1795, but the lessons had developed a different format by the 1760s. The first lesson continued to be a presentation by the 'intrant' on some aspect of surgery, such as inflammation, fistula, gangrene, or gunshot wounds. The first lesson may have been where the candidate was examined 'strictly and minutely'[73] on knowledge acquired during apprenticeship itself, for Cumberland Moffat was turned down after his first examination in 1782, and 'advised to pay more attention to the practical part of surgery',[74] before he re-applied for trials. If the first lesson went well, the candidate was given a specific topic in anatomy, such as bones of the head or pelvis, or the anatomy of the thorax, to prepare for the next lesson, usually held a week later. At the third lesson, he was expected to discuss materia medica, botany, and pharmacy generally, and also comment on two medicinal preparations. The fourth lesson was to perform a particular operation, 'if required', according to the later statute.[75] It is not clear how often operations were actually required. A restricted range of operations were assigned, most frequently trepan, cataract, and operation for hare lip. Trepan was assigned twenty-one times between 1763 and 1804, and cataract, seventeen times.[76] It is hard to imagine that 'suitable subjects' could have been procured for all of these on demand, or that the College would have wished to watch the procedure in the middle of their examination hall. Possibly candidates were simply questioned on surgical procedures. If the operations were actually performed, no clinical records have remained.

Even discussion of an operation was changed after 1804, to the public defense of a treatise on a surgical subject. A written treatise was first proposed by Dr Aitken in 1784, and became a formal requirement in 1793.[77] From 1804 the printed thesis replaced the operation, and had to be printed with the title page, 'A Probationary Essay . . . submitted by [name of candidate] by the Authority of the President and his Council to the Examination of the Royal College of Surgeons of Edinburgh . . .'.[78] The surgeon's treatises were in English, but Aitken's model was the 'Inaugural Dissertation' required for the University medical degree. The written thesis coincided with Aitken's suggestion that the College correspond with other professional bodies; it was obviously intended to further emphasize the nature of the College as a 'literary' society.

The College revised their regulations a number of times to further make this point. By 1826, the similarities with the MD examination were more obvious than the differences. The surgeon's examination was in English, but according to regulations printed in 1804, no one was to be admitted as candidate who 'has not had a liberal education',[79] and William Wood told the Royal Commission that a surgeon needed Latin and Greek, mathematics and natural philosophy, adding 'I really think the education of a Surgeon very defective indeed if it does not include these branches'.[80] Candidates were also to have studied 'Anatomy medicine and surgery in some public school and hospital for the space of three years'.[81] These were not precise course requirements, but the Fellows were dealing with a more constricted group, over which they had more direct control. Forty-three of the sixty-three Fellows who entered between 1810 and 1826 – 67 per cent – also received MDs. And the only point which distinguished the Probationary Surgical Essay from the Inaugural Medical Dissertation was that it was in English, not Latin. If it was true that most graduates wrote their theses in English and had someone else translate it for them, even that difference was eliminated.

Adopting the outward forms of the MD theses meant acquiring some of the problems, such as disagreements between the author and examiner over the contents. The College found this out in 1823, when Dr John

Mackintosh included in his essay some derogatory remarks on accoucheurs, whose 'persecution' of Sir Richard Croft, the physician treating Princess Charlotte when she died in childbirth, Mackintosh wrote, 'I shall never cease to hold it up a scandalous and infamous, because it was gratuitous as well as unjust, and unworthy of a liberal profession'.[82] Presumably the College examiners found Mackintosh's own comments gratuitous, because 'it was proposed', according to the minutes, 'that the president should wait upon Dr. Mackintosh and inform him that it seemed to be the general feeling of the College that the passages . . . should be cancelled and to enquire if Dr. Mackintosh had any object to withdraw them without the interference of the College'. Their justification for this was the same as the medical faculty's: since the essay appeared 'by the Authority of the President and his Council' the examiners had a right to regulate its contents. Mackintosh requested, according to the minutes, that he might 'be heard in defence of the passages alluded to before determining as to the line of conduct he should adopt'. The College agreed, and Dr Mackintosh 'addressed the meeting'. The minutes do not record what he said, but we may imagine his defence was similar to John Wainman's, that if he made the changes he would be 'prevented from saying what *I really believe*, to the manifest injury of my Dissertation'.[83] Afterwards the College still felt 'that the objectionable passages should be withdrawn', and Dr Mackintosh was then informed that the College wished that he 'would agree of himself to cancell [sic] the passages This Dr Mackintosh declined'. The College then voted to assert its authority and require Mackintosh to remove the passages before he would be allowed to continue the examination. Mackintosh, thus compelled, made the necessary changes; we do not know if he felt, as Robert Jones had done, that this was 'downright outrage'. We may wonder, though, whether in 1823 there were any Fellows left to sigh for the old days, when 'intrants' were mere 'prentices, and not gentlemen students.

By the 1820s, then, apprentices to Edinburgh surgeons had been transformed from 'mere mechanicks' who did not even need to attend university lectures to 'students of medicine strictly speaking'. Yet that transformation carried with it seeds of more change. As liberal education became more important for surgeons, students spent the years between fifteen and eighteen learning Latin, mathematics and natural philosophy, rather than serving indentures. Hospital training and University clinical lectures superceded those 'real clinical lectures, though not dignified by the name', in part because hospital and university lectures were dignified both with the name and with certificates of completion. After all, if apprenticeship was really just a form of study combining lectures and tutoring, and becoming a Fellow like obtaining an MD, what was there to keep a student from becoming a surgeon by attending lectures and small classes and acquiring a degree?

The advantage apprenticeship to a Fellow retained the longest was its oldest one: greatly reduced cost of entry into the monopoly over the practice of surgery and pharmacy in Edinburgh. That monopoly was still valuable in 1816, when the entry fee for apprentices who had served for the freedom was raised to £100, and for those who had not, to £250.[84] One year later, though, in 1817 – coincidentally the same year William Brown became a Fellow – another young gentleman, James Syme, described as 'student',[85] took the alternate route into surgery of becoming a Licentiate of the Royal College of Surgeons. His title conveyed no guild privileges and conferred no monopoly, as we will see in Chapter Eight. Equally, though, it did not prevent him from paying the necessary entry money to become a Fellow himself in 1825. Under Professor James Syme's presidency in 1840, the Royal College finally gave up its local monopoly in favour of a national charter. Gentlemen-apprentices, then, only really lasted for one generation. But they left gentlemen surgeons in their wake.

6

Occasional auditors

[M]y Uncle desires that I will go over to Edinburgh . . . when
I reflect on the advantages which will arise from it I am quite
overjoyed. I can finish my education completely – Oh dear it's
delightful –

Alexander Lesassier, Diary[1]

The third group of students found at Edinburgh University was both the
largest and the most elusive: they were the group who came to study and
left without any form of certification. We know of most of them only
through their signatures in the Matriculation Albums, since only a handful
turn up in any of the surviving letters and diaries of the period. The Royal
Commission described them as 'occasional auditors', and I have adopted
the term as a convenient shorthand, even though the Commissioners
assumed, incorrectly, that auditors did not intend to practice medicine.[2]
If we take occasional to mean 'as opportunity requires,' rather than
'casual',[3] the phrase is a very good description of this group of students.
The lack of information about them has made them all but invisible to
historians, but they were as important a component of the University as
the graduates, since it was the auditors who swelled the matriculation
records and filled the lecture halls. Professors may have looked to the
graduates to ensure their fame, but they relied on the auditors for their
fortune: 64 per cent of the students between 1763 and 1826 fit into this
category.

No systematic study of the auditors' backgrounds is possible, partly
because of lack of information, and partly because there were different types
of auditors. The most striking aspect of the auditors' education is its
brevity: 70 per cent studied for only one year. See Table 6.1.

One year was not much time to begin and end university medical
education, and students did so for different reason. One well-documented
group were those who came solely to take Chemistry. Students who took
only Chemistry should probably not be considered 'students of medicine
strictly speaking', or at least were not studying to become practitioners.

Table 6.1 Auditors' period of study, 1763–1826

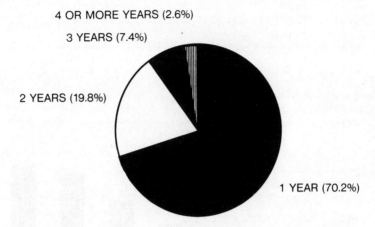

4 OR MORE YEARS (2.6%)

3 YEARS (7.4%)

2 YEARS (19.8%)

1 YEAR (70.2%)

As mentioned in Chapter Three, Chemistry in this period became a fashionable subject. Joseph Black was already giving lectures in Chemistry to a lay audience in 1775, for Sylas Neville complained that Black

> finished his lectures rather unexpectedly . . . alledging as an excuse that his health required some relaxation. But I cannot help thinking that abridging his proper course after beginning another at an early hour to a set of lawyers etc has not the best appearance.[4]

However, the major increase in auditors who attended only Chemistry came in the 1780s and after. See Table 6.2.

Many of those who attended the course came specifically to hear Dr Black, 'whose celebrity is so great', the author of the *Guide for Gentlemen Studying Medicine* wrote, 'that it is unnecessary to mention the important advantages which may be derived from attending his lectures'.[5] As discussed Chapter Three, Black's lectures provided 'general views of chemistry',[6] rather than instruction on how to compound medication. Thomas Charles Hope's numerous demonstrations were no doubt an important reason why the numbers of students who attended only Chemistry went up after 1800. Another was the increased interest in chemistry in manufacturing, and another was, that 'Chemistry is now . . . with much propriety, considered as a branch of general education'.[7] These auditors may have attended Chemistry as part of their general education, or may have been specifically interested in the science, and wanted to hear its principles discussed by a celebrated chemist. In either case, although they are important for understanding the development of chemistry in this period, they are much less useful for examining the trends in medical education. Indeed, the large increase in the percentage of

Table 6.2 Auditors attending chemistry only, 1765–1820

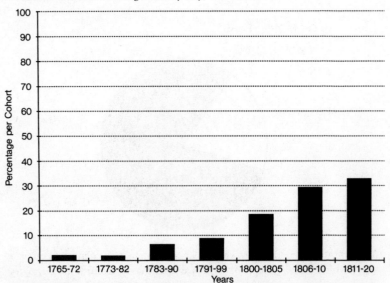

students who took only Chemistry masks some of the other changes in the auditors' education in this period.

Let us, then, peel away the students who took only Chemistry from the rest of the auditors, in order to examine the educational patterns of the latter group. The *Guide* mentions two such groups, students who had no previous training, but who 'intend to complete their education at London or Paris', and students who had come from other universities, and 'attend the college of Edinburgh for the purpose of acquiring the opinions of the several professors in the different medical subjects'.[8] These students were on either the beginning or ending stages of a medical 'Grand Tour', and by the end of their education would have studied in several different universities or hospitals.

Many of the American students fit into these categories. Thomas Parke, for example, had received his MB from Philadelphia College of Medicine in 1770, and came to Britain to study in London and Edinburgh. He spent two summers in the London hospitals and went to Edinburgh for more formal training. Though Parke went to hear the opening lectures of several courses, he ended up only attending the lectures on Medical Practice and the Clinical Lectures at the Infirmary. Since he had had considerable background in medicine prior to coming to Edinburgh, he felt there would be little point in attending the rest of the lectures.[9] Jane Rendall has suggested that students from New York and Philadelphia were especially likely to study for one or two years, since they had taken medical courses for several years at home. [10] James Rush's study at the University of Pennsylvania medical school led him to be highly critical of the Edinburgh faculty when he went there in 1809. He took tickets for Medical Practice, Chemistry, and Anatomy and Surgery, but grew so disgusted with them that he gave up attending them. [11] He, like other students in this group, spent much of his time improving himself as any gentleman on a Grand Tour would, through travel, attention to manners and customs, and polite entertainment.

A different pattern was established by Oxford and Cambridge students who came to Edinburgh to 'find physic' they could not get at their own universities. [12] Thirty per cent of the 179 Fellows who joined the Royal College of Physicians of London over the period studied at Edinburgh, generally for one year. Table 6.3 gives their course of study.

Table 6.3 Course attendance, Fellows of the Royal College of Physicians of London, 1763–1826

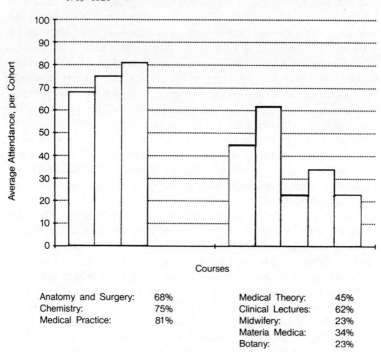

Anatomy and Surgery:	68%	Medical Theory:	45%
Chemistry:	75%	Clinical Lectures:	62%
Medical Practice:	81%	Midwifery:	23%
		Materia Medica:	34%
		Botany:	23%

Their attendance at Anatomy and Surgery, Chemistry, Medical Practice, and Clinical Lectures is especially high. Attending Clinical Lectures would make a great deal of sense for this group, because Fellows frequently did obtain positions at the London hospitals. The 23 per cent who attended

Midwifery is also noteworthy, because Fellows of the London College of
Physicians were prohibited from practicing midwifery; either this group
of students did not definitely intend to practice in London, or they were
simply interested in 'medical improvement' of all kinds.[13]

The largest group of auditors, however, would have been 'Those',
according to the *Guide*, 'who wish to practice as surgeons or apothecaries
directly after leaving the college', or 'Those who wish to perfect themselves
in the knowledge of the practice of physic and surgery, after having served
a regular apprenticeship to a surgeon or apothecary'.[14] These were the
prospective surgeon-apothecaries, whose function as general practitioners
has been thoroughly analyzed by Irvine Loudon.[15] Although it is impossible to trace the later careers of all of them, many do turn up as medical
practitioners in the 1779 *Medical Register*.[16] Thirty-eight per cent of the
120 men listed practicing in Scotland without MDs studied at Edinburgh
University.[17] More may have done so prior to 1762, when medical
matriculation records begin. English general practitioners also studied at
Edinburgh, for 18 per cent of practitioners without MDs listed for
Yorkshire,[18] and 56 per cent of those in Cumberland had been auditors
between 1762 and 1779.[19]

Apprenticeship followed by courses in medical subjects was indeed one
of the most prevalent forms of medical training. Andrew Marshall,
advising an unnamed lord on the education of his lordship's illegitimate
son, recommended that the young gentleman first 'be put to a short
apprenticeship with some respectable country surgeon, till he be fit to
enter on the study of anatomy'. Next, he was to spend two years or so
attending lectures on anatomy and chemistry, and perform dissections and
'walk an hospital as physician's pupil'.[20] Marshall, like many writers,
especially recommended London for its dissecting and hospital facilities.[21]
Edinburgh University lectures, though, fulfilled the same function for
students whose family or professional connections led them, like Alexander
Lesassier, nephew of Professor James Hamilton, to 'think of Edinburgh'
when considering further study.[22] The many problems associated with
apprenticeship led more and more prospective practitioners to augment
their education with further study. '[N]otwithstanding it is so expensive,
no Young Fellow ought to set up in our Branch without attending it some
time' Thomas Ismay wrote to his father after only a few weeks at
Edinburgh. 'I'll assure you in this little time I have found that, as I have
seen so many things which a Person in our Branch may, if he has not been
at any of these Places, make a fatal Blunder in.'[23]

As Ismay's comments make clear, the expense of attending classes and
living away from home were limiting factors in auditors' education. We
know very little about the social backgrounds of the auditors, but the
handful we can trace would have fallen into the lower part of the middling

ranks. Thomas Ismay was the son of a Yorkshire vicar, and Job Harrison, of a prosperous yeoman farmer from outside Chester. According to James Lucas, in *Education . . . of a Surgeon-Apothecary*, 'Many practitioners bring up their sons to the profession',[24] and sons of surgeons or apothecaries no doubt accounted for many of the auditors. Marmaduke Hewitt junior who was an auditor in 1799, was almost certainly the son of the Mr Marmaduke Hewitt who was listed under the heading 'Surgeons and Apothecaries' at Beverly in the *Medical Register* for 1779.[25] Alexander Lesassier was the son of a rather unsuccessful physician in Manchester.[26] All but Harrison would readily have been described by contemporaries as 'gentleman's sons of very moderate fortune', to borrow David Skene's phrase.[27] The presence of auditors like Harrison suggests that this route into medicine was one of the more accessible ways for prosperous farmers, tradesmen and artisans to make their sons gentlemen.

Since their fortunes were moderate, auditors had to carefully consider which courses to attend. Their assumptions were succinctly stated by Ismay, who paid '£20 and some Shillings' for his classes: he wrote to his

Table 6.4 One-year auditors' course attendance, 1763–1826, excluding students who attended chemistry only

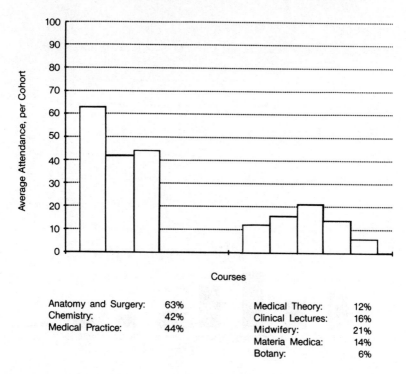

Courses

Anatomy and Surgery:	63%	Medical Theory:	12%
Chemistry:	42%	Clinical Lectures:	16%
Medical Practice:	44%	Midwifery:	21%
		Materia Medica:	14%
		Botany:	6%

father 'as I am not certain of staying another winter I now attend the most
material ones'.[28] Rendall found that American students in Edinburgh for
only a short period of time made similar decisions about the most
important courses to attend, concentrating on Anatomy and Medical
Practice;[29] James Rush, studying at a later period, added Chemistry to
those two classes. Other students must have made the same choice, for as
Table 6.4 shows, the 'most material' courses for one-year auditors were,
overwhelmingly, Anatomy and Surgery, Chemistry, and Medical Practice.

It is not surprising that an average of 63 per cent of the one-year auditors
attended Anatomy and Surgery, for we have already seen writers like the
author of the *Guide for Gentlemen Studying Medicine*[30] and Andrew Marshall
discuss its importance. James Lucas similarly stressed the necessity of
knowing the structure of the body in health in order to treat its diseases.[31]
Lucas also remarked that he had

> often heard my late Preceptor, Mr Pott, observe, that the superior
> skill of modern Surgeons, depended chiefly on their being better
> Anatomists, and that, unless integrity was wanting, fallacious predic-
> tions might be imputed to ignorance in Anatomy.[32]

Indeed, for some Edinburgh auditors, Monro's Anatomy and Surgery
constituted their entire university education. See Table 6.5.

Table 6.5 Auditors attending anatomy only, 1765–1820, excluding students who
attended chemistry only

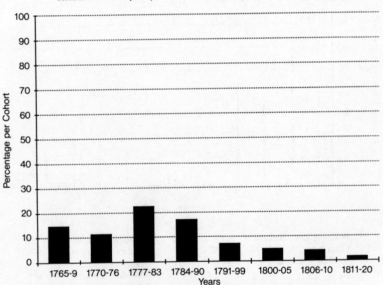

Anatomy and Surgery never became a fashionable subject outside of medicine in the same way as Chemistry did, and so presumably even those who took no other courses did intend to practice medicine. As Table 6.5 indicates, an average of 13 per cent of auditors in the 1760s and 1770s came only to take Anatomy and Surgery. Between 1777 and 1783, the figure rose to 23 per cent, no doubt because of the American War. The war increased the demand for surgeon's mates, and would-be mates would have hurriedly come to Edinburgh to attend Monro's course for a year, in order to take advantage of the opportunities in the army and navy. The figure stayed high in the 1780s, but dropped significantly after 1790. The Napoleonic wars from 1793 on did not produce the same influx of Anatomy and Surgery students; as we shall see, by that time there were new educational opportunities for army and navy surgeons and surgeons' mates.[33]

It is less obvious why Chemistry had the comparatively high enrollment – 42 per cent – of the one-year auditors. Lucas asserted that 'A Practitioner cannot be an accurate, and neat compounder of medicines, without some knowledge in this practical branch of science',[34] but we know from Neville and the *Guide* that Black and Hope did not teach their Chemistry class as an aid to pharmacy. Instead, they concentrated on general principles. Lucas, indeed, went on to insist on the importance of a knowledge of chemical principles, so that the student could

> distinguish between mechanical, and chemical mixtures, understand the simple substances contained in compounds, comprehend elective attractions, and the properties of factitious airs . . .[35]

But what he seems to have in mind is that the surgeon-apothecary should know enough chemistry to make sure he could mix his preparations, not that he needed to have a detailed knowledge of, for example, latent heat. The *Guide* gave contrary advice: it recommended that those intending to set up practice as surgeon or apothecary not take Chemistry, as it was 'to be considered rather as an ornamental than a necessary study'. Only if the surgeon-to-be studied for three years did the *Guide* feel he had time to take the course.[36] Why, then, did so many one-year auditors take Chemistry? Why not attend Materia Medica, a far more practical course, instead?

Auditors may, of course, have agreed with John Gregory, that the Chemistry class was necessary to understand the changes brought about in the body 'in consequence of chemical principles'.[37] Or they may simply have considered it part of their general education. Most likely, though, their high enrolment in Chemistry was a consequence of the strengths and limitations of apprenticeship. Lucas insisted on the importance of a course in Materia Medica to a surgeon-apothecary, and suggested it be taken at the same time as Anatomy.[38] But the *Guide* flatly stated that Materia Medica 'will be well enough understood by every one who has served some time in a shop'[39] and Ismay mentioned that Home's course on Materia

Medica 'is a thing not very necessary to a Person, that has been acquainted with medicine before'.[40] That explained why only 14 per cent of the one-year auditors took Materia Medica: a student who had just completed his apprenticeship would have felt it hardly worth the money to take a course in compounding medication.

Chemistry, however, was a different matter. Few masters would have had the equipment or knowledge to introduce their apprentices to the subject; it was indisputably a topic which required a university or private lecturer to explain. Even Lucas suggested that if a student's family did not have enough money to pay for all the necessary courses,

> a Pupil must content himself with gaining information from the best authors on [Materia Medica], and pay particular attention to all the instruction on this head communicated by a Professor of Chemistry.[41]

In other words, all surgeon-apothecaries should take both Materia Medica and Chemistry, but if money was tight, they should take Chemistry, and read up on Materia Medica on their own. The one-year auditors' course attendance suggests they followed similar advice, opting for Chemistry rather than Materia Medica. They could learn about compounding drugs anywhere, but what better place to hear the principles of chemistry than under the celebrated Dr Black, or the ingenious Dr Hope?

Medical Practice was the third course which attracted a large number of one-year auditors, an average of 44 per cent over the period. Lucas was very definite about its importance for the surgeon-apothecary, for, he said,

> except a student make himself thoroughly acquainted with the history of maladies, he cannot expect to have proper discernment in distinguishing them, or success in their treatment.[42]

The histories and treatment of diseases were the main topic covered in Medical Practice under all the Edinburgh professors. We might have expected students to take Medical Theory first as an introduction, since it dealt with 'the principles upon which the practice of physic is founded', according to the *Guide*.[43] However, as we have seen, much of the material in Medical Theory was covered in other courses as well, and students anxious to save money would not have considered it 'most material'. They may also have been following recommendations similar to the *Guide*'s that 'those branches which are absolutely necessary for the practice of medicine and surgery, should be first studied'.[44] There was no doubt that a course which systematically discussed diseases and their cures was absolutely necessary.

Some auditors also attended Clinical Lectures and Midwifery — 16 per cent and 21 per cent respectively. The low percentage of Clinical Lectures is not too surprising, for if a student had served an apprenticeship, he may have felt that there was no need to submit himself to the crowds in the Clinical Lectures wards. Again, we have no way of knowing how many brought tickets to visit the Infirmary on their own. The low percentage for Midwifery is more surprising, since surgeon-apothecaries would also often act as midwives. Both Thomas Ismay and Job Harrison attended Midwifery, but they were comparatively unusual. Irvine Loudon found that midwifery was the least paid of any aspect of general practice, and students with only enough money to spend a year at Edinburgh may have felt the rewards of Midwifery not worth the expense.[45] Far fewer one-year auditors took Medical Theory, Materia Medica, and Botany. Students would have to stay an additional three months to take the Botany class, which would have added to the expense. Job Harrison took the class, as we have seen, but then his expenses of £150 per annum were high by the standards of Ismay and Lesassier.[46]

The course attendance of the one-year auditors is a useful corrective to the idea that students always get out of a course exactly what a professor puts into it. For example, William Cullen told his students in Medical Practice that he assumed they had already attended a course in Medical Theory. 'The better you are prepared in this way,' he said, 'you will learn the more from my course.'[47] Yet the one-year auditors – the largest single group of students – at best took the courses concurrently, and probably did not take Medical Theory at all. Cullen was, indeed, 'sensible', he said, 'that from various circumstances there are many gentlemen come there, not so well prepared as I could wish', and tried to accommodate himself to their lack of prior study.[48] He was not altogether successful, though, for Thomas Ismay was not pleased to have Cullen for Medical Practice, as we have seen, because Cullen 'generally deals too much upon Theory'.[49] He went on to say that

> The Students call Dr Cullen, The Great Cullen, the Oraclete, as he generally uses some pompous Language. For instance, last week in one of his Lectures he says, I shall endeavour to obviate several Prejudices that have long subsisted in the Schools of Physics.[50]

If Ismay found this language difficult, most of Cullen's philosophical concerns would have gone right over his head. Even Benjamin Rush, who came to Edinburgh University to prepare for a career as Professor of Medicine in Philadelphia, found on his arrival in Edinburgh that he was 'less acquainted with classical and philosophical learning than was necessary to comprehend all that was taught in medicine', and spent a summer studying Latin and mathematics.[51] Ismay, and auditors like him, would not have had the same opportunity for extra study.

The one-year auditors' course of study is so limited in comparison with the graduates' and neglects so much recommended by medical writers, that it raises the question of whether they had originally aspired to the same education as graduates, but had dropped out along the way. A comparison of Table 6.4 with Table 4.4 shows that this is not the case: there were

Table 6.6 Three-year auditors, by year of study, 1763–1826, excluding students who attended chemistry only

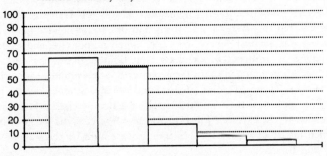

Year 1

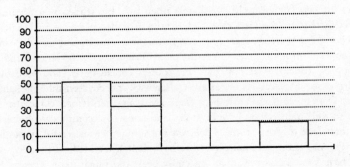

Year 2

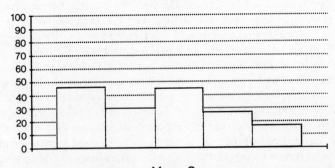

Year 3

	Anatomy	Chemistry	Medical Practice	Clinical Lectures	Clinical Surgery
Year 1:	66%	59%	16%	7%	4%
Year 2:	51%	32%	52%	20%	19%
Year 3:	46%	30%	45%	27%	17%

great differences between the groups right from the first. Similar percentages of both groups attended Anatomy and Surgery in their first year, suggesting that it was generally considered a first-year course, as we might expect. However, one-year auditors, during their first and only year of study, were much more likely to take Medical Practice, and less likely to take Chemistry, than graduates. That suggests that one-year auditors were not drop-outs who only made it through the first year of a well-defined curriculum, but instead were deliberately following the course of study discussed previously, consisting of Anatomy and Surgery, Chemistry, and Medical Practice. The practice of auditors taking the 'most material' courses all in one year persisted through the 1820s, when the faculty told the Royal Commission that it was common for students to take Anatomy and Surgery and Medical Practice the same year: they felt such students should 'be allowed to study at the same time such branches as may be most useful to them'.[52]

Did auditors really think it was a good idea to take these courses at the same time? Or would they have preferred to divide their education into a graded curriculum of beginning and advanced courses, if money had been available? Table 6.6 suggests the latter, for auditors who could afford to stay at Edinburgh for three years generally responded to the additional time by waiting to take Medical Practice in their second or third year.

They also attended a more comprehensive set of courses, suggesting that one-year auditors' education was circumscribed only by lack of funds, not lack of belief in University lectures. See Table 6.7.

Not even three-year auditors, though, attended the same number of lectures as three-year graduates, which confirms what we found in looking at graduates, that students did not necessarily follow faculty recommendations unless compelled to do so by University statute.[53]

To a great extent, auditors lived in a different world from that of graduates or apprentices, and different kinds of auditors lived in different worlds from each other. A comparison of James Rush and Alexander Lasassier makes that point very clear, for they studied in Edinburgh within a few years of each other, and each kept a full diary of his experiences. Both had been brought up to think of Edinburgh as '*the mighty in medicine*', in James Rush's phrase,[54] and before Rush arrived he might have said, as Lasassier did 'When I reflect on the advantages which will arise from it I am quite overjoyed . . . Oh dear its delightful'.[55] Both spent some time visiting the sights of the city, and both fell in love briefly.[56] Yet the two diaries might be describing two different universities. In addition to attending class, Rush experienced most of Edinburgh's other medical attractions, such as conversation with professors, access to medical literature, and membership in the Royal Medical Society, and found none of them worthwhile. Though he wrote 'It was well for me to come to this

Table 6.7 Three-year auditors' course attendance, 1763–1826, excluding students
who attended chemistry only

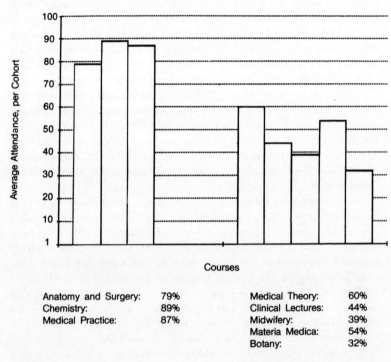

Courses

Anatomy and Surgery:	79%	Medical Theory:	60%
Chemistry:	89%	Clinical Lectures:	44%
Medical Practice:	87%	Midwifery:	39%
		Materia Medica:	54%
		Botany:	32%

country to learn the principles and experience the practice of hospitality',[57] he felt he had acquired little in the way of professional improvement and his diary paints a picture of a medical school in decline, unable to live up to its former glory. 'You knew Edinb[urg]h in her days of just and enviable celebrity, the days of Cullen and Black,' he wrote his father.[58] Alas, by the time James arrived, he said, 'The medical world here is in chaos . . . and I ask myself in vain, why Edinb[urg]h is called the seat of medical science.'[59] He much preferred medical study in London the following year.[60]

Lesassier, in contrast, registered no such complaints in his diary. He was younger than Rush – eighteen, rather than twenty-three – and Edinburgh was his first opportunity for university study. Indeed, he felt, his uncle's insistence that he attend Edinburgh medical lectures had saved him from his very brief, and completely unsuccessful, attempt at setting up his own practice. 'What do I not owe to him,' Lesassier wrote. 'Has he not saved me from poverty, disgrace nay worse has he not prevented suicide – A month longer unsuccessfully spent at Rochdale would have determined my fate'.[61] He lived with Professor James Hamilton as a member of the family, and so was more comfortable than Ismay or Harrison. He did not borrow books from the university library, though, or try to engage professors in medical discussions, or attend extra lectures, or join medical societies, and his diary gives no sign that such activities were available. Instead, he spent his time diligently attending lectures, which he clearly enjoyed, writing 'I waste but little of my note-book with scribbling at present – The truth is that I've nothing to say My life passes along in a most uniform manner But not the less pleasing on that account'. Indeed, Lesassier wrote, 'I can say with truth that I never knew more real happiness than I at present enjoy [with] Nothing to engage my attention but my own improvement.'[62] For Lesassier, it was Edinburgh medical lectures themselves which were the source of his improvement. A less critical – in both the positive and negative sense – observer than Rush, the University his diary depicted appeared a stable and flourishing institution.

However limited the medical education of one-year auditors seemed to contemporaries, or to us, there is no sign from Lesassier or Ismay or Harrison that they felt they had had anything other than an excellent preparation for practice. Lesassier, on hearing that his Uncle would sponsor him for a year of study at Edinburgh, was delighted, as he said, that 'I can finish my education completely'.[63] Part of this was naïvete, but part stemmed from this group of students defining a prestige hierarchy so as to maximize their own position in it, as discussed in Chapter Two. This involved their minimizing the distinction between one year of study and three, or an auditor and a graduate. Ismay, for example, was certainly aware that many students studied for longer than he intended to, but did not feel he was missing anything essential. Instead, he wrote his father that in their first year other students 'generally attend only some very unnecessary [classes] for a Practitioner, except he has Time enough to spend over them, and intends to graduate, they must attend them or cannot take their Degrees'.[64] In his view only classes whose connection with practice he could clearly see were really necessary; the rest were merely formal requirements for graduation, perhaps equated in his mind with pompous language.

Moreover, if auditors had only one year at Edinburgh University they may have ended up studying more than the graduates, not less, since they had to fit all their medical improvement into that one year. Even simply attending Anatomy and Surgery, Chemistry, and Medical Practice meant that auditors were at lectures from 9–11 am and 1–3 pm, five days per week. If they went to the Infirmary between 12 and 1 pm as well, that was five solid hours of lectures each day, besides time for copying or reviewing notes and Saturday lectures if Professor Monro started to run out of time. We have already seen Ismay's schedule, and Lesassier, too, spent his time 'very industriously indeed' as he described. 'I rise in the morning at 8,' he wrote

> finish breakfast, & get seated in Dr Gregory's class room by 9 – from 10–11 I hear Dr Hope on Chemistry From 11 to 12 – Dr Barclay on Anatomy – Then from 12 till 1 I attend the Infirmary. From 1 till 2 the famous Dr Monro – from 2 to 3 I go home & take a basin of soup – from 3 till 4 o'clock my Uncle's lectures on Midwifery – then from 4 to 5 Dinner from 5 till 1/2 past 6 Studying & reviewing what I've heard during the day – Tea over by a little past 7 & I go to the Infirmary to go round with the Clerk – tho' this not always quarter past 9 – Supper & to bed by 1/2 past 10.[65]

Students like Ismay and Lesassier had studied at the same eminent University as the graduates and apprentices. They had attended some of the same famous professors and had shown at least equal interest to medical subjects. Surely they were, therefore, equally entitled to consider themselves 'students of medicine strictly speaking', and share the prestige of being Edinburgh University men. Lesassier certainly thought so: he proudly reflected after his one year of study 'hereafter I can rank with the highest of them – Oh! delightful thought'.[66]

By 1806, though, that assumption was becoming less common. The proportion of auditors declined dramatically over the period, from 80 per cent in the 1760s to 54 per cent by the 1820s. Part of the change, but only a small part, can be explained by American and other foreign students choosing to study in France or Germany. Much more important was the increase in demand and opportunities for formal certification. These opportunities will be discussed in Part Two.

7

The Royal Medical Society

> The laudable and liberal views of the venerable founders of this
> Institution can never be enough admired . . . Our predeces-
> sors perceived that it was not merely the frigid plodding on
> books, nor the doctrines and precepts of age and authority;
> nor the little detail of an empirical practice, that could inspire
> that taste and spirit, and give that manly turn to our inquiries,
> which alone can render study agreeable, vigorous, and success-
> ful. They perceived, that it was in Society alone, by the
> mutual communication and reflection of the lights of reason
> and knowledge, that the intellectual as well as the moral
> powers of man are exalted and perfected.
>
> Gilbert Blane, Address . . . to the Royal Medical Society[1]

Nowhere do the keywords of Edinburgh medical students, spirit, taste, candour, and liberality, appear more frequently than in their encomia for student medical societies.[2] Gilbert Blane, in the address before the Royal Medical Society cited above, used 'liberal' and 'liberality' four times in as many paragraphs. Medical students elsewhere also founded societies, like the ones at Guy's and St Bartholomew's Hospitals who were 'desirous of improvement in medicine'.[3] In Edinburgh, though, societies had special resonance as focal points for Edinburgh literati, with members like Hugh Blair and Dugald Stewart, Joseph Black, and Adam Smith as the models for literary and philosophical discourse. Any member of the Chirurgo-Obstetrical Society, listening to John Aitken declaim that 'Association exalts the human powers, and exhibits them in a splendour almost god-like, which otherwise they could never attain',[4] could have recognized hyperbole even without attending Blair's lectures on rhetoric.[5] He would also have recognized, though, that societies were what gave polite Edinburgh its lustre.[6]

The medical societies were important vehicles for conveying and reinforcing attitudes towards medicine. They conveyed actual information as well, as we shall see. But the way in which that information was presented was as important as the knowledge itself: it transmitted a set of assumptions about the way a 'student of medicine strictly speaking' ought to behave. The main activity of all the student medical societies was discussing essays, usually called 'dissertations', written by its members. This was the main activity of all the literary and debating societies which flourished in Edinburgh in the eighteenth century. They had the aim of polishing the manners, and improving the address, of their members. The historian of the Rankenian Club, for example, described its purpose in 1771 as 'Disseminating freedom of thought, boldness of disquisition, liberality of spirit, accuracy of reasoning, correctness of taste and attention to composition'.[7] These were the goals of the medical societies as well, though members concentrated on medical and scientific topics.[8]

Thus the first lesson taught by the medical societies was that medicine was a literary activity. As James Ford remarked in his Royal Medical Society dissertation, every physician should plan to 'act in a literary character . . . and when it is not so, it must either denote indolence or want of genius, for want of opportunity can scarcely be supposed'.[9] This does not mean that students regarded medical essays as a form of imaginative literature like poetry or drama, or believed that reading and writing about medicine were more important than practicing it. I have argued elsewhere that student assumptions about the 'literary character' of medicine often went hand in hand with assumptions about the importance of experiential knowledge based on clinical observation and scientific experiment.[10] What it does mean is that students did not regard the literary form of the essay as merely incidental to the information contained therein. The ability to speak and write elegantly and to the point, to argue convincingly on a variety of pertinent topics, and to combine wit and erudition in a telling phrase, was thought to be essential to the educated medical practitioner.

Indeed, membership in a society of this kind was especially important for a medical student, for the dangers to mind and body from solitary study were well known. Too much could easily lead to melancholy and brooding, and even interfere with acquisition of professional attainments. John Bard wrote to his son Samuel, who was studying at Edinburgh, that 'the mind tied down to allow study for a considerable time is apt to give a stiffness and in some weak minds an air of pedantry', which could interfere with practice later on.[11] Gilbert Blane wrote that it

> was not merely the frigid plodding on books, nor the doctrines and precepts of age and authority; nor the little details of an empirical practice, that could inspire that taste and spirit, and give that manly turn to our inquiries, which alone can render study agreeable vigorous and successful.[12]

John Bard advised Samuel to augment his studies by 'frequenting polite easie gentile (sic) company',[13] and Blane concluded that 'it was in Society alone by the mutual communication and reflection . . . that the intellectual as well as the moral powers of man are exalted and perfected'.[14] Blane went on to appeal 'to every man's experience, if in the glow of social debate he is not conscious of a vigourous exertion of mind, of an energy of thought, unknown in the solitary hour'.[15] The debates in the Society were expected to act as a complement to the dissertations: the latter would foster insight and clarity of expression in written form, and the former would foster insight and clarity in speech. For that reason 'social debates' were an essential aspect of the Society's literary activities.

In 1792 the *Guide for Gentlemen Studying Medicine* listed the student societies holding meetings that term: the Royal Medical, the Royal Physical, the Chirurgo-Physical, the American Medical, the Hibernian Physical, the Chirurgo-Obstetrical, and the Natural History societies.[16] The Natural History society seems to have formed around John Walker, Professor of Natural History in 1785,[17] and in the same year the Chemical Society formed around Professor Joseph Black.[18] These societies appear to have been distinctive in their connection with a professor, and in their restricting the subject matter of the essays to the topic implied by their titles, Natural History and Chemistry.[19] The rest of the societies seem to have had no explicit connection with faculty, and members wrote on a variety of medical topics. Members of the Royal Physical Society, for example, did not restrict themselves to 'physic' in either its modern or eighteenth-century definition, but instead wrote 'dissertations on philosophical, physiological, medical, and chirurgical subjects', which members read and discussed.[20] The Chirurgo-Obstetrical Society was apparently founded or encouraged by John Aitken, Fellow of the Royal College of Surgeons of Edinburgh, but none of the four Annual Presidents listed in the *Edinburgh Almanack* for 1787 were Fellows or apprentices of the Royal College.[21] George Logan belonged to three societies, 'from which', he wrote, 'I have received as much improvement as from any one professor',[22] One was the Medical Society (later the Royal Medical Society), and the other the Chirurgo-Medical Society, but there is no obvious different between the kinds of essay topics he wrote for each.[23] Many students, like Logan, joined several different societies: the Annual Presidents for the Natural History Society, for example, usually also belonged to the Royal Medical Society.[24]

The Royal Medical Society is the best known of the societies, and because it is the best documented must serve as our main source of information about Edinburgh medical student society life. It was superior to the rest, the *Guide* claimed 'in being the most ancient, the best known abroad, and in possessing the most valuable library'.[25] It had been founded within a few years of the medical school itself. William Stroude, who joined the Society in 1817 and graduated in 1819,[26] wrote a history of the Society in 1820, tracing its informal origins to 1734, when six students got together to dissect the body of a woman who had died of fever. The dissection lasted about a month, and one of the students then proposed that the six of them should meet once every two weeks, at their lodgings, to read a dissertation, either in Latin or English, on a medical subject.[27]

The meetings of the original six students did not last beyond that year, but they were the inspiration for the formal origins of the Society in 1737, when a group of students began to meet weekly in a tavern, and call themselves the Medical Society. New members joined, and the Society became an established institution. In 1741 members asked for, and received, permission to use a room in the Royal Infirmary for their meetings. Growing in membership and funds, the Society collected subscriptions to build a new Hall for their weekly meetings. Andrew Duncan senior, then just beginning his career as extra-academical lecturer, may have been the prime mover behind this, for he was appointed Treasurer and placed in charge of funding for the building. The cornerstone, with the inscription 'Sacred to Medicine', was laid in 1775; the occasion was the inspiration for Blane's 'Address'. The Hall itself had 'a plain handsome front; and the roof terminates in a cupola . . . adorned with the ensigns of the Aesculapian Art'.[28] It was completed in 1776. The Hall was built on land granted by the College of Surgeons in Surgeons' Square, in the heart of Edinburgh medical life: next to Surgeons Hall, on the other side of the Infirmary and Public Dispensary from the University buildings. Once the Hall was opened, the Society also hired a housekeeper and porter.[29] It received a Royal Charter in 1779, and was known thereafter as the Royal Medical Society. That gave it the most imposing legal and physical presence among student societies, though it had rivals, for the Royal Physical Society, too, had a charter from the Crown, as well as an 'elegant hall in Hunters Park'.[30]

Royal Medical Society meetings quickly became an established part of the academic year. Meetings were held weekly during the Winter Session; though originally the members tried to meet over the summer, this soon proved impossible.[31] The meetings began at 4 pm for 'private business' such as submission of petitions and announcement of visitors, and 6 pm for 'public business', the reading and discussion of dissertations.[32] All members were required to stay until at least 11 pm, or be subject to a fine.[33] Beginning in 1764, the Society elected four Annual Presidents, whose duties were to draw up the minutes for private business of the Society and to regulate the debates on dissertations.[34] The Treasurer was likewise a member of the Society, but the position of Secretary/Librarian was given to a non-member, who received an annual salary of £25.[35] His duties were to transcribe dissertations, and of course take care of the library, which contained the best collection of medical books and periodicals in Edinburgh. Its value was attested by Andrew Duncan junior in 1794, while studying in London. 'There is nothing in the way of literature which I miss so much as the library of the Med[ical] Soc[iety],' he complained to his father. 'Students here have no access to books of value, and are therefore, in general, extremely illiterate.'[36] The library of the Royal Medical Society was an important incentive for joining it, for members then did not have to compete with professors and all other matriculated students for books. This was of special benefit if students wished to write essays for prizes announced by professional bodies, for, Andrew Duncan junior told the Royal Commission, the ones who 'foresee what books may be recommended on the subjects, get the start of others', and checked those books out of the University library.[37]

The most important activity of the Society was writing, reading, and discussing dissertations. In the first meeting in March, members had to submit to the President a case history, a medical or philosophical question, and one of Hippocrates' aphorisms each on a separate piece of paper. There were supposed to be twenty-four sets, which were then distributed to the twenty-four oldest members, who had each declared 'in person, or by a letter, his intention' of writing next session.[38] No question was to be given to its author to be answered, but students could write on subjects of their own choosing by presenting a petition to the Society since, according to Stroude, 'tasks promiscuously assigned are often alike repugnant to genius and inclination'.[39] Judging from the minutes, petitions seem to have been frequently submitted, and generally passed.[40] The Society adjourned in April for the summer, and the papers were delivered the following fall and winter. The rules for presentation were carefully worked out: on the last Saturday in October, the three senior members presented their dissertations,

> the senior, one on his Case; the second, one on his Question; and the third, one on his Aphorism. On the Saturday following, the senior, one on his question; the second, one on his aphorism; and the third, one on his Case. On the Saturday following, each his remaining dissertation. The President in office shall order the succeeding members, in sets of three, according to seniority, to deliver papers in the same order.[41]

One week was allowed for transcription of the dissertations into the Society books, and then two for the books to circulate to all members. The dissertations were finally discussed in the third week.[42] The cases and questions delivered to the Society were written in English, and only the aphorisms were presented in Latin. The custom of discussing an aphorism seems to have fallen into disuse by the 1790s, because, according to Stroude, discussions followed the rest of the Society business, 'at a late hour of the night, when the attention was already fatigued'.[43] The practice was officially dropped in the Code of Laws of 1796.[44] This is a good indication that even elite students' ability in Latin had declined by the 1790s.[45]

The activities of the society were deliberately modelled on the graduation exercises, because, as Stroude mentioned, one reason for the founding of the Society had been the desire of students to prepare themselves for graduation, 'by the performance of exercises similar to those prescribed at Universities'.[46] Certainly writing a set of dissertations for the Society would have been good practice for a student who was intending to graduate, even though they were in English rather than Latin. He would be confronted with a case history, a medical question, and, until 1796, an aphorism to comment on, just as he would be in his graduation exercises. Samuel Bard wrote that he thought the debates in the Society were very useful, 'for we are obliged to muster our whole stock of knowledge to defend our opinions, which are never allowed to pass without being thoroughly examined'.[47] His dissertations, especially, turned out to be excellent practice for his graduation examination: he wrote that his commentary on two practical cases for graduation were done 'much in the same manner as that I sent, which I wrote for the medical society'.[48]

Students would also benefit from reading other students' essays and listening to the commentaries. Over the course of a year, a member could expect to hear a commentary on most of the common diseases, whether in the form of a case history or a medical question. Between November, 1780, and May, 1781, for example, members delivered commentaries on dysentery, mania, leprosy, cholera, hydrothorax, chorea, puerperal fever, dyspepsia, enteritis, whooping cough, smallpox, scurvy, consumption, pneumonia, jaundice, cancer, rheumatism, typhus, ascites, and syncope.[49] Any of these could have turned up on a graduation examination. These were also the most popular topics for MD theses: Apoplexy and Jaundice, Dysentery, Dyspepsia, Fever, Hysteria, Pneumonia, Rheumatism, and Smallpox.[50] Students also wrote Society essays on physiology and chemistry and materia medica. The circulation of the blood, digestion, Peruvian Bark, and fixed air all appeared frequently in the bound volumes of Society essays, and probably appeared as frequently on graduation examinations.[51]

The desire to prepare for graduation, though, was not the only, or even the most important reason for joining the Society, for only 56 per cent of the members went on to graduate at Edinburgh. This is a striking example of the authority the medical faculty had in dictating the form and content of medical knowledge, even among students who did not expect to be tested by them directly. Nor was this true only in the Royal Medical Society. The Chirurgical-Obstetrical Society apparently kept the form of '*cases* or *questions*',[52] and even the Chemical Society dissertations would fit perfectly into the category of general medical questions.

The more important reason for joining societies was what Stroude called the 'general object of professional improvement',[53] for which students were willing to spend at least once a week from 4 pm until 11 pm at meetings, in addition to the time spent reading and writing essays. The success of the society depended upon students taking this form of improvement seriously, for if they ever lost interest, the meetings would come to a halt. John Aitken's address to the Chirurgo-Obstetrical Society suggests that this could happen, since he felt it necessary to remind members that 'they ought to come duly prepared with every sort of information, so that our deliberations may be mutually instructive'.[54]

The long and not always harmonious life of the Royal Medical Society shows that its members, at least, took the business of medical improvement seriously. The question is what activities they felt led to that improvement. The Society was not a scientific society, and students did not regularly carry out discoveries. Neither the cases nor the questions make for exciting reading. They were student exercises, rather than original research, and varied in quality, from the one which began with the hope that 'the Society will not reproach me with a false ostentation of erudition if I cite authors whose works I have never read'[55] to the well-researched, well-written essay like William Withering's on Apoplexy, replete with Latin quotations.[56] Yet not even the best presented much that was new. William Stroude, in his history of the Society, said that it was designed to encourage the student to put forth 'the exertion requisite to collect, to arrange, and to communicate knowledge . . .'[57] and that is an apt description of the activities required for the dissertations.

Students, then, did not join the Royal Medical Society for the purpose of engaging in ongoing medical or scientific research, though some were involved in research later in life. Though most members would have agreed with Samuel Allvey, that each member should 'contribute those observations, which he has made, and the opinions which he has formed; rather than . . . collect the facts and opinions of others',[58] this was too ambitious a plan for the majority of students. Allvey's comments should rather be seen as expressing the general student assumption that their Society essays, like their theses, should express 'what they really believed'.[59]

Students anticipated other kinds of benefits from membership besides the opportunity to present their observations and opinions. The first of these was that, by joining the Society, the student was identifying himself with an elite group of medical students, for membership was intentionally exclusive. Students arriving in Edinburgh found themselves surrounded by hundreds of others, with no way of distinguishing themselves from the 'vulgar' who crowded into Monro's anatomical theatre. Nor did they have any way of distinguishing the twenty students which, George Logan felt, a man of 'good sense and taste' would care to associate with.[60] The Royal

Medical Society provided one way of doing this. In 1792 the *Guide for Gentlemen* gave the membership fee as five guineas, in addition to a fee each year for the library, effectively restricting membership to wealthier students.[61] Membership policies were also designed to allow in only a select group, because, Stroude explained, 'it is in the power of unsuitable associates to reflect injury and discredit on the community to which they belong, and . . . their exclusion in the first instance is far preferable to their expulsion afterwards'.[62] Applicants had to be proposed for membership by an existing member, and the Society then voted on their admission. At first new members could only be admitted unanimously; later this was changed to allow one negative vote.[63] In 1799 John Allen, inspired by the egalitarian principles of the French Revolution,[64] proposed that a simple majority be enough to admit new members. In 1802, this was changed again to a three-fourths majority,[65] perhaps following the wave of anti-Jacobin reaction in Britain. From 1806, a candidate for admission needed six current members to attest his suitability.[66] How that might be defined was largely left unwritten, except for a 1781 regulation that prospective members had to have studied in a University at least six months.[67] This suggests that members of the Society, like Walter Jones, mentioned in Chapter Two, defined a student of medicine strictly speaking by his professional attainments as well as taste, sociability, and liberality. At no time did membership exceed 13 per cent of the student body. Twenty per cent studied for one year, 21 per cent for two, and 59 per cent studied for three or more. Members were thus not at all representative of the total Edinburgh student population. The one-year students were like James Rush, who joined the Society,[68] rather than like Thomas Ismay or Alexander Lesassier, who never mentioned it.

Not everyone was immediately impressed by either the gentility or accomplishments of the membership. 'I expected to see a number of well dressed men', Sylas Neville complained, after his first visit to the Society,

> but few were decently dressed and yet this Society is reckoned the first and superior to the Physico-medical or Chirurgo-Physico-Medical with others of the same kind.[69]

Indeed, he said,

> Few of the members understand the subjects on which they are to debate. The undigested matter they threw out tends more to perplex than to increase medical knowledge and as much time which might be better employed is lost in attendance, writing papers, preparing questions etc, I do not think I shall ever petition for admittance . . .
> A Mr. Goulding, who has most unaccountably been here ten years, was the only person present who spoke with any degree of grace or precision.[70]

His reasons for eventually joining are revealing: they had less to do with the benefits produced by listening to the debates of the Society than with 'the fear of being thought to want spirit if I did not solicit a seat in the assembly'.[71] As Blane implied in his oration, 'taste', 'spirit,' and 'manliness' were all characteristics of those who joined the Society. Anyone therefore who chose not to belong laid himself open the charge that he did not have those characteristics. A more positive way of making the same point is that those who did choose to belong were demonstrating that they did have them. Neville eventually became one of the Annual Presidents of the Society, and took his duties quite seriously. He was gratified to receive a letter of appreciation expressing the 'high sense, which the Society entertains of the diligence & attention with which you have discharged your office as President'.[72]

The Society also provided the initiation of young students into the company of their seniors, for Samuel Bard wrote of the Society being composed of 'a number of members who are near graduating, and Men of real knowledge' who thoroughly criticized the papers presented at the Society, so that 'we young members are not allowed, to be carried away by false reasoning, or led into Errors instead of truth'.[73] Membership was a form of induction into the world of learned physicians represented by the older, more accomplished students. Graduates themselves, if they remained in Edinburgh, often continued to attend Society meetings, as Neville did, no doubt becoming a role model for the junior members.[74] Other young practitioners who wished to become extra-academical lecturers or grinders, like John Brown, John Allen, Andrew Fyfe and Peter Reid seem to have been a particularly active sub-group within the Society, perhaps because they wished to attract students, or just to make use of the Society library. The University library was not open to graduates, precisely because, Andrew Duncan junior told the Royal Commission, the most useful books 'would almost all be taken out by teachers'.[75]

This was an image of medical education as a series of steps, where progressive years add to the student's knowledge until he becomes an older, experienced student himself and could graduate to practice. This message is so clearly conveyed by the graduated curriculum of modern medical schools, as well as most other educational institutions, that it takes an effort of imagination to realize that a similar graduated curriculum formed the experience of only a small proportion of Edinburgh medical students. It certainly would not have been the experience of students like Lesassier, who expected to 'finish his education completely' in one year.[76] Indeed, the Royal Medical Society was the only place where that message was consistently enforced, because it was the only point where a group of neophytes might move gradually from reading essays, to screwing up the courage to comment on them, to delivering their own in order of seniority.

Another important aspect of medical life reinforced by the Society, then, was the existence of a comparatively small elite group of medical men within the large body of medical practitioners. As we have seen, Lesassier's and Ismay's experience of study at Edinburgh would have led them to blur the distinction between their own education and that of the graduates, or other better-educated students. Neville's and Stroude's experience, in contrast, would have led them to draw a sharp distinction between their own education and that of the auditors intended for general practice, similar to the distinction Walter Jones had made between 'the Gentlemen . . . who apply themselves to study', and 'the vulgar', who were either 'indolent' or 'devoid of everything polite and agreeable'.[77] Membership in the Royal Medical Society would only have sharpened that distinction by reinforcing the idea of an elite defined by its 'liberal and laudable' behaviour, combining an unspecified amalgam of 'merit and address . . . with a proper degree of skill', to borrow John Bard's phrase.[78]

Another message conveyed by the Society was that individual ability could best be sharpened through competition. The other side of 'fear of being thought to want spirit', was the ambitious student's desire for a forum to distinguish himself by showing off his knowledge and understanding of medicine. Stroude, for example, wrote of the 'generous emulation to excel, the desire to honorable fame, the encouragement of mutual example, and the gratification of mutual instruction',[79] as among the benefits of taking part in the Society's activities. Making use of students' innate competitiveness and 'desire of honorable fame' to encourage them to work hard was an explicit goal of Georgian educational reforms like class examinations and prizes.[80] The Royal Medical Society offered a Latin diploma to members who had completed one set of dissertations, commending them for their literary effort; members who had not written a set of papers could receive a certificate commending them for their diligent effort in the Society.[81] In 1787 the Chirurgo-Obstetrical Society exceeded this by offering a gold medal for 'the Member who shall appear to have acquitted himself best in writing and argument'.[82]

James Rush disapproved of this flagrant self-seeking, 'the same useless debates, the same personal contention, the same electioneering ambition', which he had found in the student medical society in Philadelphia.[83] The value attached to competition, coupled with the intensity of student friendships and enmity, carried over into the debates held at the Society, only thinly disguised by the glow of self-righteousness which came from fighting in a noble cause. Stroude's 'Encouragement of mutual example' could easily become rivalry for the reputation as the most brilliant student, and 'gratification of mutual instruction' could easily become the pleasure of criticizing another member's ideas. Not all students took correction as calmly as Samuel Bard, or felt it justified, and feeling often ran high in the course of a debate. As early as 1751, George Sutherland, then President, had begged members

> to manage your disputes, with candour, discretion, and a becoming
> decency, and when you have an opportunity of correcting one anothers
> mistakes, do it in a gentle friendly manner, without the appearance
> of malice or ridicule, which would betray a low mean spirit, and be
> an evident mark of a person by no means fitt [sic] for society.[84]

He went on to admonish members,

> Never allow your passions to get the better of your reason, for if
> anyone is such a weather glass, as to be ruffled and put out of humour,
> whenever his assertions are called in question, or his favourite
> hypothesis ridiculed, he will both lose the satisfaction of giving and
> receiving instruction.[85]

Of course, though most members began their dissertations by apologizing
for their own inadequacies, they must undoubtedly have been very proud
of their efforts, and pleased at the opportunity to demonstrate their
knowledge; few would have taken kindly to receiving 'instruction' from
their fellow students. On April 6, 1776, for example, Thomas Pemberton
delivered a paper on Fevers, in which, according to Neville, '. . . he made
a violent attack on the venerable doctrine of Critical Days, as supported
by Hippocrates, and other ancients and by Dr. Cullen'. Neville seems to
have felt it his duty as one of the four annual presidents, 'to collect what
force I could to defend a doctrine which I think just and well founded.'[86]
If Pemberton had collected a similar force, the debate might well have
been violent. Neville wrote in his diary the next week that he was 'in some
danger of getting into a quarrel and having a duel on my hands for no
other reason than having done my duty to the Society over which I
preside'.[87] Much to his relief, he was never actually challenged.

Pemberton's essay was probably influenced by the ideas of John Brown.
Brown, as mentioned in Chapter Two, was a poor but gifted student who
worked his way through Edinburgh University by coaching students with
their Latin, and with the patronage of Professor William Cullen. By the
1770s, the friendship based on that patronage began to sour as Brown
began to write, and teach, his own theory of medicine. The extent of the
influence of Brunonian theory, as it was called, are outside the scope of
this book.[88] Brown's immediate influence in the Royal Medical Society
was considerable. He attracted a group of devoted followers, who supported his cause against the faculty. 'Shall truth & science, unsupported
stand', one anonymous student asked in a marginal note in the Edinburgh
University Library's copy of John Brown's *Elements of Medicine*,

> And abstract theories o'erwhelm the land?
> Shall envy, injured Brown, for e'er pursue
> Rather in immortal fame, his well-earned due.
> Him, nature taught, her secrets to display
> Him, they who study nature's laws obey.[89]

This was temperate, compared to the marginal note in William Cullen's

First Lines, which said that the 'Professors of the Edinburgh College are
the most vilenous [sic] group on the face of the earth.'[90] Brunonians in
turn found themselves opposed 'in greater numbers, and in general with
better information, but not always with equal eloquence and talent',[91] by
an equally devoted group of Cullen's supporters. National prejudice may
have played some part in this, for one of Cullen's most outspoken
supporters, Thomas Addis Emmet, was Irish. The University library copies
of Brown's and Cullen's works were filled with scurrilous comments about
'Paddy' and 'Sawney' and an Irish student, possibly Emmet, was the target
of a published account of one of the Society meetings.[92]

Pemberton's essay shows how a discussion of the doctrine of critical days
could quickly become a duelling matter. The actual question Pemberton
was set was 'Is the duration of fevers capable of being shortened by the
exhibition of medicines?' Pemberton could have chosen to say yes, and
given various examples, taken from practice or literature, where medication had been useful in fever. Cullen, in his Clinical Lectures, had given
several examples of the use of medication; he had even stated that the use
of ipecacuanha, to evacuate the contents of the stomach, was 'the first step
in the cure of most fevers'.[93] Pemberton could even have chosen to answer
the question calmly in the negative. Instead, he did, indeed, violently
attack the doctrine and those who held it, saying,

> it would have been happy for mankind, if these useless theories had
> been only chargeable with falshood [sic] and absurdity, but their
> pernicious influence has been more wide and extensive. They have
> not only misled the understanding, but have even chilled and blasted
> the effort of rising genius, and formed an opposed barier [sic] to every
> enlargement of the bounds of science.[94]

Clearly no loyal Cullen student could let such statements pass. What
Pemberton was implying was that Cullen – 'the great the unrivalled Dr
Cullen',[95] – was not only a bad physician and scientist, he was a dogmatic
tyrant as well. He was also saying that his fellow Society members who
agreed with Cullen were the opposite of 'rising genius'. No doubt Neville's
defence of the doctrine, and by implication its professor, was similarly
violent, and touched on Pemberton's clear inability to understand the
concepts he so unjustly calumniated.

Later Brunonians also attacked the concept of critical days, but their
main target was Cullen's Nosology, presented as the basis of the course in
Medical Practice. The main complaint was that in University lectures the
practice of medicine itself, as John Watson Howell wrote

> instead of being represented, as an art imperfect in its most essential
> Branches, instead of having its deficiencies pointed out with a view
> to their being supplied; is digested into a regular, and seemingly
> compleat system. In this light it is beheld by the student who

embraces hypotheses with the same facility and confidence as he would do facts established on the testimony of his senses.[96] This may be taken as the more sophisticated students' critique of what Mary Hewson praised in universities, 'all branches of science drawn together so compactly'.[97] Presenting medicine as a 'compleat system' left nothing for the would-be philosopher but to learn it unquestioningly. 'In other words Gentleman,' James Jeffray commented in disgust after reading the third edition of Cullen's *First Lines* 'you must not pretend to reason but implicitly believe.'[98]

This attack on nosology must have polarized the Society, for the ordinary structure of case histories involved, as Richard Kiernan wrote, 'that nosological definition which is requisite for a proper elucidation of the subject, and which the established custom of this society requires'.[99] Originally case histories were intended to be actual medical cases

of any Patient that shall occur . . . in Practice, or in the writings of any practical Author, provided there be sufficient Evidence that the case has really existed . . . These Histories shall be carefully narrated, as if wrote to a Physician to be consulted . . .[100]

Some case histories were. The case of Rheumatism, proposed by Richard Freer, a clerk at the Infirmary, presumably came from there: at least that was what Richard Pew, who wrote on the case, assumed, inferring the patient's situation in life 'from the residence of the worthy member who drew up the case'.[101] Another source of cases was the students' prior experience from apprenticeship or military practice. Thomas Girdlestone, for example, gave an account of hepatitis, 'as it appeared in several hundred of the men and officers, during and after a 22 months campaign, in the Carnati and Tanjore counties of India', a campaign in which he participated.[102]

Most of the case histories, though, were chosen for their clear depiction of symptoms of specific diseases, rather than the fact that they were taken from personal experience. Acute Rheumatism was the topic of nineteen dissertations between 1770 and 1826. Each case history presented the same well-known symptoms, fever and inflammation, coupled with pains in the joints. The clinical descriptions varied in length and completeness, but these two essentials were always included. It was always distinguished from chronic rheumatism by fever and inflammation, and by the fact that it tended to attack younger patients, whereas chronic rheumatism attacked the old.

Apoplexy was featured as frequently in the Royal Medical Society essays: nineteen essays were written on it between 1770 and 1826. The symptoms were, once again, clearly marked and easy to describe: patients were aged 40–60, corpulent, sedentary, used to eating and drinking well, who suddenly had a seizure which left them unconscious, with their pulse full and strong, but slow. Diabetes was another often-discussed case – twenty-one essays were written on it between 1770 and 1826 – despite the fact that it was 'a disease that is rarely the subject of our practice'.[103] However, not only was it easily diagnosed – the patient suffered from enormous thirst and his urine tasted sweet – but also Francis Home had treated the case in his *Clinical Experiments*,[104] which the Society owned, and members cited.

Discussion of causes of disease, and treatment, followed the same pattern, with a few exceptions. Students gave the history of the disease, the definition from Cullen's *Nosologia*,[105] the proximate and immediate causes, the prognosis, and treatment. In the majority of cases, most of the case histories could have been taken straight out of Cullen's *First Lines*. Often students described the appearance of the body on dissection, but usually this, too, was taken from standard written sources, or, at best, from other members. In discussing the post mortem of a gonorrhoea patient, William Spooner wrote that Andrew Fyfe, Monro's demonstrator, assured him 'that in the course of last winter, he opened the urethra of a man'.[106] Obviously Spooner himself had not done so.

Members of the Royal Medical Society, then, were studying clinical medicine 'by the book'.[107] Members do not appear to have used cases to sharpen each other's actual clinical skills, or even to try and trap one another by posing difficult or complicated cases. Charles Throckmorton was unusual in his case, for the symptoms could, he said, 'with equal propriety', be assigned to gastritis, enteritis, and ileus. He was only able to diagnose it as enteritis because he had been 'fortunate enough to procure a full and accurate account both of the subsequent symptoms, and of the phaenomena which appeared upon dissection'.[108] That allowed him to write his case history, and shows Edinburgh students were aware of the importance of pathological anatomy. It also confirms, though, that members did not consider differential diagnosis while the patient was alive to be the most important part of the case history. Instead, the point was to become familiar with the history of the disease. This was recognized in the 1790s, when the custom of proposing a case history was discontinued, and instead a member was simply given a disease to discuss.[109] This brought the dissertations closer to a learned treatise on a disease, rather than to a case history 'as if wrote to a Physician to be consulted'.

It is hard to avoid the thought that listening to these case histories, week after week, must have been extremely boring. Brown's challenge to Cullen may have come as a welcome injection of real medical controversy into the routine proceedings. Finally, members may have felt, they could discuss and defend the ultimate philosophical principles behind medical practice. By the late 1770s, between four and five of the sixty or so students who were members of the Royal Medical Society at any one time can be identified from their essays as Brunonians. Through the normal process of recruitment and admission, ten to fifteen of the members in residence each year were Brunonians by the mid 1780s. This meant that every time a member wrote a case history — twenty-four times during the Winter Session — he would have to choose whether to use Cullen's Nosology or not. If he did not, he would be attacked as a Brunonian by the more numerous, if not, in Stroude's view, more talented, Cullen supporters. If he did, he would be attacked by Brunonians, who, though a minority, were a vocal one. Edmund Goodwyn, obviously expecting opposition in his essay on Colica Pictonum, lead poisoning, turned the usual nosological definition on its head by leaving the disease without a name, 'a humble suppliant at the tribunal of nosology, amongst a numerous list of others that are daily met with in practice; to mock the pride of classification, and teach us the imperfection of our art'.[110]

Brown left Edinburgh in 1786, and Cullen died in 1790. The number of Brunonians in residence each year trailed off as members completed their studies, and the debate lost its virulence. Herbert Packe, in 1790, cited both Cullen and Brown in his case history,[111] and John Thomson, whose ideas on inflammation were heavily influenced by Brown, went on to become Cullen's devoted biographer.[112] By 1820, Stroude, while deploring the tone of the controversy, could see it as an ultimate victory for the principle of free philosophical debate. 'The ill effects of the Brunonian controversy were transient,' Stroude wrote, and even served to demonstrate the value of Society debates, where

> the love of truth, alike opposed to ignorance and prejudice, has happily united liberty of speech, and a complete exception from undue authority, with the mutual deference and courtesy, so becoming in the fellow-students of a liberal profession.[113]

Indeed, one of the most striking features of the Brunonian controversy is how it reinforced, rather than undermined, the value of academic study. The structure of the Society, and the exercises members performed, remained unchanged. Most Brunonians conscientiously wrote the dissertations based on graduation requirements despite their opposition to the medical faculty, and then went on to fulfill the graduation requirements conscientiously. As we have seen, Robert Jones did not insist that a faculty which could act as such a 'barrier to rising genius', to use Pemberton's phrase, had no authority to examine him. William Thornton, one of Brown's admirers, did graduate from Marischal College in 1784, not Edinburgh. According to the letter recommending him, though, it was because he could not stay in Scotland another year to attend Botany; the letter, apparently written by a professor, called Thornton 'one of the most respectable Medical Students in this Place'.[114] Sixty-one per cent of the Society members who wrote essays influenced by Brown between 1783 and

1791 went on to graduate at Edinburgh; only 44 per cent of the total membership in that period graduated. Brunonianism may have been an alternative medical theory,[115] but it did not provide an alternative to academic medicine.

The Royal Medical Society performed an important educational function in stimulating academic rivalry, rewarding ability, reinforcing knowledge and facilitating expression. Membership also inculcated certain intangibles about medical life: that students had an obligation to say 'what they really believed', that philosophical debate led to the progress of medicine, and that 'students of a liberal profession' formed an elite opposed to the mass of practitioners. The Society was a faithful reflector of the interests of Edinburgh students: chemistry in the 1770s and 1780s, surgery in the 1810s and 1820s,[116] and 'medicine in all its branches' throughout. It was an even more faithful reflector of student attitudes towards medicine as a literary subject, dependent for success on the same qualities that made a liberal gentleman: taste and sociability joined, as Blane said, to the 'lights of reason and knowledge'. The locus of Society activity in Edinburgh was the neo-classical hall on Surgeon's Square, fitted out with cupola, library, and meeting room. If members were aware of other possible loci, such as laboratory, dissection room, hospital, and morgue, their dissertations do not reflect it.

Part Two

Students and their regulation

Introduction to Part Two

> Why should it be thought derogatory or disagreeable to a
> young man, to find that his professor uses means to know
> whether he be present at a lecture, whether he fully compre-
> hends its various positions and arguments, or, whether further
> instruction might not be materially useful to him? Would any
> sensible professional student, desirous of information and
> improvement, regard such precautions on the part of his
> professor in the light of an insult, or as the occasion of
> annoyance?
>
> George Jardine, *Outlines of Philosophical Education*[1]

The years 1790 to 1815 saw profound changes in British society, changes
which ultimately affected Edinburgh medical education. Most directly, the
long course of the Napoleonic Wars created an increased demand for
military medical men, and the percentage of Edinburgh students entering
the Army Medical Department as surgeons and assistant surgeons reflected
this demand. Between 1763 and 1789, an average of 6 per cent of
Edinburgh medical students per cohort obtained positions. From 1790 to
1810, the average rose to 12 per cent with peaks of 15 per cent in 1795
and again in 1807 and 1808. From 1811 to 1824, the average dropped
back down, to 5 per cent. These figures only represent students who
became commissioned officers in the army. We have no way to investigate
surgeon's mates systematically, who were not commissioned, or surgeons
and surgeon's mates in the Navy, but it seems fair to assume that their
number increased in wartime as well.[2]

More important in its long-term effect, though, was the outcry against
lack of qualified medical men in the military. This was not a new problem.
Robert Hamilton, an Edinburgh MD, had complained in 1787 about the
lack of incentives for well-qualified practitioners to join the army, and had
called for reform of the medical service in order to attract them.[3] The war
made the problem more acute. Robert Jackson, another Edinburgh MD,
complained again about the lack of incentives for joining the army in
1805;[4] William Turnbull, an Edinburgh auditor, pointed out the same

problem in the Navy in 1806.[5] Under Sir Lucas Pepys, Bart., as Physician-General, the incentives decreased, for he only appointed men to the highest rank of Physician who were Fellows of the Royal College of Physicians of London, that is, who had Oxford and Cambridge MDs. That meant that an army surgeon with an Edinburgh or Glasgow MD found his path to the highest positions blocked, whatever his abilities or seniority.[6] General dissatisfaction with the management of the Army Medical Board led to its complete reorganization in 1808. In 1805, though, the demand for medical practitioners led to revision of nearly all aspects of recruitment. Promotion to all ranks was to be based on seniority and competence, determined by examination. The new Board replaced the lowly rank of surgeon's mate with the commissioned rank of assistant surgeon, and raised salaries of all positions. It began to take seriously the task of examining candidates for medical appointments on their qualifications, insisting on minimum educational requirements even for assistant surgeons. The government agreed to pay for the medical education of medical personnel.[7] The higher standards spilled over into the Admiralty as well, though naval surgeoncies continued to be the least rewarding of medical positions.[8]

In fact, the period of war, with its attendant social and economic disruptions, led to an increased emphasis on educational qualifications generally. As Sheldon Rothblatt has noted, patronage did not cease to determine who got what position, but with so many competing for scarce appointments, academic qualifications could be important in catching the eye of a powerful patron.[9] A letter written to Robert Saunders Dundas about patronage in the East India Company, illustrates this point. The letter stated

> that, there is in this county, a family connection, of four, or five freeholders . . . they have given Lord Kellie to understand, that if he can, procure a surgeoncy for India, for this season, for the son of one of the gentlemen, a young man, who is perfectly qualified, they will hereafter support his L K's line of politics in the county.[10]

This appeal to Dundas was mainly concerned with political advantage, but it is significant that the author mentioned that the young man was 'perfectly qualified'. This combination of medical and non-medical criteria for evaluating a young practitioner has some similarity to John Bard's 'merit and address, with a proper degree of skill'. It is not quite the same, however, because to be qualified is not the same as having skill: qualification implies the existence of some independent standard of accomplishment which the young man has been successfully tested for or otherwise measured against. The question still remained, of course, what being 'perfectly qualified' might mean, and the definition and measurement of qualification became an increasingly important issue.

There were other educational changes in Britain. Under a series of energetic Deans, young gentlemen at Christ Church Oxford were encouraged, cajoled, and pushed into hard academic work. [11] In early nineteenth-century Cambridge, the mathematics tripos had the same effect, so that by 1834 the 'brace of Cantabs' who put together a dictionary of colloquial Cambridge terms described a senior wrangler as the 'highest honour in the Schools'. [12] The competitive examinations set up in both Universities were intended in part to channel student energy away from the dangerous pursuit of political debate and novelty. [13] They also worked to promote that 'spirit of emulation' that was believed to lead to student accomplishment. [14] The result was that though Oxford and Cambridge still had their detractors, they began to acquire new defenders, at least for their undergraduate education. [15]

Examinations and prizes, though hardly new, aroused greater interest in Scotland as well. Their most influential advocate was George Jardine, Professor of Moral Philosophy at the University of Glasgow. His *Outlines of Philosophical Education* described what he called his 'practical system' for improving the teaching for what had been 'emphatically, though rather rudely designated *"the drowsy shop of logic and metaphysics"* '. [16] His book included a discussion of professional education, even though, he said, many professors believed that professional students would not accept the discipline of examinations or written themes. '[E]ven a class of philosophers,' he wrote, 'would give their attention more closely to a scientific discourse, did they know that they must speedily render an account of it . . . Would any sensible professional student desirous of information and improvement, regard such precautions on the part of his professor, in the light of an insult, or as the occasion of annoyance?' [17] Jardine's book was widely praised. [18]

Closer to home, the period from 1790 to 1820 saw the 'making of classical Edinburgh', as A. J. Youngson put it, which transformed the old medieval city to its new Georgian counterpart. [19] Students were directly affected by the final completion of the University buildings which replaced the 'poor irregular pile of buildings' George Logan had found in 1778. [20] Begun in 1789, the building project had come to a halt during the wars for lack of funds, and only finished in 1827. [21] A few students also began to find lodgings in the New Town, in St James or St Andrews Square or Princes Street. [22]

Again, the more influential changes were the less direct ones. Edinburgh was becoming Georgian in more than just architecture: the years 1790 to 1820 saw an acceleration of its integration into Greater Britain. [23] The massive building project that so altered the appearance of the city provided an unfortunate example of this process. The Town Council ultimately went bankrupt paying for it, and the combination of the Parliamentary Commission on Municipal Corporations of 1833 and the Burgh Reform

Act that same year ended its political autonomy and firmly subordinated city government to Parliament.[24] Contemporary observations on Edinburgh life suggest other, less drastic ways in which Edinburgh was losing its local character, and perhaps some of its traditions as well. Henry Cockburn railed against the vision of architectural improvement that had destroyed the distinctive sixteenth-century Parliament in order to erect an undistinguished nineteenth-century one.[25] John Ramsay of Ochtertyre grumbled about the 'sad landscape of modern manners'.[26]

Yet integration brought its advantages, for the city of Edinburgh benefitted from Britain's economic growth. So did the University, for it meant that more parents had more money to invest in their sons' educations. Medical students, seeing the avenues and crescents that made up the New Town − 'In justice,' Alexander Lesassier wrote, 'I must say that nothing can possibly be more beautifully picturesque'[27] − or entering the fine new University library and museum,[28] may have considered them tangible expressions of the new opportunities Edinburgh's integration made possible. The consequences of that integration for medical education is the subject of Part Two.

8

Licentiates in surgery

Candidates for Surgical Diplomas must have followed their
studies in some University or School of Medicine of reputation
. . .
Every Candidate must produce Certificates of his having
attended . . . for a period of three or more Winter Sessions,
. . . the following separate and distinct course of Lectures, viz,

Anatomy	2 Courses
Chemistry	1 do.
Materia Medica	1 do.
Institutions, or Theory of Medicine	1 do.
Practice of Medicine	1 do.
Principles and Practice of Surgery	1 do.
Midwifery	1 do.
Practical Anatomy	1 do.

Every Candidate shall, in addition . . . produce . . . a
Certificate from a Professor or Teacher of Anatomy recognised
by the College, that he has been actually engaged in the
dissection of a human body . . .
The Candidate must likewise have attended a Public Hospital for at least one year, with a course of Clinical Surgery . . .

The Medical Calendar, 1828[1]

Successful as they were in attracting apprentices, by the 1770s the Fellows
of the Royal College of Surgeons of Edinburgh clearly felt that their
authority was too limited. Education of apprentices could affect only a
small group of people, for there were only so many masters, who could
only take on so many apprentices. Control over practice in Scotland's eight
eastern counties was only local control, at a time when power and
patronage in Britain was increasingly being defined in national terms.
When Scotland lost its Parliament in 1707, the Edinburgh surgeons lost
their traditional route to national influence; the old Incorporation could
not regain it as a guild, but the new Royal College did by turning itself
into a degree-granting institution. The Diploma offered by the College
from the 1770s, together with the new surgical courses which it required,

was the most innovative feature of Edinburgh medical education in this period. The regulations listed at the head of this chapter are a measure of the College's success, because they were published in the *Medical Calendar*, which was intended to be a comprehensive survey to all opportunities for medical education throughout Great Britain and Paris. Another measure is that by the 1820s, more students were awarded the Royal College's diploma than the MD, over 100 or 30 per cent per cohort.

The Edinburgh surgeons' guild had always had the privilege of controlling the practice of surgery in the eight counties within their jurisdiction by granting licenses to country surgeons, but they do not seem to have exercised it consistently prior to 1770, when they first began to call themselves the College of Surgeons. The minutes contain no records of surgeons outside of Edinburgh presenting themselves as candidates for a license, nor of any litigation concerning surgeons practicing without one. That changed in February 1770, when the College issued a new diploma for country surgeons. The diploma testified that the candidate 'was examined upon his skill in the arts of surgery and pharmacy, agreeable to the charter granted by King William and Queen Mary . . . and Act of Parliament confirming the same . . .' and having been found fully qualified, was authorized to practice 'within the three Lothians (the city of Edinburgh and suburbs excepted) the counties of Fife, Peebles, Selkirk, Roxburgh and Berwick'.[2] On the diploma, the candidate was designated 'surgeon in ——', emphasizing that it was a license conveying the privilege of practicing in a particular geographical area. It cost 100 pound Scots, called 'merks', or £5/11/1 1/3 sterling. Thomas Cochrane from Penicuik was the first surgeon to apply for the diploma. He had been attending medical lectures in Edinburgh and presumably wished to take advantage of the opportunity to obtain formal accreditation. Several other men, some, but not all of whom were students, applied after 1770. In 1772 a motion was passed that former army and navy surgeons need pay only 7s 6d for the diploma.[3]

Even after granting the diploma, the College did not enforce its privilege in the eight counties; the main incentive for surgeons to get the diploma, then, was as a testimonial of skill from a public body. Surgery was a competitive business, with no formal title like Doctor of Medicine to help patients distinguish one practitioner from another, or practitioners to attract patients. The satirical *Aesculapian Labyrinth*, published in 1789, implied it was customary for surgeons to hang certificates from lecturers on the wall, for it advised the beginning surgeon

> to let the certificates of your professional qualifications . . . be so placed (in elegant frames) as to meet the eye in a conspicuous direction; lest . . . your patients . . . should have reason to conclude you a consummate dunce and most illiterate booby, if . . . learned

professors had not done your friends the favour to 'certify' to the contrary.[4]

The country surgeon's diploma from the Edinburgh College of Surgeons may also have served the purpose of showing off to prospective patients the surgeon's qualifications.

The outbreak of the American War, with the concomitant increase in demand for military surgeons, was probably responsible for the next development. In 1777 'George Charles and James Forsyth students of medicine', asked to be examined on their skill in surgery, and were subsequently granted diplomas. They did not intend to take up a country surgeon's practice within the jurisdiction of the College, for they only gave promissory notes for the 100 pound Scots. One of the members thereupon proposed that the College charge a two-guinea fee from men requesting to be examined for a diploma, with the balance of the 100 merks to be paid if they ever settled within the eight eastern counties,

> as they would probably have a good many obligations of this kind from the future from gentlemen who perhaps never intend to settle within the jurisdiction of the Incorporation which would create a considerable deal of trouble to the examiners without any benefit to the society.[5]

Apprentices of members were exempted from the fee.

Eight other men applied for the diploma that year, five listed as apprentices and three as 'students of medicine' in the College records. In 1778, the year the College received the Royal Charter, it drew up two new diplomas. One testified that its bearer 'being examined on his skill in surgery and pharmacy as found sufficiently qualified to practise these arts', the second declared that after examination the candidate 'was found sufficiently qualified to act as surgeons mate in His Majesty's service'.[6] The candidate was described by name, not town or county, and no mention was made of King William, Queen Mary, Parliament, or the eight counties. The sole authority for the diploma was 'The Royal College of Surgeons of the City of Edinburgh'. In 1784, the year Dr John Aitken suggested that the College 'collect memoirs and essays',[7] he also proposed that both diplomas 'be made out in Latin and engraved in copperplate'.[8] This proposal, unlike his first, was acted upon, so that subsequent candidates had the satisfaction of being examined '*In praesentia Collegii Regii Chirurgorum Edinensium*'.[9]

These were a new kind of surgeon's diploma. They were not a license to practice in any given area, gave no access to any professional monopoly, and said nothing about the holder's civic rights. Nor were they quite like eighteenth-century medical degrees, which often did convey specific privileges, like Fellowship in the Royal College of Physicians of Edinburgh. All they said was that the owner had been examined and found to be sufficiently qualified.[10] They were, in fact, much more like modern university degrees, or certificates of skill to perform a particular kind of task, than they were like the traditional guild licence whence they had derived. It is therefore ironic that from 1816 bearers of the diploma were known as Licentiates,[11] clearly by analogy to the Licentiates and Fellows of the Royal Colleges of Physicians of Edinburgh and London. For convenience I will use the term in lowercase to refer to anyone awarded a diploma from 1772.[12]

Having created a new degree, the Edinburgh College found themselves in the position of having to set formal requirements. Up until 1804, no specific course of study was required, but the specificity of the regulations increased over the period, as did their rigour, for the College of Surgeons found, as had the Medical Faculty, that 'besides following what you prescribe, students are too apt to stick to the strict letter of your statute, by not following what you do not prescribe'.[13] In 1804, the College ruled that candidates had to have attended lectures in 'anatomy, surgery and the practice of medicine'.[14] Specific requirements, including a course of study, were set in 1808, when the regulations were published for the first time. Like University graduation requirements drawn up in 1783, they were intended to impress the public with the high quality of education that licentiates had received, thus proclaiming at the same time the value of the institution granting the certification, and of the gentlemen awarded it.

The regulations began by emphasizing 'how necessary it must be for the interest of the Public, and of what importance for the future comfort and respectability of the individual, that every one who applies to the study of Surgery should have obtained the benefit of a Liberal Education'.[15] That was the characteristic which distinguished the new gentleman-surgeon, such as the Fellows of the College, from the 'mere mechanick' of the old Incorporation. The regulations did not specify precisely what a liberal education entailed, but the list of recommended preliminary studies increased over time, from Latin and Mathematics in the 1808 regulations to 'the study of the Latin, Greek, and modern languages, of the elementary parts of Mathematics and Natural Philosophy, of Natural History, and Botany' by 1826.[16] How many licentiates actually had studied these subjects is hard to say. Not as many as the College would have liked, though, for they also mentioned in their regulations that all candidates would be required to translate some medical author from Latin to English, and that 'frequent instances still occur of Candidates being remitted to their studies in consequence of their ignorance of the Latin language'.[17]

The College also began by making special provisions for students who had served an apprenticeship. Until 1822, apprentices were required to take fewer courses than other students. Even afterwards, the College continued to 'remind the Public' in its regulations 'that the profession of

Surgery is a practical art, which cannot be acquired without a long-continued and personal intercourse with the sick:' they therefore regretted 'the neglect of that practical education, which can best be obtained by serving an apprenticeship in early youth to a regular practitioner'.[18] Yet they did not require apprenticeship or test candidates on the knowledge they acquired while indentured, as they did for University study. Moreover, the preliminary education they suggested would have been easier to obtain in a secondary school than while apprenticed. However much they regretted the neglect of apprenticeship, then, their own regulations, together with the general emphasis on study, contributed to its decline.

Up until 1808, candidates who had not served a regular apprenticeship for three years had to attend classes for one year for surgeon's mates diplomas, and two for full diplomas; after that date, they had to have studied for three. Until 1820, candidates who had served an apprenticeship only had to attend classes for two. These changes make it difficult to tell from students' patterns of study at Edinburgh whether they were conforming to regulations, especially since the College also accepted certificates from London lectures and lectures approved by the Colleges of Glasgow, Dublin, and London.[19] As Table 8.1 shows, the licentiates, unlike other groups of students, did not have a distinctive period of study.

Table 8.1 Licentiates' period of study, 1770–1826

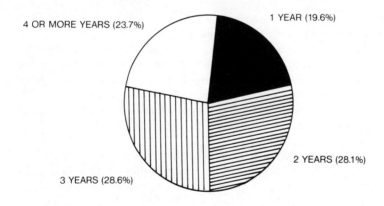

4 OR MORE YEARS (23.7%)

1 YEAR (19.6%)

2 YEARS (28.1%)

3 YEARS (28.6%)

Table 8.2 shows their course of study, which did generally fit the regulations.

The College minutes from the 1820s give frequent examples of petitions for exemption from the regulations which 'being contrary to regulations

Table 8.2 Licentiates' course attendance, 1770–1826

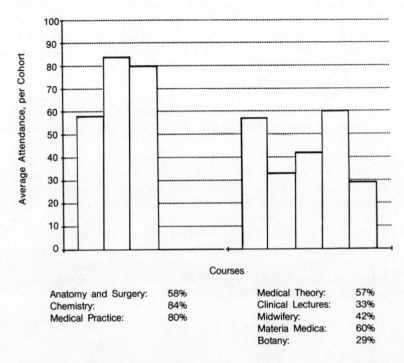

Anatomy and Surgery:	58%	Medical Theory:	57%
Chemistry:	84%	Clinical Lectures:	33%
Medical Practice:	80%	Midwifery:	42%
		Materia Medica:	60%
		Botany:	29%

were refused',[20] suggesting that the College, like the University, required compliance with its stated requirements.

Only 15 per cent of the licentiates were apprentices of the Royal College itself. A few others later became Fellows, like James Syme, showing that becoming a licentiate could be an alternative route into the surgical monopoly for 'students of medicine'.[21] The remainder were simply 'gentlemen students', with no additional affiliation to the College. Over the period, as Table 8.3 shows, the number of licentiates rose, while the number of auditors fell.

This suggests that the main appeal of the diploma was to students 'who wish to practice as surgeons or apothecaries directly after leaving the college', or 'who wish to perfect themselves in the knowledge of the practice of physic and surgery, after having served a regular apprenticeship to a surgeon or apothecary'.[22] This group would otherwise have received no certificate of their qualifications. David Birrel, for instance, studied in Edinburgh in 1805, 1806, and 1807. He attended only Anatomy and Surgery, Chemistry, and Medical Practice in his first two years,[23] and Materia Medica, Anatomy and Surgery, and Monro's Practical Anatomy

Table 8.3 Interaction of auditors and licentiates, five-year aggregates

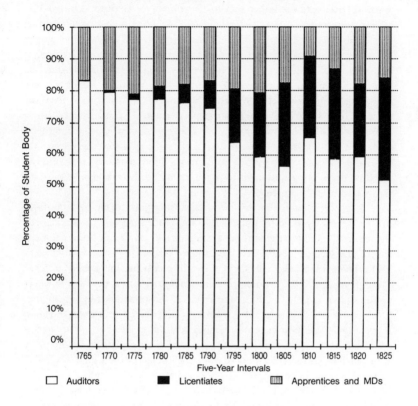

course. Professor James Home urged Birrel to attend Medical Theory as well, because, Birrel wrote

> all those who intend to graduate must have attended & he says that when Gentlemen leave the College without taking a Degree and get settled in business for a number of years they wish to have a Degree but cannot get attended the College another winter without leaving their business for two [sic] long a time.[24]

But, Birrel said, 'there is another class in Clinical lectures of Medicine w[hic]h I have not attended. But I suppose I shall have plenty of classes for this winter tho' I take none of these'. He therefore was not eligible to apply for an MD. He was, however, eligible to apply for the Royal College's diploma, having studied 'anatomy surgery and the practice of medicine', which he was awarded on June 8, 1807.[25]

The chief importance of the diploma was that it defined a new kind of surgeon, based not on what a young man did in practice, but rather on what he had studied. Once the definition was established, it became a standard that students either had to live up to, or compete with, if they wished to practice surgery, as the university MD had become a standard for physicians. For students like David Birrel, it provided a new opportunity: for others who had not studied long enough to be properly certified, it created a new limitation. The College of Surgeon's diploma was thus the first attempt at controlling what Edinburgh students other than graduates did. It seems to have been universally welcomed. To students it gave the prestige of a Latin diploma and the psychological reassurance of being 'perfectly qualified'. To parents it gave a set course of study to recommend or dictate to their sons. To patients it gave the confidence that licentiates were well-educated. The surgical diploma therefore passed quickly into the accepted range of options open to young men and their fathers looking for forms of medical education.

It was not enough for the Edinburgh surgeons to have successfully insisted on the necessity of university training for surgeons. This enhanced the reputation of both the individual surgeons, as learned professional men, and of the College, but it did nothing to change the nature of surgery itself. The student who attended courses in medicine, but learned surgery through apprenticeship, would continue to regard it as a mere art, however useful; only if it were taught in a university, and presented, like medicine, according to its first principles, could its practice be improved and gain in prestige. The Edinburgh surgeons, relying so heavily on university education as a sign of the liberal character of their profession, made every effort to have surgery introduced as a subject at Edinburgh University, and to have one of their own members installed as professor.

This was to prove an extremely hard fight. The Medical Faculty was apparently not concerned with the development of the diploma as a surgical degree, since it was not real competition for the Doctorate of Medicine. They may even have welcomed it as a means of attracting more students to medical courses, agreeing with what George Bell later told the Royal Commission, that 'There ought to be no rivalry . . . Every additional number of students attracted to Edinburgh by the Surgical School may be regarded at the same time as so many added to the University, and vice versa'.[26] However, it was one thing to have surgical students attend the University, and another to allow the College to acquire any influence there. For that reason, the Medical Faculty did all they could to prevent the College of Surgeons from having one of their members appointed Professor in the University.

The first attempt of the old Incorporation to have one of the Members, other than Monro *primus*, installed as a Professor was in 1741, when Dr Thomas Glen was proposed as Professor of Lithotomy. This was never acted upon.[27] Students could, however, watch hospital surgeons perform operations in the Royal Infirmary.[28] Members of the College also taught in extra-academical lectureships, and in 1769, the four surgeons to the Infirmary petitioned the hospital for permission to give lectures in Clinical Surgery. The Infirmary agreed to the request, and gave the surgeons a separate room in the hospital.[29]

James Rae, who gave a set of lectures in 1772, asked for, and received, the official endorsement of the College of Surgeons for his course. They therefore inserted an advertisement in the newspapers, announcing that Mr Rae would be giving a course consisting of 'a plan of lectures on the whole art of surgery, also practical discourses on the cases of importance as they occur in the Royal Infirmary'.[30] Since the course was 'founded on the practice of the hospital and delivered by a person who has been in the habit of constant observation', the College recommended it 'as useful and necessary to the students of physick and surgery'. To make it even more useful, the College was 'resolved to communicate to [Rae] such cases of importance as may occur in their practice'.[31]

The success of this venture encouraged the College to take the matter a step further by presenting a memorial to the Crown requesting the establishment of a professorship of surgery in the university, which Rae was to fill. This would enhance the education available in Edinburgh, they claimed, by insuring that surgery would be taught by a practicing surgeon.[32] This brought them directly and deliberately in conflict with Alexander Monro *secundus*, who had resigned from the College of Surgeons when appointed Professor of Anatomy because he had entered a business 'thought incompetent [sic] with the exercise of surgery and pharmacy'.[33] The *Senatus Academicus* brought the matter before the Town Council, which confirmed Monro's privileges as 'professor of medicine and particularly of anatomy and surgery',[34] effectively denying the surgeons any chance of establishing a chair of surgery in the University for one of their members during the lifetimes of Monro *secundus* or *tertius*.

The next move came in 1786, when James Russell proposed to the Royal College that Fellows be allowed to deliver lectures on surgical cases from the Infirmary, provided permission could be obtained from the surgeon in attendance.[35] Russell's course on Clinical Surgery quickly became an established part of the course offerings at Edinburgh, though an extra-academical course. According to the *Guide to Gentlemen Studying Medicine*, the object of Russell's course was 'to illustrate the practice of surgery, in the same manner as the clinical lectures delivered by the professors, elucidate the practice of physic'.[36] Russell's lectures were clearly supposed to provide a contrast to the Monros' courses of surgery. A student attending Professor Alexander Monro *secundus'* course would have seen the most common surgical operations, for which Monro gave very detailed and precise instructions. He told his students that although he had sometimes thought of arranging operations according to 'classes, and orders, and genera, as is done with other diseases',[37] he had decided it would not, in the end, be very useful. Instead, he felt, 'it is sufficient that we reduce them under general heads, that bring under the same view the similar operations tho done in different parts of the body'.[38]

Russell's course was very different. Like the lectures on clinical medicine, it was organized according to cases which appeared on the ward. According to the *Guide*, Russell 'explained the general nature and treatment of the disease, and the variety of appearance which it assumes in different cases'.[39] If an operation had to be performed, Russell explained why it was necessary, and discussed the specific reasons for the surgeon's decisions.[40] The concept of surgical disease, and of the surgeon's task as consisting most importantly of deciding when to operate, were central to the gentleman-surgeon of the late eighteenth century.[41] Indeed, the major portion of Russell's case notes, which he may have used for lecturing, were devoted to the management of the patient before and after the operation.[42] Russell discussed the examination and treatment of the affected part of the body, but he paid most attention to the face, pulse, blood, and overall condition of the body. The operations were performed by surgeons to the Infirmary, and Russell described few of the operations themselves in any detail. More frequently his comments were brief, for example, 'Dr Wardrope operated above the knee in his usual way'[43] or 'the operation of aneurism was then performed by Mr. Rae in the usual manner and the common dressings applied'.[44] Russell clearly assumed a basic knowledge of surgical techniques, the mainstay of Monro *secundus'* course of surgery; he was much more interested in the complete treatment, internal as well as external, of surgical disease.

It was probably the outbreak of the Napoleonic wars, and perhaps also the popularity of the surgeon's diplomas, that enabled Russell to finally gain a university appointment. In 1802 he petitioned the Town Council to found a chair of 'the clinical and pathological professorship of surgery'; this was created, and he appointed, in 1803.[45] Russell continued to teach his course in the same way, but now Clinical Surgery had been raised to the status of a university, rather than an extra-academical course. It was offered at 5 pm, Monday and Thursday. That gave it a position in the University course schedule comparable to Clinical Lectures, offered at 4 pm on Tuesday and Friday; it therefore seemed obvious to Alexander Bower, in his 1817 *Edinburgh Student's Guide*, to place Clinical Surgery right after Clinical Medicine in his description of courses.[46] In 1808, the Royal College made a course in Clinical Surgery a requirement for their diploma. The result of these actions was that an average of 26 per cent of the students per cohort attended Russell's class between 1810 and 1826. Sixty-three per cent of licentiates, and 62 per cent of apprentices attended it. However, 30 per cent of MDs, and 36 per cent of three-year auditors attended it as well, a sign of the growing interest in surgery among all segments of the student population.[47]

Russell's appointment as Professor of Clinical Surgery was independent action on Russell's part, undertaken without the efforts of the College of Surgeons. Although the College approved, according to their minutes, 'of both the chair and the person proposed to fill it',[48] they felt they should have 'some share in its patronage, as it was related to teaching and practice of surgery, over which they had a monopoly'.[49]

In 1804, therefore, they tried again to break the monopoly on surgery held by the Professor of Anatomy, by this time Alexander Monro *tertius*. Several members submitted a memorial to the College again stressing the dangers of having the only lectureship of surgery available in Edinburgh taught by a man who was not a practicing surgeon. The most detrimental aspect of this mode of teaching, the authors explained, was that

the attention of the student will be directed to the performance of operations and little, if at all, to what must ever in practice constitute the principle part of his duty, namely the medical treatment of chirurgical diseases.[50]

The memorial proposed John Thomson to be appointed Lecturer of Surgery. The College approved both the idea and the appointment, but decided that Thomson be given the title instead of Professor of Surgery. This again involved the College in a vigorous legal dispute with the *Senatus Academicus*, which declared that only the university could properly appoint professors. Eventually the College won, and Thomson remained an extra-academical Professor of the Principles and Practice of Surgery.

Thomson's lectures on the Principles and Practice of Surgery, like Russell's, became a requirement for the College's diploma in 1808. Thomson's lectures read like a combination of manifesto for the new, liberally-educated surgeon of the early nineteenth century, and local Edinburgh polemics. A student attending Thomson's lectures would have heard that 'The theory and practice of physic and surgery are intimately connected together and are undoubtedly one and the same science'.[51] This attack on the distinction in subject matter between the physician and surgeon was of course an attack on the social distinction between them as well, and understood as such. According to Thomson, there were three reasons why surgery 'in modern times' had been considered a 'mere mechanical art',

First by surgeons being taught by the physicians & 2dly from those following surgery having such a limited education & 3dly from the custom of surgery being taught by teachers of anatomy.[52]

This, too, was a kind of manifesto, and were current areas of concern for the Royal College. The first had been remedied by Thomson's own appointment, the second, by the requirements for the Royal College's diploma, and the third, by James Russell's course in Clinical Surgery. With clear reference to the course in Anatomy and Surgery taught by Alexander Monro *tertius*, Thomson went on to say that surgery should never be taught in the same course as anatomy, 'the surgeons attention being too much engaged in considering operations without learning the most important part which is the medical treatment'.[53] This echoed the language of the memorial recommending Thomson for the lectureship, which Thomson may have written, as well as current concerns of surgical education.

The student who attended Thomson's course would have received benefit from more than the lectures themselves. Every Wednesday, between five and six o'clock, Thomson examined his students, half of the time on surgery, the other half on 'Anatomy, Chemistry, Theory and Practice of Physic, Materia Medica and Pharmacy'. These were required for the examination for a diploma, and Thomson assured his students that his own examination 'renders the future public examinations in Surgeon's Hall much more easy & gives [students] more confidence in undergoing these examinations'.[54] Since this was not a University course, though, it did not appear in the matriculation records, and so we have no way of knowing how many students attended.

In 1806, Thomson was also appointed Regius Professor of the newly-created chair of Military Surgery in the university, but he continued his course of lectures for the College, only transferring his consideration of wounds to the new course.[55] Military Surgery attracted only an average of 10 per cent of the students per cohort between 1810 and 1826, but nonetheless quickly became an established course offering. Thomson resigned his chair in 1822; his successor was George Ballingall, who, unlike Thomson, had been an army surgeon.[56]

Unfortunately we do not have any student account of what the actual examinations for the diploma consisted of. George Bell told the Royal Commission that when he was an examiner,

> the first procedure was to make [candidates] translate two or three
> sentences . . . of Gregory's Conspectus, or Celsus, and then to write
> it down upon a piece of paper, to see if they could construe and spell;
> then they were to translate some prescriptions in the Pharmacopoeia,
> and were examined upon the composition and uses, and doses of
> medicine . . . The next Examinator took the candidate up on
> Anatomy; the third went to Surgery; and if there was any doubt upon
> the minds of any of them, the fourth examined him generally.[57]

The examinations generally lasted about thirty minutes. Archibald Robert-son, who had written *Colloquia* for prospective graduates, also published *Conversations of Anatomy, Physiology, and Surgery*, dedicated 'to the Gentlemen attending the anatomical and surgical lectures'. In the preface, he also announced an edition of *Conversations on the Principles and Practice of Surgery*.[58] William Gordon, 'Member of the Royal College of Surgeons, Edinburgh, &c. &c' published *Academical Examinations on the Practice of Surgery, intended for the use of students* and dedicated, like Robertson's 'to the Gentlemen attending surgical lectures'.[59] These books, together with Thomson's question and answer sessions, suggest that the surgeon's diploma was incorporated into the same pattern of extra-academical study and grinding as the University MD. The examinations were apparently accompanied with some ceremony as well, for David Birrel wrote to his parents,' I must have a new waistcoat before my examination – but do not know what kind yet Black silk is generally used on that day by those who can afford it.'[60]

The greater the ceremony, the greater the disappointment of rejected students. The College of Surgeons found out some of the problems that entailed in 1809, when William Waddell, who had been rejected by the examiners several months earlier, tried to forge a diploma. It was not a very good forgery since it was written in English, and the engraver, instead of affixing the seal of the College to it, had affixed the seal of one 'Mr Baird of Gilmerton'. Waddell, his friend John Cowan Paxton, who had helped him, the scribe, and the engraver were brought before magistrates. The College was inclined to think that the engraver and the scribe were the main guilty parties, since they were 'men in a public character in the city', who should have known better. The engraver was obviously culpable: he must have known he was being asked to produce a forgery, and he had certainly known he was misusing Mr Baird's seal. The scribe later made the apparently acceptable excuse that it was his business to write whatever he was given; he was 'very shocked and sorry at the use his work had been put to', and the charges against him were dropped.[61] Waddell and Paxton were also let off the charge, since it appeared that

> Waddell was a young man of weak intellect and seemed unconscious of having done any thing wrong . . . [He] acknowledged with candour that he had committed the forgery and the manner in which he had proceeded in doing it and upon his being conducted from the council chamber to his own room produced the diploma.[62]

When asked, 'what was his motive for committing so gross a crime', he replied 'that it was done to please his father'.[63] The case was not pursued, but the College drew up and printed a warning against forgeries. The College had to draw up a warning of a different kind in 1826, when one of the examiners, Dr Adam Hunter, received threatening letters from students, and was hissed when he entered the surgical amphitheatre in the Royal Infirmary. The letters accused Hunter of unfairly rejecting several candidates, including one 'unfortunate young man, who after rejection

. . . put a period to his existence on Arthur's Seat'.[64] The Royal College felt 'imperiously called on to express their decided disapprobation of such proceedings'. They did so in an announcement which defended Hunter and all their examiners. 'The Medical Students must be well aware,' the announcement stated,

> that the Value of their Diplomas depends in a great measure on the opinion entertained by the Profession & by the Public, that while the examinations instituted at Surgeons Hall are conducted with candour and impartiality, they are at the same time conducted with that degree of Strictness necessary to ascertain the Possession of an adequate professional knowledge in the individuals holding their diplomas.[65]

The strictness of the examinations was an especially important point by the 1820s, for the College of Surgeons had worked hard to have their diploma accepted throughout Great Britain as a certification of 'possession of an adequate professional knowledge. This point first came up in 1783, when the Edinburgh surgeons received a letter from Dr Alexander Stevenson on behalf of the Royal College of Physicians and Surgeons in Glasgow. The Glasgow College had the privilege of licensing surgeons in the western counties of Scotland, and Stevenson wrote to inform the Edinburgh surgeons that some gentlemen with Edinburgh diplomas had been practicing in the counties under Glasgow's jurisdiction. He wished to point out as a courtesy, of course, that possession of an Edinburgh diploma did not exempt those gentlemen from the need to acquire a licence from the Glasgow College. The tone of the communication appears to have been polite, but pointed: The College of Physicians and Surgeons of Glasgow intended to defend its traditional monopoly against the possibility of Edinburgh encroachment. The Edinburgh surgeons were quick to reply that the diplomas were not licenses, and were not intended to give the right to practice in any particular county, but simply certified that its bearer was qualified to practice surgery.[66]

From that point on, the Edinburgh College made every effort to increase the value of their diplomas by having them accepted as sufficient qualification for entry into the military and colonial services. The London Company of Surgeons, called the College of Surgeons after 1800, had the privilege of licensing surgeons for the army and navy, which meant that every candidate for a position in military or colonial service had to undergo their examination.[67] The Edinburgh College tried to get the London College to waive its right of examination, so that licentiates of the Royal College of Surgeons of Edinburgh need not submit to further examination before taking up their positions. The London College interpreted this, correctly, as an encroachment on its privileges, and opposed it every step of the way.

This became part of the battle over *ancien regime* privileges of medical corporations.[68] In Great Britain privileges were often defended by corporate bodies as legally-held property, and their legitimacy fought over in law courts and public opinion.[69] The Edinburgh College of Surgeons held on to their own corporate monopoly until 1840, as mentioned in Chapter Five. They attacked the London College's monopoly from the 1780s by appealing to the new concept of the diploma as an impartial testimonial of the bearer's ability. Not surprisingly, the Edinburgh College was initially successful only in those areas where a politically powerful ally, especially Henry Dundas, was able or chose to exert his influence on their behalf. Their first successes, the examination of surgeons for the African Slave Trade, in 1788,[70] and for the East India Company, in 1799, both came from Dundas' patronage.[71]

It took many years for the Royal College to wring similar concessions for the more traditional positions in the army and navy. In 1797 the Office of Sick and Wounded Seamen agreed that their diploma was an acceptable testimonial for navy mates. In 1803, the Army Medical Board decided to accept the diploma for army hospital mates, and in 1805, for assistant surgeons.[72] These were all secondary positions, and a diploma from the Edinburgh College was only accepted as sufficient qualification for full army surgeons in 1813.[73] Even though the majority of licentiates did not join the Imperial services, its acceptance as testimony that the bearer was 'perfectly qualified' enhanced its prestige as a form of accreditation.[74]

The new courses and new diploma of the Royal College of Surgeons reinforced each other, as they were intended to do, by ensuring students' 'possession of an adequate professional knowledge'. Taken together, all the activities of the Royal College of Surgeons of Edinburgh reinforced what George Bell called the 'Surgical School'.[75] That School was established enough by 1822 for the Lord Advocate to consult the College as to whether the University of Glasgow should be allowed to offer degrees in surgery. The College responded that the right to grant 'such diplomas or licenses' had hitherto belonged only to the College of Physicians and Surgeons in Glasgow, and to the 'Royal Colleges of Surgeons of London Dublin and Edinburgh'. The College therefore could not

> help considering the late claim made by the University of Glasgow to grant surgical diplomas as an innovation and one which if followed by the other Universities must materially affect the rights of all the Surgical Colleges.[76]

It is an indication of how completely the Edinburgh surgeons had taken on the role of an educational institution that they felt they had to power to prevent a University surgical degree. An even greater sign of their increasing independence from – and perhaps competition with – Edinburgh University came in 1823, when the College officially ruled that the surgery course offered by Alexander Monro *tertius* was too short to be

considered adequate for their diploma.[77] By 1826, Professor William
Pulteney Alison could, with justice, call the College of Surgeons a 'rival
school'.[78]

One measure of the College's impact on students is the start of surgical
subjects for Royal Medical Society essays. Up until the 1790s, the
dissertation topics had always been resolutely medical, as indeed the name
of the Society implied. Even though the Edinburgh surgeons provided the
land on which the Hall of the Society was built, there seems to have been
no suggestion that the Society incorporate any aspects of surgical training
into its activities. Some surgeons joined the Society, but their essays did
not display any particular surgical interest or outlook. Andrew Wardrop's
dissertation on 'Can the advantages expected arise from methodical
nosology?' considered medical nosology alone, and made no attempt to
apply the subject to surgical cases. Indeed, his conclusion, that nosology
was impracticable because pathognomic symptoms for most diseases did
not exist, and that the practitioner 'must have recourse to reasoning and
indications taken from the causes of the symptoms, by which means we
may diversify our practice to any diversity of symptoms',[79] seems completely inapplicable to surgical treatment. James Russell, while a member
of the Society, wrote his medical question 'On the theory of vision' and
his case on 'Combination of hysteria and epilepsy'.[80] Neither essay
displayed any distinctively surgical point of view, and both epilepsy and
hysteria were standard case history topics. Indeed all of the prospective
Fellows who wrote essays for the Society between 1761 and 1794 dealt
with standard medical topics, such as opthalmia, digestion, cold bathing,
and scurvy.[81] Even John Thomson, later to teach the Principles and
Practice of Surgery, wrote his case histories on the standard medical
subjects of 'Hectic Fever', and 'Catarrh'.[82] All these subjects were
frequently chosen for MD theses.[83]

Surgical subjects were chosen for Royal Medical Dissertations for the
first time in the 1790s. George Bell, who joined the Society in 1795,
seems to have been the first member to present a surgical dissertation,
writing on Fistula Lachrymalis, a common surgical subject and frequently
part of the Royal College's entrance examination for Fellows.[84] Most of the
other Fellows who joined the Society after 1795 wrote at least one essay
on a surgical subject. James Wardrope wrote on Aneurism, William Wood
on Cataract, James Bremner and John Turner on Hydrocele, Thomas
Lothian on Amputation, and John Gordon, James Keith and David Hay
on some aspect of wounds.[85]

The 'predisposing cause', to use eighteenth-century medical language,
of this increase in surgical subjects was the European-wide interest in
surgery, but the 'exciting cause' was the changes in the Royal College of
Surgeons. By the late 1790s, a new generation of apprentices and Fellows

would have been educated with the idea of the surgeon as a learned gentleman, and surgery as a fit subject for learned treatises. The up-swing in the number of licentiates also made surgeons a more visible presence in the University, and that affected even the purely medical students.[86] By the 1790s, they, too, would have been educated with the idea of the surgeon as a learned gentleman. The two groups shared a common course of study, and perhaps a common perception of the importance of surgery to the practitioner, since many graduates also attended James Russell's class in Clinical Surgery.

Many, but not all, of the surgical essays in the Royal Medical Society were written by either apprentices, or prospective Fellows or licentiates. Six essays were written on Amputation between 1795 and 1826, three by students associated with Surgeons Hall but three who were 'pure' MDs, that is MDs who were neither apprentices, Fellows or licentiates.[87] Seven dissertations were written on Cataract in the same period, one of which was by a Fellow, one by a pure MD, two by auditors and three by licentiates and apprentices who also graduated.[88] Six dissertations were written on Hydrocele, two by Fellows, one by a pure MD, and the other three by students affiliated with Surgeons Hall who also graduated.[89] The repetition of subjects indicates that surgical subjects had become standard enough academic fare to be routinely proposed for Cases or Questions. The fact that even pure MDs with no affiliation to Surgeon's Hall chose or agreed to write on them is another sign of how acceptable surgery had become in a University setting. George Meek, for example, seems to have had no personal contact whatever with his chosen topic: he began his dissertation by apologizing for having chosen a topic

> with which, as far as practice is concerned, I am in no respect acquainted; for I never have been so fortunate, or I may rather say, so unfortunate, as to have had the opportunity of seeing a single one during the whole course of my medical studies.[90]

His account of wounds is not nearly as impressive as James Robertson's, who described the manner in which he had himself 'drawn together the lips of a great number of simple incised wounds'.[91] That makes it all the more significant: if a Society member without experience or ability in surgery chose to write on it, it is a good sign that it had become a standard, accepted topic.

As discussed in Chapter Seven, the form of the learned essays required by the Society conveyed information about medicine as well as the topic. The surgical dissertations made it clear that surgery was a learned discipline, requiring academic study. Thomas Haines-Banning, for exam-ple, in his dissertation on amputation, gave an extensive discussion of the progress of amputation, citing numerous authors, including that old medical standby, Celsus, as well as clear, carefully-drawn diagrams.[92] John

Gordon cited his 'learned preceptor, Mr [John] Thomson, in his lectures on the principles and practice of surgery', in his discussion of 'What is the process of nature in the healing of wounds?'[93]

A common preoccupation of the dissertations was contradicting the notion that surgery 'consists in dressing sores, and hewing off limbs with the dexterity of an artisan'.[94] James Pender warned that 'From the experience of most men, we find immediate amputation seldom necessary, and not near so often as imagined'.[95] Humphrey Herbert Jones, while acknowledging the general utility of bleeding in the case of flesh wounds, nonetheless felt that even 'after a general engagement, when our hospitals are crowded with both sick and wounded, a number of circumstances should be maturely considered before we bleed in a common flesh wound'.[96] In other words, a surgeon should not behave like a 'mere mechanick', whose only skill consisted in his ability to wield sharp tools. George Meek presented this view most graphically when he said the surgeon should not

> rashly insert the probe among the viscera of the thorax or abdomen, in order to know which particular one of them is the seat of the wound . . . [one author] was particularly against this practice, for, he says, I never could bear the thought of thrusting a long pair of forceps, the Lord knows where . . .[97]

Meek went on to say that

> the judicious surgeon, instead of pursuing such a butcher business, immediately after the wound, orders his patient to be laid in bed, and there, by the course of the symptoms as they come on, he judges of his situation, and entertains a favourable, or unfavourable prognostic, as these indicate.[98]

The skill of the 'judicious surgeon', in other words, did not consist merely in knowing how to probe for the bullet, but in understanding the circumstances under which the operation should be performed.

Meek's account fits the ideas of Thomson and other Edinburgh surgeons, that the principle object of surgical study was the medical treatment of surgical disease. So did the other surgical essays written for the Society. In making a decision as to whether to bleed a patient with a flesh wound, Humphrey Herbert Jones said he would consider

> the age, constitution, and length of time a patient may have served [in the army] . . . a young and healthy recruit, may more safely be blooded, than a veteran, or one worn down by fatigue, disease, bad and scanty provisions, and the length of the campaign. I would also consider the climate and season.[99]

'[T]he surgeon . . . ought to consider attentively all the circumstances of the disease, or injury . . .' Thomas Lothian wrote. 'Attention must be paid to the age and habit of the patient, and local circumstances also, in some cases, must have considerable influence in directing our conduct.'[100] It was attention to the indications for treatment presented by the individual patient, and knowledge of the way in which individual circumstances affected surgical disease, that distinguished the 'judicious surgeon', in Meek's phrase, from the 'butcher business' of former times. And it was the presence of the judicious surgery student that distinguished members of the Royal Medical Society, still the elite of the student body, at the start of the nineteenth-century from members in the mid-eighteenth-century. In the 1790s, five or six of the approximately sixty Society members in residence each year went on to become licentiates. By 1805, the number of prospective licentiates was up to fifteen each year. By 1820, when Stroude wrote his 'History of the Royal Medical Society', there were 101 members in residence in Edinburgh that year, and thirty of them became licentiates. Stroude thus united physicians-to-be with surgeons-to-be when he described Society members as 'fellow-students of a liberal profession'.[101]

There is a more sensational example of the changes in surgical education in Edinburgh over the period covered by this book. In 1745 Sir John Clerk of Penicuik, while recommending anatomical study to his son, told him nevertheless to 'avoid the horror of raising dead bodies'.[102] This was a sentiment entirely approved of by the Edinburgh surgeons at that time. In 1771, hearing that a child's body had been taken from its grave and found at St Anthony's Chapel, the College had joined with sheriff and magistrate in offering a reward for the guilty party, 'especially as from the appearance of the body it had been cut and mangled, which would induce people to suppose it had been done by some 'prentices or students'.[103] The College offered a ten guinea reward and advertised it in newspapers. Six years later, a similar incident of 'raising dead bodies' led them once again to offer a reward and insert an advertisement in newspapers to assure the public that the College would never do anything to encourage such a barbarous practice.[104] Yet in 1828 the College published an advertisement, circulated throughout Britain, requiring prospective licentiates to produce certification 'from a Professor or Teacher of Anatomy recognized by the College, that he has been actually engaged in the dissection of the human body'.[105] That was the same year that one such teacher, Robert Knox, Fellow of the Royal College of Surgeons of Edinburgh, was involved in the scandal surrounding William Burke, William Hare, and Helen McDougal, who murdered visitors to their lodging-house and sold the bodies to Knox for his dissecting classes.[106] Despite public outcry against 'resurrectionists', the College did not alter the requirement. We may wonder whether Fellows reflected on the connection between the demand, which they had done much to create, of over 100 new licentiates per year for bodies to dissect and Burke's and Hare's attempts to fill that demand.

If so, they took no action. By the 1820s, anatomical dissection was too important a part of surgical education to be omitted, and the 'Surgical School' was too important a part of the Royal College of Surgeons of Edinburgh to be subject to lay opinion.

9

The response of the medical faculty

I. No one shall be admitted to the Degree of Doctor in Medicine who has not studied Medicine for the Space of four years . . . either in the University of Edinburgh or in some other University where the degree of MD is given . . .

II. No one shall be admitted to the Examinations required for the Degree of Doctor, who has not given sufficient evidence, –

1st, That he has studied, once at least, each of the following departments of Medical Science . . .

Anatomy and Surgery,	
Chemistry,	
Materia Medica, and Pharmacy,	During Courses
Theory of Medicine,	of Six Months
Practice of Medicine,	
Midwifery . . .	
Clinical Medicine }	During a course of Six Months . . .
Botany	During a course of Three Months

2ndly, That he has also studied . . . two at least (which he is at liberty to choose) of the following subjects, viz.

Practical Anatomy	
Natural History	During a course of
Medical Jurisprudence and Police	at least Three
Clinical Surgery	Months
Military Surgery	

3rdly, That in each year of his Academical Studies in Medicine, he has attended two at least of the Six Months Courses of Lectures above specified, or one of these and two of the Three Months Courses.

4thly, That, besides the course of Clinical Medicine already prescribed, he has attended, for at least six months of another year, the Medical and Surgical Practice of a General Hospital.

The Medical Calendar, 1828[1]

If the Edinburgh University medical faculty had had a motto in the first twenty years of the nineteenth century, it might have been *quieta non movere*, 'when a state is tranquil, it should not be unsettled by causeless innovation'.[2] Certainly it is hard to accuse the faculty of being rashly innovative: the above regulations were the first substantive change in graduation requirements since 1783. Judging by the number of students and graduates, the state of medical education was not only tranquil, but even flourishing. The total number of students matriculating rose from over 200 per cohort in the 1790s to over 400 per cohort by the 1820s. Moreover, the percentage of MDs per cohort, though fluctuating, never dropped below 17 per cent and by the 1820s was consistently well over 20 per cent. This meant that the six faculty members who examined an average of forty-five candidates for graduation per cohort in the 1790s were examining an average of 112 candidates per cohort between 1815 and 1824.

At that point the new graduation requirements cut down on the number of graduates per cohort, to an average of seventy-two in 1824 and 1825 – a reduction of forty students per year. With each student paying a graduation fee of £10, this meant a loss in income of £400 each year. This may seem an odd policy for the faculty to adopt if one assumes, as the Royal Commission later did, that the medical professorate had an interest only in regulations which would increase their fees. The explanation, of course, is that the medical faculty had always been interested in fame as well as fortune, the reputation of their degree as well as the income to be derived from it. The 1825 regulations represent their attempts to maintain the reputation of the medical degree in the face of changing conditions of medical practice and education.

Comments on Edinburgh life in the early nineteenth century were marked with a pervasive sense of the end of an era. This was caught most vividly in Henry Cockburn's *Memorials of his Time*. 'It has always been a pleasure to me to have seen some of the men of the retiring generation,'[3] he wrote, referring to Joseph Black among others. Though young at the time, he and his friends

> knew enough of them to make us fear that no other race of men, so tried by time, such friends of each other and of learning, and all of such amiable manners and such spotless characters, could be expected soon to arise, and again ennoble Scotland.[4]

The succession of the generations was marked in the medical faculty. William Cullen died in 1790, and was succeeded by James Gregory as Professor of Medicine and the Practice of Physick. Joseph Black died in 1799 and was replaced by Thomas Charles Hope as Professor of Medicine and Chemistry. Francis Home lived until 1813, and Alexander Monro *secundus* until 1817, but both resigned their chairs to their sons, James Home and Alexander Monro *tertius*, in 1798. Alexander Hamilton died in 1802; two years previous he, too, had been succeeded by his son James as Professor of Midwifery. By that time the old-timers were, in addition to James Gregory, Andrew Duncan senior and Daniel Rutherford, both appointed in the late 1780s. Between 1800 and 1819 no new men were appointed to the traditional chairs, an important reason why the state of tranquility of the medical faculty was not disturbed.

Another reason was that from the 1790s all the faculty, except for Andrew Duncan senior, were sons of professors. They had each inherited from their fathers a going concern: a professor's chair with privileges protected by law, assured status within the profession, and, with the steady increase of students, an income guaranteeing a gentleman's style of life. Even Duncan senior, though originally an outsider, had spent his early professional life as an extra-academical lecturer, and may have regarded his professorship as a kind of reward for early exertions. Certainly he showed no signs of wishing to open up the professorate to outsiders, but instead ensured that his own son, Andrew Duncan junior, would inherit his chair.[5] Duncan senior does have the distinction of being responsible for the only innovation in medical education attributable to the faculty in this period: he founded the chair in Medical Jurisprudence. He also ensured, though, that the first incumbent was his son Andrew, who held it until he could take over his father's more lucrative chair in Medical Theory.

William Pulteney Alison was appointed to the chair of Medical Jurisprudence in 1820, and Robert Christison in 1822. 'Medical Jurisprudence is of very considerable importance,' wrote Alexander Bower in the *Edinburgh Student's Guide*, 'and involves the determination of questions which are intimately connected with the peace, the happiness, and in many cases, the very existence of civil society.'[6] It was not required for graduation, however, and was scheduled first in the summer, and later at 1 or 2 pm, the same time as Anatomy and Surgery. 'What was to be looked for as the inevitable consequence?' Professor Robert Christison later asked. 'Would not the students inevitably infer . . . [that it] must be a needless branch of study?'[7] Perhaps they did, for only an average of 4 per cent of the students per cohort attended it.

All of these professors fulfilled their obligations competently, and some with real ability: all, for example, were elected Fellows of the Royal Society of Edinburgh.[8] With their accession, however, some of the brilliance of the original Faculty was dimmed. 'It has been said that the medical professors of Edinburgh are inferior to their predecessors,' Andrew Duncan junior wrote with some annoyance, '. . . if it be a disgrace to be inferior to such men, it is a disgrace which they share with all their professional brethren of this age and country.'[9] Some of the criticisms, though, were more specific. Alexander Monro *tertius*, it was rumoured, lectured from his grandfather's notes;[10] according to James Rush, 'the medical students form but a part of that crowd who know his faults; who smile at his folly, or wonder at his stupidity'.[11] Daniel Rutherford reputedly never liked Botany; Andrew Duncan senior was 'an aged, most amiable, benevolent, but by this time rather feebleminded man'.[12] Thomas Charles Hope acquired an excellent reputation as a lecturer, surpassing all others, according to Prince Adam Czartoryski, for 'the neatness of his demonstrations, his skill in the carrying out of experiments, and in his mode of expression, which is elegant to the point of affectation'. Still, Prince Adam said, Hope was 'little known for his discoveries and a man rather limited generally'.[13] He was, in other words, a good professor but not a profound philosopher like Joseph Black. The same might be said for James Gregory, though the most illustrious of this generation of professors. 'On no medical brow are grey hairs so finely contrasted with the evergreen of a laurel chaplet', wrote a reviewer in *Blackwood's Magazine* in 1818, in response to a pamphlet which compared Edinburgh unfavourably with the medical school at Trinity College, Dublin.[14] But Gregory died three years later, and was replaced, not with a new man known for his scientific contributions, but with James Home, then sixty-one years old.

Not even the appointment of Robert Graham as Professor of Medicine and Botany in 1820, and William Pulteney Alison as Professor of Medicine and Medical Theory in 1821, could change the impression that the University of Edinburgh had become a kind of medical education 'mill': it ground out a solid education for the average student, but those in search of exceptional opportunities would do better elsewhere. Scientific investigation was becoming ever more important as the mark of prestige for a medical school, but Edinburgh professors were apparently doing it less. Students interested in learning the latest techniques in chemistry had to attend extra-academical lecturers like David Boswell Reid, go to Glasgow to study with Professor Thomas Thomson, or, even better, attended lectures at the Collège de France or Jardin des Plantes in Paris.[15] Opportunities for anatomical dissection and extensive clinical experience in hospitals, generally regarded as essential medical studies by the 1800s, could also be obtained more conveniently, if not more cheaply, in London or Paris.[16] Edinburgh, then, did not so much decline as stand still, with the result that it began to be outdistanced in reputation, though not student numbers, by other institutions.

Even in the area of Edinburgh's greatest strength, 'all branches of science, regularly taught', it began to have serious rivals. By 1800, American students could attend medical schools at the University of Pennsylvania in Philadelphia and King's College in New York, each of which offered the same lectures as Edinburgh without the expenses of travel abroad. By 1825, there were fourteen medical schools in the United States, 'viz. seven in New England, three in the Middle, two in the Southern, and two in the Western States'.[17] Though study in Britain continued to be a mark of prestige for American physicians, it was no longer a necessity. Within Britain, Glasgow University and Trinity College Dublin expanded their medical faculties.[18] Glasgow was hampered by conflict between University and Regius professors, and between University professors and the Faculty of Physicians and Surgeons, which controlled access to the Royal Infirmary. For that reason there were no university lectures in clinical medicine.[19] Trinity College Dublin required students to first obtain a BA before the MD and thus had few graduates, though the Royal College of Surgeons in Dublin, like the Edinburgh Royal College of Surgeons, offered diplomas based on study. All these institutions appealed to students looking for a course of medical lectures leading to a degree; each claimed at some point to offer the best lectures. The number of lectures available at the hospital schools in London expanded as well.[20] Moreover, by the 1830s the institution of a University in London offering medical degrees had been proposed.[21] This university would have given students attending lectures, dissections and hospitals in London the opportunity to acquire a University MD at the same time. The London hospital schools were Edinburgh's rivals as it was; the projected University would have intensified the rivalry.[22]

The proliferation of medical lectures, both within and without universities, meant that Edinburgh faced more competition: it was no longer the only place offering a rigorous course of study leading to a degree. It also meant that more students had more opportunities to attend lectures than ever before. For the medical profession, and indeed for patients, that was undoubtedly a good thing. Each individual medical student, though, found that he was facing more, and better educated, competition. As the standard level of medical education rose, a kind of inflationary spiral in medical instruction developed. The success of each new lectureship provided an incentive for new practitioners to give lectures anywhere students or apprentices were to be found; the ready availability of such lectures meant that students who did not attend them were regarded as poorly-educated; students interested in lectures as a mark of distinction found they had to attend still more in order to be truly distinguished.

The Royal College of Surgeons of Edinburgh had been partly responsible for this. Their diploma brought in more students, and provided an incentive for students to attend courses for more years. However, the increase in educational attainments for surgeons and surgeon-apothecaries was a British, not merely Edinburgh, phenomena, fuelled in part by the increased competition within the medical profession on all levels.[23] It presumably was also fuelled, at least in England, by a rising birth rate, a slight increase in the proportion of young adults in the population, and the rising level of real wages which translated into more money to spend on a son's education.[24] It was promoted by the military medical services, which increased their educational requirements for appointments as a result of the Napoleonic Wars. By 1828, Army hospital assistants – the lowest rank of army practitioner – had to have spent a year walking the wards in a hospital, in addition to attending lectures in Anatomy, Practical Anatomy, Chemistry, Materia Medica, Botany, Surgery, Theory of Medicine and Physiology, Practice of Medicine, and Clinical Lectures.[25] Assistant surgeons in the Navy – again, the lowest rank – had to have attended almost as many lectures.[26] This is a striking change from Alexander Lesassier's assumption that he could 'finish his education completely' and enter the Army after only one year of study. The lowest rank of medical military service traditionally attracted men with the least education, because it paid the least. If those positions required such an extensive education by the 1820s, then surely those who aspired to higher ranks in the profession required still more.

A result of this increase in academically-trained surgeons, and the corresponding one in surgically-trained physicians, was the blurring of the traditional distinction between physician and surgeon. The eradication of that distinction altogether was promoted by surgeons like Professor John Thomson, who argued, as we have seen, that 'physic and surgery are intimately connected together and are undoubtedly one and the same science'.[27] Indeed, the gradual unification of the two branches has usually been considered by historians as one of the major developments of early nineteenth-century medicine.[28]

Contemporary observers, though, were not always in favour of it. Thomas Charleton Speer, who graduated from Edinburgh University in 1812, complained of the breakdown of the traditional distinctions. 'Between the physician, the surgeon, the apothecary, and surgeon-apothecary, the accoucheur, &c &c,' he wrote,

> there seems now established a more puzzling and discordant medley than ever; the lines and limits between them seem . . . loose and broken . . . Perpetual schism and warfare has been the consequence.[29]

Speer looked back to a medical Golden Age, when

> the line separating each branch had at least something clear and definite about it . . . divisions of the profession then seemed to belong to the divisions of the human body; the physician claimed the interior and the trunk, the surgeon claimed the exterior and the limbs . . .[30]

This division had the benefit not only of simplicity, but also in promoting amity among the different branches, for 'the arguments of each were plausible, each felt strong in his own province, and soon resented any encroachments'.[31] Speer's arguments, though couched in medical terms, have the same import, though not the same style, as Alexander Pope's *Essay on Man*:

> God, in the nature of each being, founds
> Its proper bliss, and sets its proper bounds:

But as he fram'd a Whole, the Whole to bless,
On mutual Wants built a mutual Happiness.
So from the first eternal Order ran,
And creature link'd to creature, man to man.[32]

Speer's arguments, like Pope's, were socially conservative, arguing for a just gradation of ranks, as well as against ambition that tried to eliminate those ranks.[33]

Speer's depiction of the medical profession was hopelessly out of date by 1823, when his book was published, and reflect his concern about encroachments on his own MD. But other, more forward-looking writers also argued against the merging of physicians and surgeons. Edward Barlow, for example, was interested in dignifying the general practitioner, a term which was gradually supplanting the varied labels for the provincial surgeon and surgeon-apothecary.[34] In 1818, however, when trying to delineate the different branches of the profession, he wrote that the physician, surgeon, and general practitioner

> may be regarded as in some measure forming the gradation of rank in the profession, by which it accommodates itself to the corresponding gradations in general society; the physician being suited more particularly to the higher orders; the surgeon holding an intermediate place between the physicians and general practitioner; and these latter embracing the whole community, from its highest to its lowest degrees, their utility rendering them necessary to the former, while their humility and habits of active industry fit them for extending their services to the lowest extreme.[35]

As late as 1840, a reviewer in the *Quarterly Review* wrote that he could 'discover no wisdom,' in all medical practitioners being 'admitted at one door, so as to form one society – the individuals of which are supposed to be equally qualified by their education to undertake one or another branch of practice'.[36] Instead, he felt, the division of physician, surgeon and general practitioner were exactly suited to the needs of society, because 'the extension of [medical] knowledge introduced the necessity of a division of labour'.[37]

Appeals to the 'needs of society' were frequently invoked in arguments against legislative reforms, for surely if society needed, as in this case, a different type of medical practitioner, then society would have produced one. What this particular set of arguments shows is that for the general public, and much of the profession, the physician kept his traditional place at the head of medicine, whether on the traditional grounds of rank in society or because of more modern notions of medical specialization. Alexander Lesassier, who had been sure that his one year of study would let him 'rank with the highest of them' in 1806, had learned better by 1816, when he returned to Edinburgh to obtain an MD.[38]

Yet the phenomena of men like Lesassier getting medical degrees illustrates the problems caused for Edinburgh University by the blurring of traditional distinctions. Lesassier had been an army surgeon, and obtained his medical degree in order to set up civilian practice. Many other former military practitioners did the same, with the result, according to Speer, that 'the redundancy of practitioners is increased and increasing every day'. Speer blamed the increase squarely on educational institutions: students had flocked to medical lectures in order to take advantage of the opportunities offered by the war, and continued to do so in peacetime, even though 'now there scarcely seems any vent for the overstock which our laid-up fleets and armies have diffused over society'.[39] At Edinburgh University alone, Speer wrote, there were over 2000 students, three-quarters of whom were medical students.[40]

Speer's figures were inaccurate and his arguments often wandered. But his assumption, that universities like Edinburgh were making more education available to more students, thus facilitating the blurring of ranks and intensifying competition, was correct. It was certainly widely accepted by contemporaries. From 1815 on, the accessibility of lectures and, even more important, of medical degrees at the 'Scotch Universities' came under attack. Professor John Burns of Glasgow University attributed the increase in MDs 'in the first place, to fashion'[41] and saw no problem with it, but 'it is the appendage of M.D. which has become the order and decoration of the day', Speer complained.[42] 'Medico-Chirurgus,' who wrote 'A Letter Addressed to the Medical Profession, on the encroachments on the practice of the surgeon-apothecary, by a new set of physicians,' complained, like Speer, of the overabundance of practitioners, and also placed the blame on military men obtaining MDs and then presuming to set up practice at a higher rank than the honest surgeon-apothecary. These men 'assume to themselves the style and title of physicians . . .' the author said,

> obtained by the remittance of fifteen pounds to a Scotch University – a title which may be conferred on any farrier, at the pleasure of any two individuals inclined to indulge in such a joke.[43]

This was of course a reference to St Andrews or Aberdeen, not Edinburgh or Glasgow. The author, however, wrote only of 'Scotch Universities', and thus gave the impression that all were equally guilty of selling degrees. The spokesperson for the Society of Physicians of the United Kingdom, a society apparently made up largely of Edinburgh graduates, also complained that

> It is now the common practice with the most ignorant and illiterate pretenders in medicine, to furnish themselves with a medical diploma from one of those Scotch Universities, who, to their eternal disgrace, traffic in degrees, and bestow them, without examination, on persons the most unqualified to possess them. The public unfortunately

confounds [all Scottish graduates] together; and a Scotch physician is become almost a term of degradation.[44]

This is unfair to St Andrews and Aberdeen; there is in fact no evidence that their MDs were going to 'ignorant and illiterate' practitioners.[45] It should, instead, be seen as testimony to how widespread the assumption had become that a set course of study, and a rigorous examination, were necessary evidence of medical skill.

Edinburgh graduates assumed that their own degree was immune from criticism, but English public opinion, especially, was not so sure. The general inflation in medical education made the Edinburgh MD less elite and more accessible, and that alone tended to lower its value in the eyes of some contemporaries, especially in comparison to Oxford and Cambridge MDs. Attempts to regulate the English medical profession only reinforced that impression. The Licentiates of the Royal College of Physicians of London, many of them Edinburgh graduates, challenged the privileges of the Fellows several times, especially in the 1790s. In each case the result was only to confirm the traditional privileges of the Fellows and of Oxford and Cambridge graduates.[46] Licentiates responded with a host of pamphlets, and the medical profession outside of London supported them, but lay periodicals were less sympathetic. 'The disputes which have so long subsisted between the fellows and licentiates of the College of Physicians . . .' a reviewer wrote, 'have never excited much interest, except among the disputants themselves . . .'[47]

Even worse, in 1815 Parliament passed the Act for Better Regulating the Practice of Apothecaries throughout England and Wales, better known as the Apothecaries Act, the first attempt at national regulation of the English medical profession. It stated that every English practitioner outside London had to serve a five-year apprenticeship and undergo examination by the Society of Apothecaries. The Act provoked widespread animosity from all English practitioners, but was especially resented by Edinburgh graduates practicing in England, who found themselves thus relegated to the same status as the surgeon-apothecaries whose 'vulgar' company they might have scorned while students. They may even have found the value of their expensive education diminished. Since the attitudes of prospective patients was so important to practitioners,[48] regulation tending to diminish the prestige of their education was a serious matter. None of the Edinburgh medical faculty made a public statement against the Act until 1826;[49] not living in England, after all, they were not directly affected by it. It did, however, affect the status of their MD, and within a few years of its enactment, Edinburgh graduates, like Edward Barlow, called for its reform.

Those calls for reform provoked one of the most pointed attacks on Edinburgh medical education, 'Observations on Medical Reform', by 'A

member of the University of Oxford'.[50] The author argued against those
reformers who wished to eliminate the privileges of Oxford and Cambridge
graduates by describing in insulting detail the social and intellectual
inferiority of Edinburgh to English MDs. Like other conservative medical
writers he combined the argument for division of labour, produced by the
complexity of medical knowledge, with portrayal of the unwholesome
effects of ambition which seeks to subvert social order. 'Those who think
must govern those who toil,' the author wrote. The physician, by virtue
of his superior education, should therefore govern the surgeon, who
practiced a 'manual art'. That did not make the latter any less useful: it
merely meant that he should cultivate his manual dexterity, not claim that
his education was equal to the physician's. 'Let us not deceive ourselves,'
the 'member of Oxford' continued, 'there must be gradation of rank, even
to ensure the performance of the commonest offices of society.' Any
argument to the contrary in politics was 'only fitted for the Marat Club of
Paris;' the argument in medicine was just as pernicious.[51] The great crime
of Edinburgh University was that it facilitated the blurring of ranks, for,
the author said, 'A Scotch physician so easily gets the degree of Doctor,
and a Scotch Surgeon is so much upon this level, that his next aim is to
be on a level of the English Physician'.[52]

What distinguished this attack from Speer's was the cogency and
accuracy of the member of Oxford's analysis. Edinburgh medical degrees
were not, as we have seen, intended to be egalitarian, but rather were
always framed so as to be accessible only to an elite. This need not have
been a social elite, though in practice it frequently was, but it certainly
was to have been an intellectual elite, with the high status traditionally
accorded a physician. By 1817 that was no longer true. The inflation
in medical education meant that even an Edinburgh MD was much
easier to obtain than fifty years previously, and as we have seen, students
with surgeon's diplomas often studied for as many years, and passed almost
as rigorous an exam, as University graduates. Indeed, by the 1820s 10 per
cent of students per cohort obtained both diplomas and medical degrees;
that meant that an average of forty-five students per cohort obtained both
degrees, with an additional sixty 'pure' MDs and 60 'pure' licentiates.
Students with both degrees could be taken as a sign that surgeons had
risen to the academic level of physicians, that an Edinburgh surgeon was
a man of 'liberal mind and endowment'.[53] Or a hostile observer might
conclude instead that Edinburgh graduates had sunk to the level of the
'manual art' of surgery. Even Lawson Whalley, who graduated in 1804
and wrote a *Vindication of the University of Edinburgh* against the member
of Oxford, retained the traditional view of gradation of ranks which
supported the status of his own degree. Whalley explained at some length
why the claim of Edinburgh graduates to be on a level with English

physicians was justified, but made no mention of the status of the Scottish surgeons. He certainly did not argue that they deserved to be on the same level as physicians, stating that he was 'equally zealous as the Gentleman whose opinions I have been combating, that each individual should keep within the sphere in which he has been educated'.[54] The blending of ranks between physician, surgeon, and general practitioners lowered the prestige of the medical degree, and led graduates to look for other marks of distinction, like consulting practice. The Society of Physicians of the United Kingdom, mentioned earlier, did in fact limit its membership to consultants in order to protect its prestige.[55]

Whalley also had difficulty responding to another of the points made by the member of Oxford, ostensibly as a commendation of Edinburgh. '[T]hat school is highly useful and necessary to the empire at present,' the latter wrote,

> Were the School of Edinburgh on the footing of the English Universities, few would be the laborers going out to harvest. For what highly accomplished Physician would depart and sit down contented to be frozen in Newfoundland, Hudson's Bay, or the Orkneys; or broiled for a pittance in the West Indies; or starved in a little dirty Scotch, Irish, or Welsh borough; or waste his health, his vigour, and his talents, among the outcasts and convicts of New Holland. Men are always wanted to fill subordinate as well as high station . . . and fortunate such persons are, in having the power of resorting to appropriate places of education.[56]

This was insulting, but it was also apt. The writer spoke in terms of highly or less accomplished physicians, but this is really a version of the economic reasoning presented in Chapter One: practice in many parts of Britain or the colonies was not worth the cost of the English Universities or study abroad. Part of the attraction of an Edinburgh degree had always been that it provided a lower-cost alternative.

By 1817, though, lower-cost, in this context, carried with it negative connotations quite apart from the unpleasant tone of the member of Oxford's remarks. The French medical profession had been reorganized after the Revolution, and the best medical education was provided by the *écoles de santé* of Paris, Montpellier, and Strasbourg. The creators of this system had recognized, however, that provincial practice paid too little to attract men who had undergone such an expensive education. They had therefore created the position of *Officiers de Santé*, the '*médecins de deuxième classe*' who were not required to have such an extensive education.[57] In Germany, Johann Christian Reil had suggested a similar classification system for medical men, one class of 'scientific physicians' and one. class of '*routiniers*'. It was based upon the assumption, the reviewer in the *Edinburgh Medical and Surgical Journal* wrote, that in 'society, there are rich and poor citizens; individuals who practice medicine as a science, and others, who exercise it as a trade; universities, and less dignified seminaries'.[58] Since the German government provided universities to train scientific practitioners, who treated the rich, Reil said, surely it should also provide seminaries 'in which *routiniers* should be educated for the service of the multitude'.[59] If carried out, Reil's recommendations would have created a permanent underclass of practitioners who could never aspire to become scientific physicians, something the member of Oxford, and perhaps even some Edinburgh MDs like Speer might have approved of. Both the *officiers de santé* and Reil's suggested *routiniers* were ways of dealing with the problem of great variations in practitioners' incomes. Presumably the medical faculty were familiar with French conditions; if they read the *Edinburgh Medical and Surgical Review*, they would have been familiar with Reil's suggestion.

In order to protect the value of their degree and their own reputation, Edinburgh medical professors had to ensure that their graduates were the scientific physicians, not the routiniers. The legal reinforcement of the privileges of the Fellows of the Royal College of Physicians of London made that more difficult; so too did the increasing numbers of graduates at Edinburgh itself. The large number of graduates took up more and more time: by 1824 there were so many that the faculty had to hold examinations 'three hours a-day, for ten weeks'[60] prior to graduation. The duty of examining was 'more laborious . . . than the giving of lectures', according to Professor Andrew Duncan junior; it kept faculty in Edinburgh for much of the summer, and Duncan, at least, did not consider 'the emolument as at all a compensation for the consumption of time, the labour, the responsibility, and the interference with professional success'.[61]

The number of graduates also made it more difficult to control their quality. There were so many that the faculty had to examine two candidates at the same time in the first oral examination, by dividing into two groups of three professors. Each group examined one candidate for half of the test; they then changed places for the second half, so that 'each professor hears half of the examination of every candidate'.[62] This diluted the original rigour of the examination, where the candidate was supposed to defend his knowledge before all the professors. The public defense of theses, too, had become 'a mere farce', according to Professor James Home,[63] since more than 100 graduates had to be questioned on their theses each year. It was thus much more difficult for the faculty by the 1820s to become familiar with the candidate's 'character, conduct, and diligence in prosecuting his studies', or decide if a thesis was '*bene eleganter et erudite scripta*', as Sylas Neville's had been. Nor does it seem likely that many students by that time could write in their diaries the equivalent of Neville's proud comment, 'When my friend Cullen came to me, he said with usual affability, "I must not forget you, Mr Neville" ',[64] for there were too many graduates for each to be personally known to the professors. Graduation therefore lost some of the symbolic value of the candidate's entry into the world of learned academic medicine, as represented by the full Faculty. With the loss of that personal contact, George Bell told the Royal Commission,

> One great incentive to exertion, and a powerful preventive of idleness, the approbation or disapprobation of the Professor, is lost to the pupils; and every one, who has paid any attention to the education of young men, knows how much talent and zeal often lie hid under apparent frivolity, idleness, and dissipation, which might be reclaimed by a little attention being paid to their *morale* by those who are placed over them.[65]

The professors themselves worried that their students were not what they once were. Indeed, they may not have been: more candidates for degrees did not necessarily mean better-prepared candidates. 'In former times, regular instruction in the fundamental branches of the Medical Science was rare, and not easily obtained,' Professor William Pulteney Alison explained the change, 'and those men who had a regular instruction in Anatomy and the other fundamental branches of Medicine were few in number, and they formed a kind of aristocracy.'[66] Graduates were no longer that aristocracy. Professors Alexander Monro *tertius*, Thomas Charles Hope, and James Home felt that 'our students nowadays are not so well prepared in the elementary branches as they formerly were'.[67] When Monro was asked by the Royal Commissioners if he felt theses were 'in general as well composed now as in former times' replied 'I am sorry to say I do not . . . I do not think the same pains are taken with them'.[68] The faculty apparently debated the possibility of offering two degrees to distinguish between good and merely adequate students. According to Andrew Duncan senior's proposal of 1824, one degree would have been for physicians and one for surgeons.[69] The two-degree system proposed to the Royal Commission was slightly different, and more obviously influenced by English criticism: an ordinary MD for the ordinary physician, and Doctorate of Medicine and Philosophy as a higher degree for medical men with an extensive literary education.[70]

In the end, the faculty proposed nothing so radical. Their first attempt to increase their standards was to require students to take at least two courses each of their three years of required academic study.[71] They tried to tighten up attendance at lectures by requiring every medical student to sign the matriculation album once per month during the Winter Session, though the only sanction was that students could otherwise not receive certificates of attendance.[72] And in December, 1824, they increased the rigour of the existing degree by requiring an additional year of study, six months of hospital practice, and attendance at two out of five elective courses. These new regulations were published in January 1825, and were intended to affect all graduates who began their studies after that date.

These regulations were intended to restrict medical degrees once again to an elite, and represented an adjustment to the delicate balance between the medical faculty's fame and its fortune first embodied in the *Statuta Solenna* of 1783. Their impact was much greater than that, however. In the 1825 regulations, Midwifery was not required for graduation, and the Professor of Midwifery, James Hamilton, was not a full member of the medical faculty. This meant he was not entitled either to make decisions or share in graduation fees. Hamilton petitioned the Town Council to force the faculty to require Midwifery for graduation. The faculty complied, but said it should affect only students who entered the University after the regulations were promulgated in 1825. Hamilton and the Town Council argued that it should take effect immediately, beginning with students who graduated in 1825. The result was a law suit. The *Senatus Academicus*, hoping for outside help in freeing themselves from the Town Council's control once and for all, called for a Royal Visitation to investigate the matter. The Royal Commission to Investigate the Universities of Scotland was the response.

The medical faculty of St Andrews and King's College and Marischal College, Aberdeen, reacted with some alarm to the proposed investigation, and passed new regulations requiring a strict course of classical studies leading to the master of Arts degree, in addition to rigorous medical studies, prior to examination for the Doctorate of Medicine.[73] The result was to eliminate entirely their attraction for medical graduates, and they were listed in the *Medical Calendar* as places students could attend for general education prior to beginning medical studies. Another result, complained Robert Brigg, Professor of Medicine and Anatomy and University Librarian at St Andrews, was that the library could no longer be maintained, since it had been largely supported by fees from medical graduation.[74]

In contrast, the medical faculty at Edinburgh University seemed to have almost been looking forward to the investigation. In April, 1826, Andrew Duncan junior wrote a review of the Apothecaries' Act in which he seems to have had one eye on the approaching Commission. 'The character of first medical school in the empire, a character which we still keep unsullied, first got us a share in the supply of English practitioners;' he wrote, 'long possession and upright management have given us a solid title to that share . . . [we] are quite ready to submit to scrutiny and reform.'[75] That scrutiny is the subject of the following chapter.

10

The Royal Commission

The following Course of Study to be observed by Candidates
for the Medical Degree, in whichever of the [Scottish]
Universities that Degree may be taken.
1st Year, Winter. – Anatomy, Chemistry, Materia Medica.
Summer. – Practical Chemistry, and Practical Pharmacy,
which may be taken with a Private Teacher or Lecturer.
2nd Year, Winter. – Anatomy, Practice of Medicine, Theory
of Medicine.
Summer. – Clinical Medicine, and Attendance on such
Hospitals as the Medical Faculty may deem sufficient.
3rd Year, Winter. – Surgery, Midwifery, and either Clinical
Surgery or Clinical Medicine, or attendance on the ordinary
Physicians of the Infirmary, when there is no Professor of
Clinical Medicine or Surgery giving Lectures in the Infir-
mary.
Summer. – Clinical Surgery or Clinical Medicine, in such
Hospitals as the Medical Faculty may deem sufficient.
4th Year, Winter. – Practice of Medicine, Infirmary, Clinical
Medicine.
One Course of Practical Anatomy in either of the last three
Winters; one Course in the second or third Summer.
Two Courses of Clinical Medicine, and one of Clinical Surgery,
to be required. The other Clinical Course may be either
Clinical Medicine or Surgery, as the Student may prefer.
Botany to be attended in the University during any Summer
of the Course.

Report of the Commissioners on the Universities
and Colleges of Scotland, 1830[1]

The Royal Commissioners for Visiting the Universities and Colleges of
Scotland, to give them their full name, received their commission in July
and September, 1826. This was the first General Visitation in 130 years
– the first, therefore, that the Edinburgh medical faculty had ever
undergone. *The Senatus Academicus* had called for a Visitation in hopes
that the Commission would become their ally in the dispute between the

Town Council and the Faculty. Since the Town Council was legally patrons of the University, the faculty could do nothing directly to abrogate their control; only a higher authority, based on the Crown's 'undoubted prerogative of Royal Visitation', could tilt the balance of power in the faculty's favour.[2] In fact, the Commissioners decided they could not address the specific dispute, since it was still in court. Though they did make recommendations for the future governance of the University, it was not free from Town Council control until the Universities of Scotland Act of 1858. To the faculty's dismay, however, the Commissioners – men of 'high rank, talents, and character', according to the *Quarterly Review*[3] – did much more. They took their charge seriously as educational reformers 'to inquire into . . . irregularities, disputes, and deficiencies, and to remedy the same'.[4] Their *Report*, published in October, 1830, contained detailed plans for reform of the curriculum leading to all University degrees; an abstract of the medical curriculum is given at the head of this chapter.

The *Senatus Academicus* were taken aback. They had hoped for allies, and instead found themselves the focus of an exhaustive investigation. The commissioners spent from September, 1826 until November, 1827 taking evidence in Edinburgh, inviting testimony not only from professors but from students and other professional men. They spent similar amounts of time at the other Scottish Universities. The Commission reconvened in January, 1830 to collect still more evidence. The result for the medical faculty was a series of recommendations that would have severely limited student access to the medical degree. The Commissioners called for candidates to undergo a preliminary examination on their classical knowledge to be administered by the Faculty of Arts, a set curriculum for all candidates for the degree, institution of roll calls, examinations, and prizes in all classes, and fees for the medical degree to go into a general fund, from which professors would be paid a set amount each year. In short, the slow encroachment on student control over their own medical education was abruptly accelerated. Under this system, students would still have had the option of graduating or not, but if they chose to graduate they relinquished all further choices as to their medical education at Edinburgh.

The Edinburgh medical faculty seems to have believed, and certainly behaved, as if they were the victims of a surprise attack, the reasons for which they did not understand. No doubt their opinions were expressed by the *Senatus Academicus* in 'Considerations' presented to the Commission, which pointed out that the University was, in fact, flourishing, and hardly required such an exhaustive investigation. The faculty had not realized what the Commissioners were after, they said plaintively: 'had the professors been previously made aware of the points to which their several examinations were to be directed,' they could have responded, and defended themselves, much more effectively.[5] They responded to the inquiry itself by preparing a statement purporting to express the views of the entire faculty. This discussed the virtues of their medical education at some length, and pointed out insuperable difficulties the proposed curriculum presented.[6] The Glasgow faculty, though more divided in its testimony, was equally direct about its inability to conform to the proposed regulations.[7] All the universities adopted the same strategy for dealing with the *Report*: public protest and private inaction in hopes that it would simply go away. In fact the specific proposals did: Parliament, caught up in reforming itself in the 1830s, was too busy to get back to the Scottish universities until 1858.[8] Still, the 1826 Commission was the first extensive inquiry into Edinburgh medical education from an outside body. Authorized by the Crown, its findings carried with them the possibility of actual intervention, the 'sanction of legislative enactment', as the Commissioners put it.[9] Once published, the *Report* raised issues which dominated Scottish education for the rest of the century.[10] The Edinburgh medical school had — at their own request — entered the public arena and could never go back to their former insularity.

From our standpoint, neither the Commissioners nor the medical faculty seem particularly progressive in their attitudes towards education. The Royal Commission has been aptly described as 'giving little thought to the advancement of science or learning as a university function. Its aim was, above all, to make the universities more systematic and efficient educational institutions, turning out doctors, lawyers and ministers with a love of the classics and the manners of gentlemen'.[11] There is certainly no sign in their *Report* that a love of scientific research might be an important attribute of a physician. For example, though they included a requirement for a course in Practical Chemistry, they made no provisions for laboratory space, apparatus, or even enough time to carry out experiments.[12]

Neither does the medical faculty come across very well. What the Commissioners were proposing was no more than the ideal curriculum that has frequently been associated with Edinburgh medicine, where the student begins with basic sciences, moves on to more strictly medical courses, and ends with extensive clinical experience in a hospital. The graduates already followed a similar course of study, as Table 4.4 shows. At no point did any member of the faculty argue that a student who followed that course of study would receive a bad or incomplete education. Nor could the faculty argue that preliminary education would be bad for a student; even Professor William Pulteney Alison, despite his position as spokesman for faculty opposition, had to grudgingly admit that it 'could do no injury'.[13] Considering the fact that the reforms would only have affected graduates, and left income from other students' fees intact, we might have expected the faculty to give the proposals more consideration. The reasons why they did not are worth investigating.

The Commissioners arrived in Scotland with a definite agenda with respect to the Universities. Though they found many things to admire, most of their recommendations were designed to make undergraduate education at the Scottish universities more like the English tradition of classical education. As both L. J. Saunders and G. E. Davie have noted, they persistently undervalued Scottish academic traditions, particularly with respect to the arts curriculum, in favour of the English.[14] Nor was this due solely to the presence of Englishmen on the committee: instead, as Anderson has shown, it can also be attributed to the Lowland Scots lawyers and clergymen who carried out the bulk of the Commission's work.[15] This kind of bias was most pointedly expressed by a writer in the Tory *Blackwood's Magazine*, who wrote

> that Scotland has long had good reason to be proud of her own Universities, and of the rapid advancement of her natives from barbarism to civility, is indeed most true; but . . . their own reputation . . . is already on the wane.

The English Universities, in contrast,

> had received the sanction of the approval of an older and far more cultivated nation, a nation that had 'taken the start of this majestic world', and stood on the very summit of renown.[16]

Scottish Universities, in other words, had served the purposes of a less advanced society, but were simply not as good as the English. However offensive this attitude might have been for Scots proud of their academic heritage, it was shared by several professors who gave testimony. Thomas Thomson, Regius Professor of Chemistry at Glasgow, when asked if he had any suggestions which would improve the Scottish Universities, replied 'No, I have not. I conceive, from the state of the Scotch Universities, any improvement is quite hopeless'.[17] James Hamilton explicitly compared Edinburgh with the English Universities, saying 'we seldom send away good scholars from this University'.[18] And a paper presented to the Commission in 1829 claimed that 'the degree of MD from Edinburgh is not held in the same estimation with the same degree from Oxford or Cambridge, and . . . it is not without reason this distinction is made'.[19]

The comments in *Blackwood's Magazine* were almost certainly directed in part at the Whig *Edinburgh Review*, which had published a series of articles attacking Oxford education. Both Thomson and Hamilton had reason to be disappointed in their position within the Universities, which certainly coloured their testimony. Still, the Commissioners were clearly sympathetic to these opinions. More diplomatic than *Blackwood's*, they nonetheless gave as a reason for proposing changes the fact that since the seventeenth century a 'material change' had taken place in the 'wealth and population of Scotland, the manners and pursuits of its inhabitants, and the state of public opinion'.[20] The Universities, therefore, had to improve with the times, however painful change might be to its faculty. 'Time is the great innovator,' wrote the *Quarterly Review*, in an article on the Universities Commission:[21]

> When we consider how many causes may affect, and insensibly pervert the original spirit and intent of academical institutions, it may safely be asserted, that a century can rarely elapse without some considerable modifications becoming indispensable.[22]

The most important change which had occurred is one we have encountered earlier: Scotland and England were now more closely integrated than ever before, and Scottish universities had a much greater impact on Great Britain as a whole in the nineteenth than the seventeenth century. This was of course especially true in medicine, since Edinburgh degrees were taken by Englishmen as well as Scots, and Edinburgh graduates practiced in England as well as Scotland. Edinburgh graduates had been claiming for years that their degree was as good or better than that of the English Universities; as discussed in the last chapter, they had challenged the privileges of the Fellows of the Royal College of Physicians of London on that basis. In the case of medicine, then, the Commissioners' comparison between Edinburgh and the English Universities, however biased, should not have been unexpected. Edinburgh graduates had been making the same comparison for years, though of course drawing different conclusions from it.

Yet another change had to do with the difficult issue of how to ensure that young men really were qualified to practice. The Commissioners claimed that they greatly admired the Scottish universities for their tradition of education, and had therefore suggested only those changes 'compatible with the interests of the Professors and the means of the Students, and sanctioned by enlightened and impartial opinion'.[23] The smooth phrases mask an inherent conflict. Concern for the interests of professors and means of students had been built into Edinburgh medical education from the start, and the former, at least, had not changed dramatically from the day William Cullen began lecturing. 'Enlightened and impartial opinion' had, however: by 1826 it declared unequivocally that medical education existed for the benefit not of professors nor students but rather the public, 'persons who require Medical advice'.[24] Since a man became a physician as soon as he received a medical degree, and was entitled to practice under that name, the Commissioners insisted that

> the Degree of Doctor shall only be granted to persons who are ascertained to possess the knowledge and qualifications necessary for the safe and beneficial exercise of the office of Physician. The privilege of conferring such degrees necessarily implies this duty.[25]

Universities, in their view, were not just in the business of turning out graduates, but also were responsible to their future patients for their conduct.

So far, there seems to be nothing objectionable in all this, but Alison did, in fact object to it. 'We should be deceiving the public,' he said,

> if we were to hold out that, by enforcing any course of study, we could at once send our graduates from the University, fitted to take the lead in all cases of men already habituated to medical practise . . . We can no more pretend to make great physicians than we can pretend to make great lawyers or great divines. No school of medicine can do more than give the elementary education, upon which the character of each practitioner must be formed subsequently for himself.[26]

This is still a source of tension in medical education: the public expects MDs to be 'perfectly qualified', but medical faculty consider education to be a life-long process.[27] Alison's assertion sounds remarkably like Adam Smith's comment to Professor William Cullen that 'A degree can pretend to give security for nothing but the science of the graduate; and even for that it can give but a very slender security'.[28] Smith had asserted that all medical degrees merely conferred a kind of monopoly, and should be eliminated to provide a free market in medical care. Cullen had disagreed. Now, ironically enough, it was Cullen's successors who adopted Smith's line of reasoning, and argued that medical degrees should be left to the free market. Enforced regulation, they maintained, would only price degrees higher than the market could bear. The Commissioners completely disagreed with this application of market principles. 'It has been thought' the *Report* stated,

> that without any regulation relative to the Course of Study, the country would have the same security for the business of education being conducted on the very best plan, which, in ordinary trade, free competition affords for the supply of the best quality.

This was simply wrong, the Commissioners felt.

> It does not appear to us that the principles applicable to trade can with propriety be extended to the education of a country, . . . without any provisions being made by Public Institutions for a good course of study for those who may desire it. Under any such system, instruction . . . will not be adequately provided.[29]

If principles of free trade were followed to their logical conclusion, after all, all universities should be abolished, and all education left to private teachers. If, however, the medical faculty wished to assert that there was something in the institution of a University that made it different from merely a collection of private teachers, if there was some justification for six of those teachers to call themselves Professors and charge ten guineas for awarding medical degrees, then those Professors and that University had an obligation to the public to provide the best medical education possible.

But who should decide what constituted the best medical education? Surely the successful professors of medicine, the faculty said. Andrew Duncan junior cited George Jardine's *Outlines of Philosophical Education*, 'that whatever changes for the better shall be made on our system of education, they must begin with the teachers themselves'.[30] The Commissioners disagreed. As Anderson has noted, the Commissioners were generally hostile to faculty,[31] and treated them throughout as incapable of unbiased testimony, declaring even that their reputation for academic excellence might render their opinions suspect. 'Eminent teachers,' the *Report* said,

> are not always the best qualified to determine the course of instruction most suitable to the general interests of society, or to the preparation for particular professions. A person may be most eminent and successful as a Professor, profound and ardent in his own studies, eloquent as a Lecturer, inspiring much enthusiasm and interest in the students, and have much of the observation and knowledge of character requisite to convey instruction to their minds . . .[32]

But his opinion of a particular course of study was not necessarily correct, the *Report* continued, because it 'can scarcely be expected that he should be an impartial judge of the utility of the study in which his life may have been spent'. The Commissioners therefore collected testimony wherever possible from eminent men from outside the University medical faculty, such as James McGrigor, Director-General of the Army Medical Department. If this conflicted with the professors' opinions, the Commissioners invariably weighed outside testimony more heavily.

There were indeed many areas in which the faculty was vulnerable to the charge of 'interested' behaviour, that is, protecting their own interests as the expense of their students or the public. They owed their positions to patronage, rather than to free elections on merit, as Sir William Hamilton pointed out in his article in the *Edinburgh Review*.[33] Alexander Monro *tertius* refused to consider having his professorship divided into two courses, anatomy, which he would retain, and surgery, which would be taught by a practicing surgeon, despite the nearly unanimous opinion in favour of this separation. By his commission of appointment, he said, 'a legal and definite right was granted to me, to perform the duties of the Professorship of Anatomy and Surgery, which the law would protect against any new arrangement calculated to interfere with or diminish its value'.[34] The Commissioners must have become very tired of that particular issue: Professors Robert Freer and Charles Badham of Glasgow also refused to have their professorship of the Theory and Practice of Medicine divided into two courses, because, as Badham stated bluntly, 'I shall lose directly the amount of fees'.[35] None of this impressed the Commissioners as disinterested behaviour.

The Commission scored a particularly telling point against the faculty in noting that though the faculty insisted their degree 'should be possessed by the great bulk of practitioners', they had refused to allow the course in midwifery as a requirement for graduation until 1825. That was, of course, the original cause of the dispute with the Town Council. Since, according to the Commissioners, 'the exclusion of the class of midwifery appears to have been wholly at variance with the very objects for which the system of instruction is said to be designed',[36] it seemed obvious to them that Midwifery had been excluded simply because the Professors did not wish to share the fees for graduation. The Professors had, in other words, put private interest ahead of their own stated educational goals.

Even the not-unreasonable position of the Edinburgh and Glasgow faculty – that the requirements, by reducing the number of students, would reduce faculty income, and make the position of professor less appealing for 'men of eminent talent and extensive knowledge or acquirements',[37] – might have seemed unduly mercenary to the Commissioners. The Glasgow professors assumed that medical professors were 'earning their bread' from their fees from students, and that if that income went down,

> The respectability of the Medical Professorships would sink, and they would soon come to be filled by an inferior set of men, destitute of the education of the present, and incapable of conveying the same quantity of information to their pupils.[38]

The Commissioners may have felt that the universities might be better off if professors had other sources of income, either private funds or professional practice, though they did not say so explicitly. They did say that the Universities should not lower their standards of preliminary education or length of courses just to admit poorer students, since 'both the usefulness of the Universities, and their character as learned societies, may be essentially impaired, if undue sacrifices are made, in order to enable persons to attend a University who really cannot bear the expense, even on the most moderate scale'.[39] They may also have felt that the usefulness and character of the universities would also be impaired if persons became university professors who would be forced by poverty to sacrifice public benefit for 'the personal interest of the Professors, both as to esteem and emolument'.[40]

The most damaging piece of evidence against the faculty, however, was one they insisted on themselves: that the value of their degree was shown by the large number of students who annually received it. This was, in fact, Alison's main line of defence against the proposed changes. 'The Medical Degree in the University is at present held in such estimation,'

he said, 'that there does not appear to be any occasion for a considerable
change in regard to it.' The proof of this was 'the number of gentlemen
applying for the Medical Degree here, which is much greater than in any
other University in the British dominions'.[41] Not so, according to the
Commissioners. 'It appears to us,' said the *Report*, 'that the reputation of
a University does not depend on the *number* of the degrees which are
granted by it, but must depend entirely on the nature of the qualifications
which the possession of such Degrees implies in the persons on whom they
are conferred.'[42] Indeed, the Commissioners showed a general distrust of
student numbers as evidence for the value of an educational program, for
exactly the same reason as Adam Smith once commended it: that professors'
fees came from students.[43] The Commission, therefore, were concerned
that the faculty had every incentive to adopt policies which would increase
student numbers, whatever their educational value.

The Commissioners were especially critical of the fact that the faculty
received payment for graduation examinations. '[I]t is . . . scarcely to be
doubted' the *Report* said, 'that there must be a natural reluctance in
Professors to reject candidates, to many of whom the fees paid to the
examiners may be a very serious sacrifice'.[44] The Commissioners found
evidence for this reluctance in the figures for medical students and
graduates presented by the faculty themselves. In 1806, 37 students had
graduated, in 1816, 76, and in 1826, 118. The increase from 1806, to
118, the Commissioners felt, 'is very great, and is not accounted for by
an increase of Medical students, for in 1806 the number was 764, and in
1826 only 896, that is, there was an addition of 132 Students; but this
bears no kind of proportion to the multiplication of Degrees from 37 to
118'.[45] This analysis comes from the numbers given by the medical faculty
themselves; how unfair it must have seemed that the careful record-keeping
which allowed professors to demonstrate the popularity of their courses in
memoranda and law suits was in this case used against them! Several
witnesses testified to the reasons that might account for the increase in
graduates: Alison, for instance, said that 'Of late years a much greater
number than formerly of the general practitioners, both of this country
and of England, have taken the Medical Degree in addition to their
education as Surgeons and Apothecaries'.[46] The Commissioners, however,
were convinced that the increase 'cannot be accounted for from any external
cause'.[47] Their implication was plain: the medical faculty had not exercised
proper control over its students, and had been flooding the profession with
unqualified MDs.

This was, as discussed in Chapter Nine, a frequent complaint about
Scottish medical education. The writer in the *Quarterly Review*, otherwise
sympathetic to Scottish Universities, made no exception for Edinburgh
when he wrote that

it is well known that, until recently, when new regulations were
passed on this subject in Scotland, the title of physician, intended to
protect the public against the impositions of empirical practitioners,
afforded no security whatever when its bearer was a Scottish
graduate.[48]

The Commissioners investigated this question closely, focusing on evidence of improper practices such as students missing classes, buying theses,
and memorizing set answers to graduation questions. The testimony they
received confirmed their fears that the medical faculty exercised too little
control over students and awarded degrees too easily. 'The complaints
against the Scotch Universities,' contained in an memorial submitted to
the Commission,

> is that they manufacture a baser article than Oxford and Cambridge
> – affix the same stamp to it – and introduce it in such quantities into
> the market that the whole cargo is depreciated – and when their
> coinage happens to be of sterling worth, that its value is lessened by
> the plated and Brummingham articles that have issued from the same
> mint.[49]

The Commissioners were in any case convinced that fewer, and more
liberally-educated physicians, would only benefit the medical profession.
They may have shared the nostalgia of T. C. Speer, mentioned earlier, for
distinct ranks in the profession, with the physician at the head. More
likely, they had in mind the same kind of professional reform that
motivated the General Medical Council in 1858: decreasing the number
of physicians to increase the incomes of those who were left.[50] For example,
the Commissioners asked Professor John Burns of Glasgow whether he
thought that 'any such disadvantage, if disadvantage it be, of diminishing
the number of persons who take the degree of Doctor of Medicine, would
be more than compensated to the University, and the public at large, by
a greater degree of eminence and respectability attending those who did
take it?'.[51] They asked Professor Thomas Thomson of Glasgow whether 'at
present, a greater number of persons take the degree of Doctor of Medicine
than are likely to find respectable employment?'.[52] And they no doubt
approved of the opinion of Professor John Towers, that it was 'essential for
the respectability of the profession that the degree of Doctor of Medicine
should be made more difficult of attainment'.[53]

The medical faculty had come to a similar conclusion several years
earlier, as discussed in the last chapter. They had not, however, proposed
to deal with it in a similar manner. The faculty proposed new courses,
which could, not incidentally, be most easily attended in Edinburgh, and
an additional year of study, but left undisturbed student decisions made
according to individual circumstances. The Commissioners felt this was
not enough to stem the production of the 'baser article'. Andrew Duncan

junior came in for especially stern questioning. 'Is there no risk', the Commissioners asked, 'that by enlarging the number of medical graduates beyond the demand for physicians, the profession may be ultimately degraded by having in the list of members many persons in a state of absolute indigence?' Did Dr Duncan not agree that 'it would be an advantage to the public and profession to have the individuals, who are graduated, of a superior order?'. Those two assertions being admitted, what, in Dr Duncan's opinion, was

> more for the reputation of this University and for the advantage of the public, that a very great number should annually graduate here, moderately versed only in scientific and literary attainments, or that there should be a smaller number, with very superior qualifications of that sort?[54]

The Commissioners' own opinion was clearly that the latter was vastly preferable. It is possible that what they had in mind was a degree that would attract men 'of a superior order' like themselves to the medical profession.

The way to ensure that students had those superior qualifications, to ensure that all Edinburgh graduates was of 'sterling worth' was, according to the *Report*, to increase university control over the medical curriculum, and end individual student choice. This opposition to student independence was entirely deliberate, and made in accordance with 'enlightened and impartial opinion'. Attitudes towards university education had changed in the nearly 100 years since the Edinburgh medical faculty had been founded, probably due to the fact that more and more students attended medical lectures. University medical students no longer formed 'a kind of aristocracy', as Alison had noted, and medical education came to be regarded less as improvement in knowledge, and more as part of 'the formation of the mind, the regulation of the heart, and the establishment of the principles'.[55] 'The greater number of the students who attend the professional classes,' George Jardine wrote,

> are far from being of mature years; and many of them . . . have not enjoyed so complete a preparatory education, as to justify the neglect of all those means by which the intellectual faculties are strengthened, and regular habits of application generated and confirmed.[56]

In this respect, too, Edinburgh medical professors had been influenced by Adam Smith, going as far as paraphrasing Smith's *Wealth of Nations* in their response to the Commissioner's *Report* 'Provided the master does his duty, force or restraint can hardly be necessary to carry on any part of education',[57] Smith had said, and that was certainly assumed in Edinburgh lectures. 'The great body of medical students in this university have arrived at years of discretion,' the Faculty wrote. 'All of them are perfectly aware that the business in which they are engaged, is to be the foundation of their character and fortune in future life.'[58] The cost of medical studies was also supposed to keep students diligent; as Thomas Ismay had said, 'When I consider the Money that it will cost me during my Stay at this place, it makes me confine myself too close to my Study; more so than is conducive to my Health'.[59]

Of course, professors must have known that not all students were like Ismay. William Cullen had said that although students might be expected to study hard in medicine in order to prepare for a career, 'it happens sometimes otherwise. Young men are often too little influenced by these distant views'. It was therefore 'necessary also to render the Way towards it pleasant and agreeable', in this case by requiring the study of chemistry, 'one of the most agreeable and engaging [subjects]'.[60] Cullen did not say how he intended to treat students who were not enamoured even of chemistry. The 1825 regulation requiring students to sign the matriculation record at the beginning of each month also indicates concern over attendance hardly compatible with the image of zealous students insisted on by the faculty.

Mostly, however, the faculty had ignored the problem of ensuring that students really did benefit from lectures. They may have felt what many a lecturer has felt, that students 'may be compelled to have opportunities for study, but they cannot be compelled to learn'.[61] Instead, professors had developed informal means of determining merit discussed in previous chapters. They had developed informal networks of the best students, by taking in boarders, sending and receiving letters of introduction, and maintaining contact with the Royal Medical Society. They had developed extra courses, and provided opportunities for students to excel in theses. All of these had enabled them to exert moral force over their best students at least. The rest had been left to learn or not, as they wished.

In the early nineteenth century that attitude towards students increasingly came under attack. 'Gentlemen students were under no sort of restraint' the Edinburgh surgeons had complained in 1770, and this complaint was echoed in 1826 when the *Quarterly Review* noted that 'there are improvements in the discipline of the Scotch universities, for which the public mind is prepared'.[62] The most important of these had to do with the use of lectures as a pedagogical tool. Since professors received fees directly from students, they were vulnerable to the accusation that they had a great incentive to replace content with performance in order to attract more students. John Robison, Professor of Natural Philosophy, complained that his courses were not popular 'because too honest I cannot pretend to teach mathematical Science without mathematics, nor submit to the low task of a Showman'.[63] A later Professor of Natural Philosophy, John Leslie, described Thomas Charles Hope as the 'showman in the other corner'.[64] A reviewer in the *Quarterly Review*, pursuing the matter further, wrote that in those universities which are still kept together by the fame of public lectures, the constant object of the professor is to aim at some striking novelty, either in the arrangement of his materials, or in the leading principles of the subject which he professes to explain. He cannot expect to secure the attention of his class, except by some contrivance of this kind.[65]

He will thus be tempted to say whatever new thing he can in order to get students' attention. This 'system of public education,' the reviewer went on which excites a thirst for novelty, which tempts the instructor to pamper this appetite, and to engraft upon it his own hopes of fame and emolument, is vicious and corrupt in the highest degree.[66]

This is an extreme statement of what other educational commentators discussed more soberly: that public lectures as the sole means of instruction were not suitable for the education of young minds.

The disadvantages of lectures, even if taken seriously as a means of disseminating information, were best expressed in a later debate by William Whewell, writing against Charles Lyell, who had compared North American universities favourably to English universities. Lyell's insistence that lecturers had only to present knowledge for students to acquire it, according to Whewell, resulted in

a confusion of two things, which any one who has been really engaged in the responsibility of Education, is in no danger of confounding; — the teaching of those who are eager to learn, and the educating of those who are averse or passive.[67]

Lyell, according to Whewell,

has in his mind the image of a Lecture-room crowded with eager listeners . . . But still to him the question will occur, What is to come of his *less* intellectual hearers? or of those who do not choose to hear? Of those who having heard a little, have no desire to hear more? I do not know in what manner Mr Lyell proposes to deal with these classes of persons; or whether he would be content to leave them to themselves. If he did so, I think he could hardly call this treatment an Education.[68]

Still less did the Royal Commission consider Edinburgh medical lectures Education. They expressed concern that

the important and primary object of the instruction of Youth may be in part overlooked; that the aids, attention and discipline, necessary for the training of regular Students, may not engross much of the time of the Professor.[69]

The Commissioners were especially interested in George Jardine's methods of incorporating examinations into his classes, an interest they shared with other writers on education. They found little sign that class examinations similar to Jardine's had engrossed much of the time of the medical professors hitherto. Andrew Duncan junior even went as far as to say that

'Class examinations . . . lead to routine questions, and have a tendency to contract rather than enlarge the mind'.[70] That opinion, like many others expressed by Duncan, the Commissioners ignored.

The Commission also recommended other aids for the undisciplined student, such as calling attendance in medical classes. 'It is indeed true,' the *Report* stated,

> that Medical Students have so strong a motive for being assiduous in their attendance, . . . that in all probability the great majority of them will not be materially deficient in their attendance on the classes.

Nonetheless the Commissioners. unintentionally echoing Cullen, pointed out that

> there were so many exceptions to this, and indolence and carelessness are so frequent in young men at the period of life at which the Medical Classes are generally entered, that . . . it has appeared to us that some effectual step is necessary to prevent the admitted abuse.[71]

The *Report* recommended that 'Catalogues', that is, lists of students' names, be called in each class, and where classes were very large, that some portion of the class be called in an order that students could not predict. Another aid was the granting of Certificates by Professors based on both attendance and on examination, 'First to enforce attendance, and then to ascertain the diligence, application, and progress of the Students'.[72] These certificates would have to be presented by candidates before they could be examined for a degree. Yet a third aid was the suggested institution of class prizes and University Honours, modelled on the English Universities, to 'bring young men into public notice, and open to them at once the brightest prospects of success and eminence in life'.[73] The prospect of acquiring distinction would awaken 'the spirit of emulation, energy and ardent application'[74] among students, and encourage their academic progress. So would prescribing a set course of study. The Commissioners ignored the testimony of the Faculty that it was beneficial for students to take courses in whatever order they wished, since it encouraged them to spend part of their training at other institutions, such as the London hospitals, which offered better facilities for clinical study. Instead, they said in the *Report*, '[w]e are satisfied that a particular order of attendance on classes ought to be enjoined'.[75] The reason for this was that students, left to themselves, would not necessarily take classes in the right order, and, the *Report* said, 'many of the branches of medicine cannot be successfully studied . . . unless the Student shall have been previously well grounded in other departments, which are admitted to be the foundation of the science'. Anatomy, chemistry, and materia medica, in the Commissioners scheme, were the basic sciences necessary before students could go on to the more advanced courses.

This, too, was an educational issue that had been the subject of discussion at Edinburgh and elsewhere. Thomas Turner, in his book *Outlines of a System of Medico-Chirurgical Education*, began by saying that under the current system of attending separate lectures in each subject, students 'spend a great portion of their time unprofitably; perplexing themselves with individual parts, without considering the relation those parts bear to each other'.[76] Professor Robert Christison, too, had said it was a 'matter of regret that . . . [o]ne science drives out the last, just as [the student] passes from one class-room to another . . .'[77] The Commissioners believed that the best way to deal with this was to require a graded curriculum, and they frequently questioned the faculty about the best order for medical studies. Andrew Duncan junior's response, that 'there is no branch . . . of medical lectures that does not presume a certain degree of knowledge of every other branch; it is a perfect circle of science',[78] seems especially unhelpful. But William Pulteney Alison also claimed that this was not a problem the University had to deal with, because students could always ask their parents, or professors, what course of study they should follow to get the maximum benefit.[79] As we have seen, this informal system could deal effectively with students in different circumstances, such as Sylas Neville and Thomas Ismay. Of course in this area, as in all others, the Edinburgh faculty assumed eager students, anxious for instruction, who asked advice from professors and then followed it. The Commissioners, who did not make that assumption, found the opinion of Dr J. H. Davidson, President of the Royal College of Physicians of Edinburgh, much more convincing. Davidson said 'that the course and succession of classes should not be left to the discretion or caprice of the Students, nor even to the judgement of their parents and friends'.[80] 'I have often been consulted by young men as to the course they should follow in Medical study,' Davidson told the Commission, 'and I found they had no views of their own. They were often anxious to begin at the wrong end.'[81] Of course, if students were anxious to begin at what Davidson considered the wrong end, it could not be true that they had 'no views of their own.' What is more likely is that they came wishing to take Medical Practice and Clinical Lectures without having taken Medical Theory and Materia Medica, and Davidson felt this was the wrong order. Under the existing regulations, as we have seen, that could and did happen; under the regulations proposed by the Royal Commission, that would be impossible.

The most controversial reform, however, was the recommendation that candidates for medical degrees be required to undergo an examination in Greek, Latin, Mathematics and Philosophy, administered by the Arts Faculty, before their medical examination. Three of these subjects, Latin, Mathematics, and Philosophy, were, the *Report* said, 'universally admitted' as necessary.[82] Greek was not, though the *Report* claimed that it would help the student in understanding medical nomenclature, and in reading classic works of medicine. Several of their witnesses, including William Wood and John Thomson from the Royal College of Surgeons, gave testimony supporting this judgement.[83]

The necessity of any preliminary examination was disputed by the medical faculty, and they were particularly opposed to requiring the study of Greek. A fluent knowledge of Greek had never been common among the majority of physicians, and in the preceding century had become much less so. In 1745, Sir John Clerk of Penicuik could still tell his son that '. . . a man may be a great physician without the knowledge of the Greek language but yet he will never have the honour of being reputed a scholar, without it'.[84] By 1826, however, few physicians read Hippocrates for information to apply in their practice, though they might for an inspirational example of a great physician. Instead they read modern authors, either in books or in the growing medical periodicals, such as the *Lancet* or the *Edinburgh Medical and Surgical Review*. Why, then, the medical faculty asked, should students be tested on their knowledge of Greek, a language they would have no use for in practice? Requiring them to learn French or German would make much more sense, so that they could keep up with new developments in medicine on the Continent.[85]

Yet as Greek had lost its value for purely professional reading, it had gained stature as part of liberal education, and the Commissioners did everything they could to encourage the study of the classics. They were 'intimately persuaded', the *Report* said, 'that no other studies are better fitted, either to improve the taste and exercise the faculties of youth, or to create a love of freedom and a spirit of generous and manly independence'.[86] This had already become a commonplace in writing on education.[87] The *Monthly Review* in 1810 derided the 'half-witted outcry that has lately been raised against Greek and Roman literature'.[88] The *Quarterly Review* stated, apparently without fear of contradiction, that 'an acquaintance with the Greek and Latin languages has everywhere been considered as an essential part of a liberal education, and indispensable to the able prosecution of all the learned professions'.[89] Though the English universities spent too much time on classical studies to the exclusion of all else, the reviewer said, 'The leaning of the public mind seems to be to the opinion that . . . in Scotland it has been most culpably slighted'. Even in Scotland some parts of the public mind shared that opinion: Henry Cockburn also wrote of the need for classical education.[90] He praised, especially, the founding of the Edinburgh Academy for raising the quality of instruction in the classics.

However little use the study of Greek and Latin might be in curing diseases, then, the physician who practiced among the English or Lowland Scots gentry had to conform to the idea that the classics provided a liberal education. Whether he believed that study of Latin and Greek literature produced men 'of enlightened minds, accustomed to exercise their intellectual powers, and familiar with habits of accurate observation and cautious reflection' or not, he would have been convinced by the *Report*'s other, more pragmatic argument: that physicians 'should be possessed of such a degree of literary acquirement as may secure the respect of those with whom they are to associate in the exercise of their profession'.[91] The idea that a physician must be a liberally-educated gentleman to practice among gentlemen was hardly new. What was new was the insistence that it was the business of the medical faculty to enforce this idea through examination.

The Commissioners' ideal of the liberally-educated physician was not necessarily bad. It combined what they clearly felt was the best of the English with the best of the Scottish academic traditions: the enlightenment and discipline provided by classical education, and the knowledge of science and medicine conveyed by lectures and examinations from men distinguished in their scientific disciplines. What more could 'persons requiring medical assistance' want?

The only problem was that this kind of education appeared impossible and unnecessary to the only men in a position to implement it, the medical faculty. For all the changes in curriculum the Commissioners proposed, they had no power to change the conditions which had brought about the almost-free market in education they so disapproved of. They could not compel Glasgow and Edinburgh to co-operate in their education, instead of competing. They could not provide salaries, or endow chairs, to ensure that the new courses they proposed could actually be taught, or make professors independent of student fees. Their proposal that certain courses be offered every summer, was a practical impossibility from the start, because, as the Glasgow medical faculty wrote, if summer courses were offered, 'very few students would be likely to attend them'.[92] The Commissioners could provide no money for better classrooms or the Anatomical or Natural History museums, or provide more cadavers for dissection or laboratory facilities for practical chemistry. Nor could the Royal Commission improve the position of the universities with respect to the Apothecaries Act, other than point out its deficiencies and transmit a request to Parliament that it be changed.[93]

Even more to the point, the Commissioners had clearly based their proposals on the assumption that the most important products of the Scottish Universities were their graduates, as they were for the English Universities. They must have been aware of the proportion of medical students who did not graduate from their analysis of the increasing numbers of MDs. In Glasgow, they were informed straight out that only a small percentage of students graduated. However, the Commissioners

paid almost no attention to this. Students who did not graduate, according
to the Commission, were merely 'occasional auditors':[94]

> men advanced in life, who attend some of the classes for amusement,
> or in order to recal [sic] the studies of early years, or to improve
> themselves in professional education, originally interrupted; or per-
> sons engaged in the actual occupation of business, who expect to
> derive aid in their pursuits from the new applications of Science to
> the Arts; or young men not intended for any learned profession, or
> even going through any regular Course of University Education, but
> sent for one or more years to College, in order to carry their education
> farther than that of the schools, before they are engaged in the
> pursuits of trade or of commerce.[95]

Only the graduates were 'regular students', in need of University discipline; all others, presumably, could be left to work hard or not, as they
pleased. Nowhere do they acknowledge that the medical students who did
not graduate were, in fact, 'students of medicine strictly speaking', that
Job Harrison, Alexander Lesassier and Francis Augustus Bonney were as
intent on setting up practice as Sylas Neville and Samuel Cleverly. By
separating university students into 'students of medicine strictly speaking'
and occasional auditors, the Commissioners overlooked the fact that all
medical students were regular students on different paths, based on
different career expectations.

The neglect of the auditors is ironic given the Commissioners' expressed
concern to protect the public from unqualified practitioners. Graduates
were the best-educated and best-disciplined of the students, and most
inclined to follow professors' advice. The type of student the Royal
Commissioners were concerned about, well-meaning, perhaps, even intelligent, but all too apt to follow his own ideas about what courses were and
were not 'most material', were students like Ismay and Lesassier. Yet they,
according to the Commission's classification, would have been occasional
auditors, not subject to the University's control.[96]

Given students like Lesassier – as indeed they were – the Faculty
believed they knew well what the result of the new regulations would be.
Students might indeed need all the guidance the Commissioners claimed.
Without any incentives to obtain it, however, they would continue to
choose the education which would most readily set them up in practice.
Edinburgh professors had based their fame and fortune upon that fact for
some eighty years and had no reason to doubt their conclusions. The Royal
Commission could not arrange for Scottish MDs to obtain special privileges
like the Oxford and Cambridge MDs. They could not eliminate the
disadvantages of the Apothecaries Act, or require an MD for practice
everywhere in Britain. Under those circumstances, both Edinburgh and
Glasgow professors were sure that, the most likely result of the regulations

was that students who might otherwise have graduated would '*content themselves with the inferior education* requisite for inferior diplomas'; thus the new regulations, if adopted, would '*lower instead of raising the general attainments of practitioners* throughout the country'.[97]

The most obvious beneficiary of the new regulations, the faculty thought, would be the Royal College of Surgeons of Edinburgh. Ever since the surgeon's diploma had been instituted, the University and the Royal College had competed for the education of the general practitioners who made up the bulk of British medical practitioners. The competition had usually been friendly, in contrast to the competition between the University and Faculty of Physicians and Surgeons of Glasgow. The reason both for the competition and its friendliness was that the courses of study and regulations for the MD and Diploma were very similar, so that students could switch easily from one to another; as we have seen, the university tended to certify students with slightly more years of study, while the Royal College of Surgeons of Edinburgh tended to certify those with less. The Commission, though, was proposing to institute an entirely differently-structured path for graduates, based on the assumption that would-be physicians were different from would-be surgeons. No wonder the faculty was dismayed: they would see the only kind of student they were familiar with decide to take the surgeon's diploma rather than the MD, and be left with the remainder. It may have been especially galling that the Commissioners paid close attention to testimony from representatives of the Royal College of Surgeons of Edinburgh and resolutely ignored the fact that the Royal College was, in effect, a 'rival school', as Alison pointed out.[98] John Thomson's *Observations on the Preparatory Education of Candidates for the degree of Doctor of Medicine* was even praised by the *Quarterly Review* for its 'disinterested zeal',[99] presumably the author was unaware that Thomson had been instrumental in promoting the Royal College of Surgeons' 'school'. The Royal College of Surgeons did raise its own standards the following year, but it did not institute Thomson's or William Wood's recommendations for compulsory preliminary education.[100]

The medical faculty was clearly bewildered by the *Report*, and not unreasonably felt it singled out their MD for special treatment. Their main defense was to insist, 'anxiously', as the Commissioners accurately described it, on the MD as a 'Working Degree', that is, a degree for practicing physicians, not scholars,[101] and their system of education as 'purely professional'.[102] This was in part a continuation of the argument that what made Edinburgh medical education distinctive was 'all branches of science, regularly taught'. Even more, though, it is an attempt to return to the definition of medical students as gentlemen attending classes for medical improvement, rather than Youth in need of education. They insisted on the diligence, zeal and responsibility of students, insisting that they were 'uniformly assiduous, well-informed, and anxious to improve every opportunity of gaining information'.[103] They also pointed out the bad effects of subjecting students who 'have arrived at years of discretion' to regulation and restraint. Under the present system, they said, 'the utmost harmony subsists' between professors and students,

> but the Professors cannot look forward to the permanency of this mutual good feeling, if they are to be made the instruments of enforcing a system of discipline . . . to which the medical students are quite unaccustomed, and which they will undoubtedly regard as an arbitrary encroachment on their time . . .[104]

The additional time spent in lectures under the new regulations would make it impossible for students to join professional societies, 'established with great effect for their mutual improvement'.[105] Finally, there was the practical problem of requiring students to reside in town during the summer. The 'most meritorious' could not afford the additional expence; many others would benefit more from attending hospitals or dispensaries; and for all 'the period of vacation is extremely useful, as then only they have leisure for reading books, and pursuing various branches of study, which are recommended in the lectures'.[106] In other words, the Faculty argued, the most likely result of the regulations would be to do away with just the kind of accomplished physician the Commissioners wanted to produce.

Neither side convinced the other. In some areas, the Commissioners had already won its case, for 'enlightened and impartial opinion' did prefer classical education for its physicians, as well as examinations and a set course of study. All became standard features of medical education.[107] But the medical faculty had also already won its case, for public opinion agreed that though a classical education might make a gentleman, 'purely professional' studies defined a physician.

Conclusion

> Classes concluded yesterday, when I got my certificates, etc.,
> all good. The capping takes place on Wednesday and I am
> glad to say that the number of graduates far exceeds that of
> any year for the past ten, it is a good sign that the University
> is not losing ground so rapidly as some would make us believe.
>
> Samuel Lewis to Mrs Hinds, 1838[1]

Even though the Royal Commissioners' recommendations did not take effect, their *Report* exposed the University to what must have been highly unwelcome public scrutiny. Andrew Duncan junior wrote that it had

> become customary to accompany and enforce the various recommendations of reforms in our medical school, with which we have been lately favoured, with terrible denunciations of the fate that awaits us, if we obstinately adhere to our old institutions, and neglect the warning voice.[2]

Sir William Hamilton took the publication of the *Report* as an occasion to publish an article in the *Edinburgh Review* criticizing the role of patronage in professors' appointments.[3] Other criticisms directed at the medical faculty came out in pamphlet wars over faculty appointments in the 1830s and 1840s. The new regulations of the Royal College of Surgeons, published in 1829, contained an implied criticism of the University curriculum, or lack of it, for the surgeons raised their requirements to four years of study and recommended to their licentiates a graded curriculum, beginning with Anatomy and Chemistry in the first year, and moving on to Clinical Surgery by the third year and Clinical Medicine in the fourth.[4] Even though prospective licentiates were not required to follow it, the curriculum gave the College of Surgeons the moral high ground in educational reform. The moral high ground of course required fewer sacrifices for the surgeons, because their income did not rest directly on student fees. But surely that only confirmed what the Royal Commissioners had implied, that the surgeons, not the medical faculty, could be best relied upon for disinterested behaviour. The medical faculty did not even institute a graded curriculum in their 1833 regulations for medical degrees. They did encourage one, however, by allowing students to be tested on the elementary branches of Anatomy, Chemistry, Botany, Institutes of Medicine and Natural History in their third year, and the more advanced medical courses in their fourth.[5]

The medical faculty's insistence on using numbers of students as a criterion for success had been severely criticized by the Royal Commission, but it continued to dominate discussion of Edinburgh education. In 1840, Professor James Syme opened what became a prolonged debate over the propriety of accepting extra-academical courses towards a degree with a letter that began 'For several years there has been a progressive diminution in the number of Students . . . it is therefore incumbent . . . to inquire into the cause of diminution, and, if possible, to devise means for its remedy'.[6] Samuel Lewis, who came from Barbados to study at Edinburgh in the 1830s, also accepted the idea that decreasing numbers of students was a sign of ill-health, for he wrote to Mrs Hinds of Philadelphia that he was 'glad to say that the number of graduates far exceeds that of any year for the past ten, it is a good sign that the University is not losing ground so rapidly as some would make us believe'.[7]

It is appropriate to end with Lewis' perceptions, because the system of medical education I have described rested on students' perceptions of the relationship of their medical education to their later practice. Students came to Edinburgh University in the late eighteenth and early nineteenth century in part because of the prestige of a degree – medical or surgical – awarded after hard study and a series of examinations. They came as well because of the accessibility of medical classes even to those who did not intend to take a degree. The combination of the two resulted in access to medical education for the many, with the preservation of elite status for the few.

This was not an egalitarian system: it assumed that better-educated practitioners would cater to the wealthy, while lesser-educated men ministered to the bulk of the population. It also meant that students whose families could afford a more extensive education had an advantage over others. For this reason, as R.D. Anderson has shown, access to University education in Scotland was not precisely democratic.[8] Yet if Edinburgh University had not removed inequalities in medical education, it had done the next best thing: it had promoted the mechanism by which they were, ultimately, to be eliminated. Classes and examinations became the only criteria for certification. Of course, distinctions still existed: between physicians and surgeons; between consultants with MDs and general practitioners with MDs; between Fellows of the Royal College of Surgeons and Licentiates; and between all these groups, and practitioners without diplomas of any sort. The lines dividing them, however, could be crossed by study and examination, means that were accessible to any young gentleman seeking medical improvement.

The Royal Commission marks the end of the student's-eye-view of medical education, because it heralds the end of the flexible system of course attendance that made that view possible. It also marks the beginning of University dominance of medical education. In 1760, as we have seen, there was a wide variety of possible ways to study medicine: apprenticeship 'for the freedom' or just for training, London hospitals, classical education at Oxford and Cambridge, study or MDs at Edinburgh and Glasgow. Each institution, lecturer or master exploited a different aspect of the demand for medical education, and innovators tended to consolidate their positions, leaving new innovations to others. By the 1820s, all these forms of education were still available, but there were fewer innovations, and over the next thirty years, the Universities slowly took over the others. In London, the new University acquired the right to grant degrees in medicine in 1836 over the strenuous objections of the established hospital schools.[9] The Universities of Dublin and Glasgow succeeded in wresting degree-granting privileges in surgery from the Royal College of Surgeons and College of Physicians and Surgeons respectively. At Oxford and Cambridge, informal connection with London hospitals became ever more formal, though medical teaching was not completely integrated into requirements for medical degrees until the end of the century.[10] And at Edinburgh, as George Bell, the first member of the Royal Medical Society to write an essay on a surgical subject, had remarked, 'surgical students tend to become medical students'.[11] Professorships and degrees in surgery, anatomical dissections and surgical theses all became part of the University curriculum, though not without a fight from the Royal College of Surgeons.[12]

The universities won in part because of the traditional prestige accorded graduates: as Mary Hewson had said, 'a University gives a man a name.'[13] They also won because they were best equipped to provide the 'aids, attention, and discipline' that contemporary opinion believed the increasing numbers of medical students required, a College bell to summon them to class, examinations and prizes to inspire a spirit of emulation, diplomas to certify their knowledge. Mary Hewson had also extolled the value of 'all branches of science, regularly taught', and that became even more important in the later nineteenth century, as secondary schools funnelled students intended for the professions to universities, not private lectures.

By the 1860s the universities they went to were very different places from those they had been 100 years earlier. For that was another reason the universities could dominate medical education: they could adapt to change. The universities benefitted, ironically enough, from the very success of the competition, which pushed and prodded them into adopting high standards and innovations in medical education or abandoning it altogether, like St Andrews and Aberdeen Universities in the 1820s. Edinburgh University in the later nineteenth-century is a tribute both to the entrepreneurial ability of the Royal College of Surgeons and to the flexible university structure that made such entrepreneurship possible. Neither the College nor the University survived nineteenth-century reforms unaltered, but both had a part in creating the standards reformers adopted.

Edinburgh University could survive the first round of criticism and reform in 1826 because it rested on a firm institutional base; the 500 students per cohort who came to attend classes. Andrew Duncan junior owed the confidence with which he could call Edinburgh 'the first medical school in the empire',[14] to the approximately 17,000 students who had come for medical improvement in the preceding seventy years. Let the final testimonial, therefore, rest with one of those 17,000, John Bell. 'Education is useful to those who have, and to those who have not, genius;' he wrote, 'the latter it teaches to act safely, the former it inspires with inventions, and enables them, in every unprecedented case, to contrive new and successful methods of cure.'[15] Edinburgh University educated those who had, and those who had not, genius; those who had, and those who had not, taste or polish or classical languages or surgical apprenticeship. It was the study of medicine alone that united 'students of medicine strictly speaking' at Edinburgh, as it was ultimately to unite the medical profession.

Appendix A:

Analysis of matriculation data

Much of the quantitative work for this book is based on my analysis of course attendance for matriculated students at Edinburgh University. As I discussed in Chapter Three, medical students came to the library each November and told the clerk what courses they intended to take that year. Since those records were kept carefully and consistently throughout the period, the matriculation records, consisting of the Matriculation Albums, 'Medical' Lists, and 'General and Medical' Lists, are important sources for student course attendance.[1] They present a number of problems, however, and so some caution is necessary in interpreting the figures I present.

In order to use the matriculation records most effectively, I have reorganized the information around individual students, rather than the number of names which were listed each year. This is necessary to get an accurate picture of the number of students who attended courses at Edinburgh in this period. Since Sylas Neville, for example, matriculated for three years, he signed the Album three times. Counting up all the names for each year, and adding them together, would give much too high a figure for the total number of students, since many of them would have been repeaters, who signed the Albums more than once. This has been the usual way of estimating student numbers from the eighteenth century. Andrew Duncan senior, for example, published a table 'shewing the number of Students at the University of Edinburgh, for the last Ten Years of the Eighteenth Century, . . . extracted from its records'.[2] He appears to have obtained his figures simply by counting the number of names each year. The figures presented to the Royal Commission to Investigate the Universities of Scotland were derived in the same way.[3] A more recent example of the same method is Alexander Morgan, who carefully calculated the number of names which appear on the matriculation records each year. His work thus gives a good picture of the number of medical students in residence in Edinburgh each year between 1763 and 1858. However, he then added up the number of names each year and so ended up with a total of 56,000 matriculates for the period, which is much too high.[4]

Counting up all the names also makes it impossible to compare the total number of names in the Albums with other lists of students, such as the list of graduates, in order to find out what percentage of the student body did in fact graduate. The dangers of this are apparent in L. Agnew's article on Scottish medical education, where he compared the number of MD degrees awarded by Edinburgh university from 1790–1800, 229, with the total number of students obtained by adding together the numbers listed in *Annals of Medicine*, 5,592. This comparison gives much too low a figure for the percentage of Edinburgh students who graduated.[5] We can see this clearly if we again examine the case of Sylas Neville. His name appears three times in the matriculation records, but only once on the list of graduates. Counting the signatures in the Album without noting that they belonged to the same person leads to the numerically precise, but obviously wrong conclusion that the ratio of matriculates to graduates was 3:1.

To avoid these difficulties, and most usefully exploit the matriculation records as sources, I reorganized the information they contained. I created a computer database of each individual who appeared in the records, noting the number of years of study and courses attended. I also noted whether the student appeared on other lists, such as the list of graduates, the records of the Royal College of Surgeons, the lists of members of the Royal Medical Society, and the published rolls of the Army and East India Company medical services.[6] In reorganizing the information in this way I had to make certain assumptions. Many students had the same name – there were numerous William Sinclairs from Caithness, not to mention John Smiths and Alexander Scotts – and it was not always clear whether two students with the same name were in fact the same person. My solution to this problem was to make the arbitrary assumption that the two names were the same person unless separated by five years or more, or I had information to suggest otherwise. For example, I assumed the two John Scotts, one of whom studied in 1793–4 and 1794–5, and another from 1803–7, were different people. I assumed, however, that the three entries for Henry Dewar, in 1797–8, 1798–9, and 1803–4, were the same person, because there was a Henry Dewar who joined the army as surgeon in 1801 and a Henry Dewar who graduated MD from Edinburgh in 1804. Since it was a fairly common pattern for a student to attend courses for a few years in order to join the army, and then to return later to take more courses in order to graduate, it seemed most likely that all the Henry Dewars referred to the same person.

Once I had organized the information in this way, I was able to analyze it effectively. First I arranged the students according to cohort, that is, according to their first year of study. This enabled me to study changes in the student population, since I could arrange all students according to a common starting point, and see how their later progress differed. Unless otherwise specified, all the years listed in tables in this book are the cohorts. All quantitative analysis and all computer work is my own, unless specifically cited. I have calculated percentages as precisely as possible, but because of the possibility of errors in the database itself I do not feel that differences of single percentage points are revealing. The differences I have emphasized in the book are, of course, considerably larger.[7]

This usage necessitates some words of caution when comparing the numbers in the book with numbers from other sources. The first point is that the 'students in the cohorts 1763 to 1805 who graduated' are not precisely the same as 'students who obtained their degrees from 1763 to 1805'. Clearly if a student began taking courses in November of 1763, he was unlikely to have graduated the preceding summer. He would have received his degree in 1764, 1765, or 1766. Similarly, students who began taking courses in 1805 did not graduate in that year, but several years later. This is true for other degrees or appointments as well: it must be remembered when reading the book that dates refer to the cohort, not the year of the degree or appointment.

Matriculation records were kept more carefully at Edinburgh University than at many other universities in the period. Nevertheless, they still present many of the problems of interpretation which have been discussed by Lawrence Stone, in his study of the Oxford student body, 1580–1919,[8] and Richard Kagan, in his study of the universities in early modern Spain.[9] Both have analyzed the possible inaccuracies of the matriculation records on which they based their research. Stone was primarily concerned to estimate the numbers of students who attended classes but did not sign the matriculation register; Kagan devoted more attention to the issue of the accuracy of information contained in the records.[10] Their discussions are a salutary reminder that care must be taken in interpreting figures based on matriculation records. However, these records are such valuable sources that both conclude, in Kagan's words, 'to accept these registers as they are, albeit, of course, with caution'.[11]

A comparison of Edinburgh matriculation records with student letters and diaries makes it clear that the Matriculation Albums did not include everyone who ever studied at Edinburgh, since there were students like Nathan Smith, who wrote home to his wife that he attended Anatomy and Chemistry, but whose name cannot be found in the matriculation records.[12] Since matriculation required a fee, it is reasonable to assume that at least some students, presumably the poorest, would choose to save money by not matriculating, and instead make a private arrangement with a professor to attend his class. Lawrence Stone found at Oxford, in the period 1510–1669, that richer students were more likely to evade matriculation, since fees were graduated according to social status, but there is no evidence that this was the case in Edinburgh, where all students paid the same fee of half a crown.[13]

Just how many non-matriculating students were there at Edinburgh?

One way to find out is to compare a professor's class lists for a given year with the students in the Matriculation Album who are listed as attending his course that year. One would expect the class list to be the most complete listing of students in the class, since it was a way to keep track of who paid their fees. Either the Edinburgh University Library or the medical faculty apparently also took an interest in this question, because a separate list of medical students and courses was kept from 1791 in bound volumes titled 'Medical'. That list seems have been based on professors' class lists rather than matriculation records, since it is a more complete list of students than in the Albums.

After the new matriculation regulations of 1811, the University sub-librarian, Nicholas Bain, seems to have collected professors' class lists in December or January each year. He, or a clerk, checked those lists against a main list of medical students compiled from the Matriculation Albums, writing down the courses that students on the main list attended and noting those students who had not matriculated. The main list was then bound together with the class lists in 'General and Medical' volumes, which thus give course information previously provided by the old Matriculation Albums.[14]

For the regulations to be effective, professors had to cooperate. At matriculation in November, students received a ticket with their matriculation number from the library. Professors were not supposed to let students into courses unless they had a ticket: in a note at the bottom of the 'List of students attending the Rhetoric Class session 1813–1814', the professor wrote 'I find that in a few instances I have omitted to take the number of the library ticket, but am persuaded that in every case the student was possessed of one'.[15] In some cases professors wrote down students' matriculation numbers on their class lists. Bain even tried to keep track of students who came too late to matriculate. Andrew Duncan senior sent a letter on 30 January 1821 presenting 'best compliments to Mr Bayne [sic] – begs to inform him that Mr Benjamin Lauder Brown is enrolled in his list as a pupil of the Institutions of Medicine his number is 199'.[16]

From 1811, then, I have been able to find out how many students attended classes without matriculating that year by taking advantage of the careful record-keeping of Nicholas Bain. I have been able to do the same for the period 1791–1808 by building on the work of Alexander Morgan, who, in the 1930s, checked the 'Medical' lists for that period against the Matriculation Albums and noted students who had not matriculated. I have entered the non-matriculates into a separate database, arranged them by cohort, and compared them with the matriculated students.

The results of this comparison are revealing. Fifty per cent of the non-matriculates prior to 1811 had never matriculated; the rest had matriculated in other years. The number of non-matriculates began at 113 in the early 1790s, and rose to 306 in 1808. In the same period, the number of matriculating student averaged 208 per cohort in the early 1790s and only rose to 279 in 1808. From 1792 until 1808, only 54 per cent of the students who attended medical lectures in Edinburgh in any given year had matriculated that year; only 78 per cent had ever matriculated. No wonder the University Library tightened up their matriculation policy. In 1811, the number of non-matriculates was reduced to 98, while the number of matriculated students in that cohort jumped to 452. The number of matriculated students averaged 444 per cohort from 1811 to 1826, and the number of non-matriculates never again rose above 100. Fifty-four per cent of the non-matriculates from 1811 to 1826 never matriculated. The result of the new regulations was that, from 1811, 87 per cent of the students attending medical lectures in Edinburgh in any given year had matriculated that year; 93 per cent had matriculated at some point.

Prior to 1808, students who never matriculated followed certain patterns. Eighty-seven per cent studied for only one year, and 33 per cent attended Chemistry only. The latter group seems comparable to the one-year auditors who attended Chemistry only, discussed in Chapter Six. It is not clear why one group matriculated and one did not, but if the students were interested in Chemistry as a science, or as a branch of general education for gentlemen, they would not have needed to matriculate. Even for the remainder of the never-matriculated students, Chemistry appears to have been an important reason for their attending classes, since 60 per cent took the course. Thirty per cent attended Anatomy and Surgery, and 30 per cent attended Midwifery. Medical Practice attracted 22 per cent, Botany, 20 per cent, Clinical Lectures, 14 per cent, and Medical Theory and Materia Medica, each 7 per cent.[17] The majority of these students attended two courses only, one usually being Chemistry. What this course of study suggests is that older students were attracted by the celebrity of the professors or interest in course content, rather than by other advantages derived from being at a university.

Students who matriculated in some years, but not others, followed a different pattern in the years they did not matriculate. Midwifery attracted 51 per cent of this group. Clinical Lectures attracted 22 per cent and Botany, 20 per cent. Anatomy and Surgery attracted 19 per cent, Chemistry and Medical Practice, each 16 per cent, and Medical Theory and Materia Medica, each 4 per cent. This pattern also suggests older students, but here they appear to be filling in gaps in their previous education. That is also suggested by the fact that 45 per cent of the graduates in the cohorts 1792–1808 attended classes for at least one year without matriculating. The majority of those – 30 per cent of the graduates – did so after they graduated. University graduates were not allowed to take books out of the University Library, and they no longer needed an official record of their studies. Why, then, bother to matriculate?

After 1811, the non-matriculates become harder to characterize. Ninety-four per cent of those who never matriculated studied for one year only; 15 per cent attended Chemistry only. Only 19 per cent of the remainder attended Chemistry; 25 per cent attended Anatomy and Surgery; 13 per cent attended Botany. Less than 10 per cent attended the rest of the courses.[18] It is also hard to discern patterns among the students who had matriculated in other years. Midwifery still attracted the highest percentage of this group of students, but that was only 17 per cent.[19] Thirteen per cent attended Chemistry, 11 per cent, Anatomy and Surgery and Botany, and under 10 per cent attended the rest of the classes. Only 7 per cent of the graduates attended classes without matriculating; only 3 per cent attended classes after graduation without matriculating.

To summarize, the non-matriculates prior to 1811 seem to have been attracted to particular courses or professors; perhaps the Royal Commissioners' description of 'occasional auditors', discussed in Chapter Ten, would best fit this group. It is possible that students who wished to take Chemistry as a branch of general education, or Midwifery after completing other medical studies, simply decided not to matriculate. It is equally possible, though, that the professors of those courses, applied to for advice, told this group of students that there was no reason for them to matriculate. After 1811, that advice would have gone directly against University statute, and it may have been harder for students to find professors who would let them into classes if they did not matriculate. We would expect, for example, that Professor Andrew Duncan junior, as University Librarian responsible for the new regulations, would be especially unsympathetic to students attending his classes without matriculating. This assumption is supported by the fact that Clinical Lectures, taught regularly by Duncan junior, attracted 35 per cent of the non-matriculates prior to 1808, but only 4 per cent after 1811. The new regulations, then, seem to have been effective in forcing nearly everyone who wished to be considered a 'student of medicine strictly speaking', or even a plain 'student', to matriculate.

The chart of student groups in Appendix D, and the numbers I have presented throughout the book, are based on an analysis of the matriculation records only. I have not attempted to incorporate information on non-matriculates into it. That means that the sharp increase of students between 1805 and 1810 is caused in part by the more accurate system of record-keeping, rather than underlying changes in student population. Incorporating non-matriculates into the chart, however, would only have moved that sharp increase to the period 1790–1795, since we do not have systematic records of non-matriculates until 1791. It therefore seemed to me most useful to keep the sharp increase where it in fact appeared in University record-keeping, and to use the separate lists to elucidate, rather than obscure, differences between matriculated and non-matriculated students.

Finally, I should clarify the extent to which I have checked the information in the database which comes from the matriculation records. It has not been possible for me to check my records of course attendance per cohort with the original matriculation records. I have, however, checked the information taken from all other lists of students, such as graduates or Fellows, against the original lists. It is therefore as accurate as I could make it. It is too much to hope that there are no transcription errors in the database, but I have done my best to ensure that there are no systematic errors which would distort the figures I have derived.

Appendix B:

Schedule of classes, winter session

Materia Medica	8–9 am
Medical Practice	9–10
Chemistry	10–11
Medical Theory	11–12
Royal Infirmary open to students	12–1 pm
Anatomy and Surgery	1–3
Midwifery	3–4
Clinical Lectures (Tuesday and Friday)	4–5
Clinical Surgery (Monday and Thursday)	5–6
Military Surgery	2–3
Medical Jurisprudence	1–2

Schedule of Classes, Summer Session

Botany
Clinical Lectures
Clinical Surgery

Taken from *Edinburgh Evidence*, Appendix, p. 207. The courses were occasionally given in a different order over the seventy years covered by this book, but this was the most usual arrangement. For a discussion of each class, see Chapter Three.

Appendix C:
Chart of professorial appointments, 1760–1826

Information in this chart is taken from J.D. Comrie, *History of Scottish Medicine* (London: The Wellcome Historical Medical Museum, 1932), 2:628–631. Parentheses indicate that the professor was appointed before 1760.

Year	Anatomy and Surgery	Chemistry	Medical Practice	Medical Theory	Midwifery	Materia Medica	Botany	Clinical Surgery	Military Surgery	Medical Jurisprudence
1760	(Alex. Monro II)	(William Cullen)	(Robert Whytt)	(Robert Whytt)	(Thomas Young)		(Charles Alston)			
1761							John Hope			
1766		Joseph Black	John Gregory	William Cullen						
1768						Francis Home				
1770										
1773			William Cullen	[Alex. M. Drummond]						
1776				James Gregory						
1780					Alex. Hamilton					
1786							Daniel Rutherford			
1789										Andrew Duncan sen.
1790			James Gregory							

Year	Anatomy and Surgery	Chemistry	Medical Practice	Medical Theory	Midwifery	Materia Medica	Botany	Clinical Surgery	Military Surgery	Medical Jurisprudence
1795		Thomas C. Hope								
1798	Alexander Monro III									
1799										
1800						James Home				
1803					James Hamilton					
1806								James Russell		
1807									John Thomson	Andrew Duncan jun.
1810										
1819				Andrew Duncan jun.						
1820							Robert Graham			William P. Alison
1821			James Home	William P. Alison		Andrew Duncan jun.				
1822										Robert Christison
1823									George Ballingall	
1830										

Appendix D:
Student groups, five-year aggregates

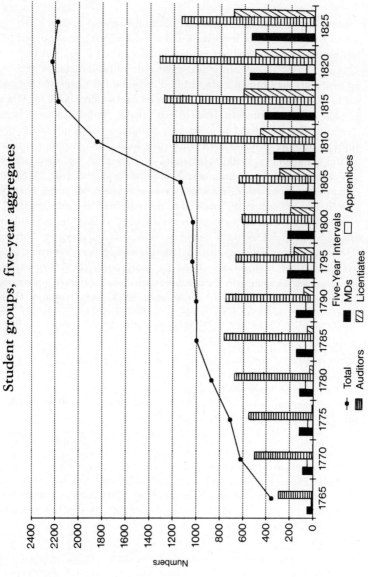

Notes

Introduction

1. Adam Smith, *An Inquiry into the Nature and Causes of the Wealth of Nations* (London: Ward, Lock, & Co., [nd]), p. 610.
2. N.T. Phillipson and Rosalind Mitchison, *Scotland in the Age of Improvement* (Edinburgh: Edinburgh University Press, 1970). T.M. Devine, ed. *Improvement and Enlightenment* (Edinburgh: John Donald Publishers Ltd., 1989). Asa Briggs, *The Age of Improvement 1783–1867* (New York: Longman, Green, 1959).
3. George Crabb, *English Synonyms Explained, in Alphabetical Order; with Copious Illustrations and Examples Drawn from the Best Writers*, 3rd ed. (London: Baldwin, Cradock, and Joy, 1824), s.v. 'Improvement', 'Progress'. In tracking down contemporary usage of certain important words, I have also used the following references: Samuel Johnson, *A Dictionary of the English Language*, 2 vols. (London: J. Knapton, C. Hitch and L. Hawes, A. Millar, R. and J. Dodsley, and M. and T. Longman, 1756); James Buchanan, *Linguae Britannicae Vera Pronunciatio: or, A New English Dictionary* (London: A. Millar, 1757; reprint ed., Menston, England: The Scolar Press Limited, 1967). The model for this kind of analysis is Raymond Williams, *Keywords. A Vocabulary of Culture and Society* (New York: Oxford University Press, 1976).
4. Johnson, s.v. 'Education'.
5. Certificate of Samuel Cleverly, Letter book of the Society of Friends in Edinburgh, 1791–1825, SRO CH 10/1/65.
6. Smith, p. 610.
7. Some women did attend classes offered by medical professors, but, as I will discuss in Chapters One and Three, they were not really considered part of the university population. For that reason I will use the male pronoun 'he' when referring to a student, not 'he/she' or some other variant.
8. There is no recent full-length history of the Edinburgh University medical school, but see J.D. Comrie, *History of Scottish Medicine*, 2 vols. (London: The Wellcome Historical Medical Museum, 1932), Alexander Grant, *The Story of the University of Edinburgh during its First Three Hundred Years*, 2 vols. (London: Longmans, Green, and Co., 1884) and A. Logan Turner, *Story of a Great Hospital. The Royal Infirmary of Edinburgh* (Edinburgh: Oliver and Boyd, 1937) supplemented by Guenther Risse, *Hospital Life in Enlightenment Scotland: Care and Teaching at the Royal Infirmary of Edinburgh* (Cambridge: Cambridge University Press, 1986). C.J. Lawrence has dealt with the 18th century medical faculty in 'Medicine as Culture: Edinburgh and the Scottish

Enlightenment', (Ph.D. Dissertation, University of London, 1984); his recent article 'The Edinburgh Medical School and the End of the "Old Thing" 1790–1830' *History of Universities* 7 (1988): 259–286 is an excellent brief account of the later period.

9. Jane Rendall, 'The Influence of the Edinburgh Medical School on America in the Eighteenth Century', in *The Early Years of the Edinburgh Medical School*, ed. by R.G.W. Anderson and A.D.C. Simpson (Edinburgh: Royal Scottish Museum, 1976) pp. 95–124; William Brock, *Scotus Americanus*, (Edinburgh: Edinburgh University Press, 1982); Wyndham B. Blanton, *Medicine in Virginia in the Eighteenth Century* (Richmond: Garrett & Massie, Incorporated, 1931) pp. 71–92; George W. Corner, *Two Centuries of Medicine. A History of the School of Medicine, University of Pennsylvania* (Philadelphia: J.B. Lippincott Company, 1965).

10. Wilfrid R. Prest, *The Inns of Court under Elizabeth I and the Early Stuarts, 1590–1640* (London: Longman, 1972); Lawrence Stone, ed., *The University and Society*, 2 vols. (Princeton: Princeton University Press, 1974); Richard Kagan, *Students and Society in Early Modern Spain* (Baltimore: Johns Hopkins Press, 1974); Charles McClelland, *State, Society and University in Germany, 1700–1914* (New York: Cambridge University Press, 1980); Willem Frijhoff, *La Société Néerlandaise et ses Gradués 1575–1814: Une recherche sérielle sur la status des intellectuels* (APA: Holland University Press, 1981); L.W. Brockliss, *French Higher Education in the Seventeenth and Eighteenth Centuries. A Cultural History* (Oxford: Oxford University Press, 1987); W.M. Mathew, 'The Origins and Occupations of Glasgow Students, 1740–1839', *Past and Present* 33 (1966): 74–94.

11. Howard S. Becker, Blanche Geer, Everett C. Hughes, Answlm L. Strauss, *Boys in White. Student Culture in Medical School* (New Brunswick, NJ: Transaction Books, 1977). Many articles in the *Journal of Medical Education*, published by the Association of American Medical Colleges, have to do with students' perceptions of medical education and their implication for educational policies.

12. The quote is from J.B. Morrell, 'The Edinburgh Town Council and its University, 1717–1766', in Anderson and Simpson, p. 51.

13. In fact, according to J.R.R. Christie, the Edinburgh medical school was 'the adoption, in precise and specific terms, of a foreign model of scientific education', which involved the teaching of anatomy, chemistry, medical theory and practice, and clinical lectures in a hospital. J.R.R. Christie, 'The Origins and Development of the Scottish Scientific Community, 1680–1760', *History of Science* 12 (1974): 130–1; For similar assumptions, see W.R.O. Goslings, 'Leiden and Edinburgh: The Seed, the Soil, and the Climate', in Anderson and Simpson, pp. 1–18. The idea that Edinburgh medical teaching was only a copy of Leyden has been modified by Rosalie Stott, who argues that many aspects of later Edinburgh teaching already existed in Edinburgh under the auspices of the Incorporation of Surgeons prior to the founding of the medical faculty. She, too, however, assumed a curriculum based on the teaching of all branches of medicine, and clinical lectures at a hospital. Rosalie Stott, 'The Incorporation of Surgeons and Medical Education and Practice in Edinburgh 1696–1755,' (Ph.D. Dissertation, University of Edinburgh, 1984).

14. Corner, pp. 1–48; Deborah C. Brunton, 'The Transfer of Medical Education:

Teaching at the Edinburgh and Philadelphia Medical Schools', in *Scotland and America in the Age of Enlightenment*, ed. by Richard B. Sher and Jeffrey R. Smittan (Edinburgh: Edinburgh University Press, 1990); John Morgan, *A Discourse upon the Institution of Medical Schools in America* (Philadelphia, 1765).

15. James Coutts, *A History of the University of Glasgow from its Foundation in 1451 to 1909* (Glasgow: James Maclehose and Sons, 1909), pp. 204–5, 237–8.

16. Some points of comparison are provided by Konrad H. Jarausch, 'The Sources of German Student Unrest 1815–1848 in Stone, 2:533–570 and James C. McClelland, *Autocrats and Academics. Education, Culture and Society in Tsarist Russia* (Chicago: University of Chicago Press, 1979), pp. 95–113 and Samuel D. Kassow, *Students, Professors and the State in Tsarist Russia* (Berkeley: University of California Press, 1989). See also Julius R. Krevans and Peter G. Cundliffe, eds., *The Effect of Student Unrest. A Colloquium Sponsored by the John E. Fogarty International Center for Advanced Study in the Health Sciences, National Institutes of Health, and the Board of Medicine, National Academy of Sciences. April 9–11, 1969.* (Washington DC: National Academy of Sciences, 1970).

17. 'Transcription of documents relating to the dispute between managers of the Royal Infirmary of Edinburgh and the medical students in 1785', p. 84, RMS Library.

18. *Ibid.*, p. 68–9.

19. See Sheldon Rothblatt's essay review, 'Supply and Demand: The "Two Histories" of English Education', *History of Education Quarterly* 28 (Winter 1988): 625–644.

20. J.B. Morrell, 'The University of Edinburgh in the late Eighteenth Century: Its Scientific Eminence and Academic Structure', *Isis* (1970): 161; J.B. Morrell, 'Practical Chemistry in the University of Edinburgh', *Ambix* 16 (1969): 66–70. Susan Lawrence, 'Entrepreneurs and private enterprise: the development of medical lecturing in London, 1775–1820', *Bulletin of the History of Medicine* 63 (1988): 171–192.

21. Adam Smith to William Cullen, London, 20 September 1774, cited in John Thomson, *An Account of the Life, Lectures, and Writings of William Cullen, MD*, 2 vols. (Edinburgh: William Blackwood and Sons, 1859), 1:475. Smith's letter to Cullen, though not Cullen's reply, has been printed in Adam Smith, *The Correspondence of Adam Smith* ed. by E.C. Mossner and I.S. Ross (Oxford: Clarendon Press, 1987), pp. 173–179.

22. Smith, *Wealth of Nations* p. 604.

23. More recent commentators have tended to stress the way in which Edinburgh professors 'marketed' their courses to attract large audiences, whether students or the local educated elite. See Morrell, 'Practical Chemistry', pp. 66–7; Steven Shapin, 'The Audience for Science in Eighteenth Century Edinburgh', *History of Science* 12 (1974): 110–113; Christie, pp. 134–136; C.J. Lawrence, 'Medicine as Culture', p. 217, noted that the relationship between student demand and professorial response was a complex one.

24. Thomson, 1:477–8.

25. William Cullen, 'Lectures on Chemistry', *circa* 1755, William Cullen Mss # 11, RCPE Library.

26. Thomson, 1:482. Thomson took this from a speech Cullen made at graduation, but felt it could be considered a response to Smith's letter.

27. Derek Dow and Michael Moss make a similar assumption in 'The Medical Curriculum at Glasgow in The Early-Nineteenth Century', *History of Universities* 7 (1988): 227–257.
28. *Edinburgh Evidence.*
29. See Appendix A for a fuller description of the data.
30. See Thomson, *Life of William Cullen*; C.J. Lawrence, 'Medicine as Culture'; R.E. Wright-St.Clair, *Doctors Monro: A Medical Saga* (London: The Wellcome Historical Medical Library, 1964); Arthur L. Donovan, *Philosophical Chemistry in the Scottish Enlightenment: The Doctrines and Discoveries of William Cullen and Joseph Black* (Edinburgh: Edinburgh University Press, 1975); Robert French, *Robert Whytt, the Soul, and Medicine* (London: The Wellcome Institute for the History of Medicine, 1969).

Chapter One

1. Samuel Bard to John Bard, Edinburgh, 29 December 1762, Bard Papers, New York Academy of Medicine Library.
2. J. Johnson, *A Guide for Gentlemen Studying Medicine at the University of Edinburgh* (London: J. Robinson, 1792).
3. Edinburgh Evidence, p. 316.
4. Elborg Forster, trans., 'Curriculum Vitae of Dorothea Christiana Erxleben, appended to her doctoral dissertation submitted to the Faculty of Medicine of Halle University'. See Londa Schiebinger, *The Mind Has No Sex? Women in the Origins of Modern Science* (Cambridge, MA: Harvard University Press, 1984).
5. Great Britain, Parliament, House of Commons, *Report from the Select Committee on Medical Education: With the Minutes of Evidence, and Appendix.* 1834 (602, I, II, and III), Part 1: Royal College of Physicians, London, p. 17.
6. For a discussion of upward social mobility among London surgeons, see Susan Lawrence, 'Science and Medicine at the London Hospitals. The Development of Teaching and Research 1750–1815', (Ph.D. Thesis, University of Toronto, 1985), pp. 184–188. Margaret Pelling has discussed the social status of medical practitioners in the sixteenth and seventeenth century in 'Medical Practice in Early Modern England: Trade or Profession?' in *The Professions in Early Modern England*, ed. by W. Prest (London: Croom Helm, 1987), pp. 90–128.
7. The phrase is from John Bell, *Letters on Professional Character and Manners: on the Education of a Surgeon, and the Duties and Qualifications of a Physician: addressed to James Gregory, M.D* (Edinburgh: John Muir, 1810). See below, Chapter Five.
8. *Ibid.*
9. *Edinburgh Evidence*, Appendix, p. 262. One of the most interesting discussions of stress among young adults in Early Modern Europe is in Michael McDonald, *Mystical Bedlam, Madness, Anxiety and Healing in Seventeenth-Century England* (Cambridge: Cambridge University Press, 1981), pp. 72–112.
10. Thomas Alcock, 'An Essay on the Education and Duties of the General Practitioner in Medicine and Surgery', *Transactions of the Associates Apothecaries and Surgeon-Apothecaries* 1 (1823): 8.

11. Alexander Lesassier [later Hamilton], 4 April 1805, Alexander Hamilton Collection, Box 11, Folder 72, Library of the Royal College of Physicians of Edinburgh, Edinburgh. I have corrected Lesassier's spelling.

12. See below, Chapter Six.

13. Richard Lovell Edgeworth, *Essays on Professional Education* (London: J. Johnson & Co., 1812).

14. [Thomas Denman, Baron Denman,] '[Review of] *Essays on Professional Education'*, *Monthly Review* series 2, 62 (May–August 1810): 9. For less sympathetic reviews, see [John Davidson], 'Edgeworth's Essays on Professional Education', *Quarterly Review* 6 (Aug–December 1811): 166–191; 'Edgeworth's *Professional Education' Edinburgh Review* 15 (Oct. 1809–Jan. 1810): 40–53.

15. *Edinburgh Evidence*, p. 298.

16. [Davidson], p. 171. This assumption is implied in James Parkinson, *The Hospital Pupil; or Observations Addressed to the Parents of Youths Intended for the Profession of Medicine and Surgery* (London: Sherwood, Neely, & Jones, 1817); James Lucas, *A Candid Inquiry into the Education, Qualifications, and Offices of a Surgeon-Apothecary* (Bath: S. Hazard, 1800); William Chamberlaine, *Tirocinium Medicum, or a Dissertation on the Duties of Youth Apprenticed to the Medical Profession* (London: Sherwood, Neely, & Jones, 1812).

17. The phrase is from *The Spectator* #108, Wednesday, July 4, 1711, but see especially #21, Tuesday, March 6, 1710–11.

18. Edward Hughes, 'The Professions in the Eighteenth Century', in *Aristocratic Government and Society in Eighteenth-Century England. The Foundations of Stability*, ed. by David A. Baugh (New York: Franklin Watts, Inc., 1975) pp. 183–203; W.J. Reader, *Professional Men. The Rise of the Professional Classes in Nineteenth-Century England* (London: Cox and Wyman Ltd., 1966), pp. 1–24.

19. W.M. Mathew, 'The Origins and Occupations of Glasgow Students, 1740–1839', *Past and Present* 33 (1966): 89.

20. Adam Smith, *The Correspondence of Adam Smith*, ed. by E.C. Mossner and I.S. Ross (Oxford: Clarendon Press, 1987), p. 76.

21. *Dictionary of National Biography*, s.v. Monro, Alexander, s.v. Monro, Donald.

22. Skene Papers, Mss # 40, Aberdeen University Library.

23. Samuel Bard to John Bard, Edinburgh, 29 December 1762, Bard Papers.

24. The phrase is taken from the 'The London University', *Quarterly Review* 33 (December 1825–March 1826): 266.

25. For a Glasgow opinion, see Professor Thomas Thomson's comments, in *Glasgow Evidence*, p. 154; *A Comparative View of the Schools of Physic of Dublin and Edinburgh* (Dublin: Hodges & McArthur, 1818; see also the review, 'Medical Schools of Dublin and Edinburgh', *Blackwood's Magazine* 4 (October 1818–March 1819): 439–441.

26. *Committee on Medical Education*, p. 9.

27. *St Andrews Evidence*, testimony of Dr Robert Briggs, pp. 17, 158. In fact St. Andrews and Aberdeen degrees were never simply sold, and candidates took seriously the task of obtaining necessary testimonials. P.J. Anderson, ed. *Fasti Academiae Mariscallanae Aberdonensis. Selections from the Records of the Marischal College and University MDXCIII – MDCCCLX*, 3 vols. (Aberdeen: New Spalding Club, 1898). Vol. 2: *Officers, Graduates, and Alumni*, pp. 111–159; P.J. Anderson, ed. *Officers and Graduates of University and King's College,*

Aberdeen MDV–MDCCCLX, (Aberdeen: New Spalding Club, 1893) pp. 131–160. For a general discussion of this, see also Joseph Kett, 'Provincial Medical Practice in England, 1730–1815', *Journal of the History of Medicine* 19 (1964): 17–29; Lisa Rosner, 'Students and Apprentices: Medical Education at Edinburgh University 1760–1805', (Ph.D. Thesis, The Johns Hopkins University, 1985), pp. 14–16.

28. Joan Lane, 'The Role of Apprenticeship in Eighteenth Century Medical Education in England', in *William Hunter and the Eighteenth-Century Medical World*, ed. William Bynum (Cambridge: Cambridge University Press, 1985), pp. 57–104.

29. Samuel Powell Griffitts to Benjamin Rush, London, 10 Aug. 1783, Rush Mss, cited in Whitfield Bell, 'Philadelphia Medical Students in Europe, 1750–1800]', *The Pennsylvania Magazine of History and Biography* 67 (1943): 15.

30. *The Medical Calendar: a Students' Guide to the Medical Schools in Edinburgh, London, Dublin, Paris, Oxford, Cambridge, Glasgow, Aberdeen, and St. Andrews.* (Edinburgh: MacLachlan and Stewart, 1828), p. 414–7.

31. Lawrence, 'Science and Medicine'.

32. Guenther Risse, *Hospital Life in Enlightenment Scotland: Care and Teaching at the Royal Infirmary of Edinburgh* (Cambridge: Cambridge University Press, 1986), pp. 240–278.

33. For teaching at the Public Dispensary, see Andrew Duncan, *Medical Cases, selected from the Records of the Dispensary at Edinburgh with Remarks and Observations, being the substance of Case-Lectures, delivered during the years 1776–7* (Edinburgh: Elliot, 1778); *Medical Commentaries* 4 (1776): 460–461, 5 (1778): 221–223; Lisa Rosner, 'Andrew Duncan MD, FRSE, 1744–1828', *Scottish Men of Medicine Series*, Edinburgh: History of Medicine and Science Unit, 1981.

34. James Coutts, *A History of the University of Glasgow from its Foundation in 1451 to 1909* (Glasgow: James Maclehose and Sons, 1909), pp. 519–20; *Glasgow Evidence*, pp. 126–7.

35. Lesassier, 20 March 1805.

36. Alcock, p. 71.

37. R.W.I Smith, *English-Speaking Students of Medicine at the University of Leyden* (Edinburgh: Oliver and Boyd, 1932); W.R.O. Goslings, 'Leiden and Edinburgh: The Seed, the Soil, and the Climate', in *The Early Years of the Edinburgh Medical School*, p. 1–18, ed. by R.G.W. Anderson and A.D.C. Simpson (Edinburgh: Royal Scottish Museum, 1976).

38. John Cross, *Sketches of the Medical Schools of Paris* (London: J. Callow, 1815); *Medical Calendar*, pp. 150–160. See also Russell C. Maulitz, *Morbid Appearances. The Anatomy of Pathology in the Early Nineteenth Century* (Cambridge: Cambridge University Press, 1987).

39. *Dictionary of National Biography*, s.v. 'Duncan, Andrew, the Younger'; Andrew Duncan junior, 'Letters, 1794–1798', Mss. Dc.1.90, Edinburgh University Library. Extracts from these were published in the *Caledonian Medical Journal* 9 (1913–4): 203–208, 262–265, 307–315, 370–377, 426–429, 456–470 and 10 (1914–15): 23–27, 84–90, 104–114, 129–146, 165–178, 194–200.

40. Francis Augustus Burnett Bonney, 'Diary of F.A.B Bonney, LRSCE, 1827–36', Mss. Gen 782/4/3, Edinburgh University Library.

41. 'Early Papers of Arthur Lee', in *The Southern Literary Messenger*, 29:63, cited in Wyndham B. Blanton, *Medicine in Virginia in the Eighteenth Century* (Richmond: Garrett & Massie, Incorporated, 1931), p. 86. Blanton added, 'Lee decided that a lifetime was enough and graduated from Edinburgh in 1764.'

42. *Glasgow Evidence*, Appendix, p. 562.

43. Brock, pp. 13–14.

44. Rendall, p. 101.

45. This summary is taken from Rendall, pp. 95–124. The pattern of southern students studying for a shorter period of time than Philadelphia ones carried over into patterns of study at the University of Pennsylvania.

46. The phrase is taken from Great Britain. House of Commons. *Report Made to His Majesty by a Royal Commission of Inquiry into the State of the Universities of Scotland*, (October, 1830), p. 9.

47. Mary Hewson to her son, Thomas Tickell Hewson, 7 July 1795, Hewson Papers, B H492, vol. 2, # 31, American Philosophical Society Library, Philadelphia.

48. *Ibid.*

49. Parke to Owen Biddle, Edinburgh, Jan 13, 1772, Friends Historical Library, Swarthmore College, cited in Whitfield Bell, 'Thomas Parke's Student Life in England and Scotland, 1771–1773', *The Pennsylvania Magazine of History and Biography* 75 (1951): 246.

50. Pelling, 'Medical Practice'. A useful summary of the medical profession in England is in Ivan Waddington, *The Medical Profession in the Industrial Revolution* (Dublin: Gill and MacMillan Humanities Press, 1984), pp. 1–28.

51. Dorothy and Roy Porter, *Patient's Progress. Doctors and Doctoring in Eighteenth-Century England* (Stanford: Stanford University Press, 1989); Roy Porter, *Health for Sale. Quackery in England 1660–1850* (Manchester: Manchester University Press, 1989). Roy Porter, *Disease, Medicine and Society in England 1550–1860* (Houndsmills, Basingstoke, Hampshire: Macmillan Publishers Ltd., 1987) is a useful introduction to medical practice in the period.

52. Neil Cantlie, *A History of the Army Medical Department* 2 vols. (Edinburgh: Churchill Livingston, 1984), pp. 180–1.

53. Parkinson, p. 36.

54. 'Medical Reform', *Quarterly Review* 67 (December 1840–March 1841): 59. See also Irvine Loudon, *Medical Care and the General Practitioner 1750–1850* (Oxford: Clarendon Press, 1986); Joan Lane, 'The Medical Practitioners of Provincial England in 1783', *Medical History* 28 (1984): 353–371; Kett, 'Provincial Medical Practice'; M. Jeanne Peterson, *The Medical Profession in Mid-Victorian London* (Berkeley: University of California Press, 1978), pp. 5–40.

55. [Taplin, William], *The Aesculapian Labyrinth Explored; or, Medical Mystery Illustrated. A Series of Instructions to Young Physicians, Surgeons, Accouchers, Apothecaries, Druggists, and Practitioners of Every Denomination, in Town and Country*, (Dublin: Zachariah Jackson, 1789).

56. Thomas Percival, *Percival's Medical Ethics*, ed. by Chauncey D. Leake (Baltimore: Williams and Wilkins Company, 1927), p. 80–81.

57. Porter, *Disease, Medicine and Society*, p. 40.

58. John Thomson, *An Account of the Life, Lectures, and Writings of William Cullen, MD*, 2 vols. (Edinburgh: William Blackwood and Sons, 1859), 1:220–1,

2:564–5. Cullen does not seem to have been a successful improving landlord, however, and on his death Adam Smith applied to Henry Dundas for a pension for Cullen's daughters. Adam Smith, *Correspondence*, pp. 323–4.

59. As it was described by his nephew Lesassier, 27 April 1806.

60. Porter, *Disease, Medicine and Society* p. 40.

61. Irvine Loudon, 'The Nature of Provincial Medical Practice in Eighteenth-Century England', *Medical History* 29 (1985): 18.

62. Taplin, p. 1.

63. Dorothy Porter and Roy Porter, pp. 117–132.

64. Dr John Murray to William Murray, Charleston, South Carolina, 6 November 1747, Murray of Murraythwaite, SRO GD219/284/1.

65. R. Campbell, *The London Tradesman*, (London: 1797), cited in Loudon, 'Provincial Medical Practice', p. 3.

66. Dirom Grey Crawford, *A History of the Indian Medical Service 1600–1913*, 2 vols. (London: W. Thacker & Co., 1914), 1: 363–4.

67. Lisa Rosner, 'Education and Interest: 18th Century Edinburgh Medical Students and the Armed Forces' in *Edinburgh Health and Medicine*, ed. by. Malcolm Nicolson (London: Croom Helm, forthcoming).

68. G.J. Bryant, 'Scots in India in the Eighteenth Century', *Scottish Historical Review* 64 (1985): 28.

69. Adam Smith, *An Inquiry into the Nature and Causes of the Wealth of Nations* (London: Ward, Lock, & Co., [nd]), p. 99.

70. John Ramsay, *Letters of John Ramsay of Ochtertyre, 1799–1812*, ed. Barbara L.H. Horn (Edinburgh: T. & A. Constable Ltd. 1966), p. 260.

71. The pay scale in the army depended on the regiment, and in the navy, on the rate of ship; both salaries increased with length of time in the service. The variations in pay make systematic comparisons between services difficult. In addition, the pay and rank of both army and navy surgeons was improved as a result of the Napoleonic Wars. Information on salaries is included in Robert Jackson, *A System of Arrangement and Discipline for the Medical Department of Armies* (London: John Murray, 1805), pp. 99–110, and William Turnbull, *The Naval Surgeon; Comprising the Entire Duties of Professional Men at Sea* (London: Richard Phillips, 1806), pp. ix–xiv.

72. Lesassier, 2 October 1805. See also the review of William Cullen Brown, *A View of the comparative Advantages and Disadvantages of the Navy and Army-Surgeon* (London: Underwood, 1814), in *Monthly Review* series 277 (May–August 1815): 432–3.

73. Adam Smith, *Wealth of Nations*, p. 224.

74. Dr Robert Dalrymple to his brother Sir High Dalrymple, Bart., Leyden, November 1738, Hamilton-Dalrymple of North Berwick, SRO GD 110/915/3.

75. The surgeon's mate daily allowance in 1783, after the army deducted a certain amount for duties. Robert Hamilton, *The Duties of a Regimental Surgeon Considered: with observation on his general qualifications; and hints relative to a more respectable practice, and better regulation of that department*, 2 vols. (London: J. Johnson, [1787]), 2:173.

76. *Guide*, p. 64.

77. Alcock, pp. 47–48.

78. Porter and Porter, pp. 33–95.

79. John Bard to Samuel Bard, New York, 11 Dec. 1765, Bard Papers.

80. Porter, *Health for Sale*, pp. 68–73.
81. G. Clark, *A History of the Royal College of Physicians of London*, 3 vols. (Oxford: Clarendon Press, 1972); Zachary Cope, *The History of the Royal College of Surgeons of England* (London: Anthony Blond Ltd., 1959) Clarendon Hyde Creswell, *The Royal College of Surgeons of Edinburgh. Historical Notes from 1505 to 1905* (Edinburgh: Oliver & Boyd, 1926); Alexander Duncan, *Memorials of the Faculty of Physicians and Surgeons of Glasgow 1599–1850* (Glasgow: James Maclehose and Sons, 1896); R.P.Ritchie, *The Early Days of the Royall Colledge of Phisitians, Edinburgh*, (Edinburgh: George Johnston, 1899); Charles Cameron, *History of the Royal College of Surgeons in Ireland, and of the Irish Schools of Medicine* (Dublin: Fannin & Co., 1886); J.D.H. Widdiss, *The Royal College of Surgeons in Ireland and its Medical School, 1784–1984*, (Dublin: Royal College of Surgeons of Dublin, 1984).
82. Olin Mackenzie to Henry Dundas, Jan. 1783, Melville Castle, SRO GD51/4/3.
83. Lesassier was never successful in attracting patients. Joy Pitman, 'Alexander (Le Sassier) Hamilton: An Eventful Life', *Proceedings of the Royal College of Physicians of Edinburgh* 17 (October 1987): 286–290.
84. Smith, *Wealth of Nations*, p. 97.
85. This estimate is based on the figures presented by A.H.T Robb-Smith, 'Medical Education at Oxford and Cambridge Prior to 1850', in *The Evolution of Medical Education in Britain*, ed. by F.N.L. Poynter (Baltimore: The Williams and Wilkins Company, 1966). Recent work on Oxford and Cambridge have confirmed the view that lectures on science in the English Universities were not intended for medical practitioners. John Gascoigne, *Cambridge in the Age of the Enlightenment. Science, Religion, and Politics from the Restoration to the French Revolution* (Cambridge: Cambridge University Press, 1988), pp. 9–14; E.G.W. Bill, *Education at Christ Church Oxford 1600–1800* (Oxford: Clarendon Press, 1988), pp. 314–326.
86. William Baillie to Mrs. Hamilton, London, 9 January 1806, Edinburgh, RCPE, Hamilton, Family of, Mss # 1, 'Letters to Thomas Hamilton, and to his son William, c. 1778–9'.
87. Lawrence, 'Science and Medicine', p 184.
88. For an excellent presentation of the changes in a typical Cambridge medical student's career, see Ruth G. Hodkinson, 'Medical Education in Cambridge in the Nineteenth Century', pp. 79–106, in *Cambridge and its Contribution to Medicine*, ed. by Arthur Rook (London: Wellcome Institute of the History of Medicine, 1971).
89. Lawrence, 'Science and Medicine', p. 646. These figures are for St Thomas', St George's, Guy's, and the Middlesex hospitals from 1780–1815, and St Bartholomew's hospital from 1808–1815.
90. Parkinson, p. 45.
91. These figures are based on R.B. McDowell and D.A. Webb, *Trinity College Dublin 1592–1952* (Cambridge: Cambridge University Press, 1982), pp. 88, 524.
92. *Comparative View*, p. vi.
93. Derek Dow and Michael Moss 'The Medical Curriculum at Glasgow in The Early-Nineteenth Century', *History of Universities* (1988): 239.
94. The numbers fluctuate widely. *Glasgow Evidence*, Appendix, p. 533.
95. *Report*, p. 55.

96. P.J. Anderson, ed. *Officers and Graduates of University and King's College*, pp. 131–160.
97. P.J. Anderson, ed. *Fasti Academiae Mariscallanae Aberdonensis*, p. 111–159.
98. *St. Andrews Evidence*, Appendix, p. 256.
99. *Historical Sketch and Laws of the Royal College of Physicians of Edinburgh, from its Institution to 1925* (Edinburgh: Royal College of Physicians, 1925), pp. 1–9.
100. *List of the graduates in medicine in the University of Edinburgh from MDCCV to MDCCCLXVI* (Edinburgh: Neill & Co., 1867), pp. iii–iv; Alexander Morgan, 'Matriculates in the Faculty of Medicine Prior to 1858', *University of Edinburgh Journal* 8 (1936–7): 124–5. I have chosen not to use student numbers per cohort in this case, because Morgan's figures and those from the *List of graduates* are more directly comparable to the numbers for London hospitals, Dublin, and Glasgow.
101. John Morgan, p. 29.
102. Andrew Duncan junior, 'English Apothecaries Act', *Edinburgh Medical and Surgical Journal* 25 (1826): 424. See Chapter Nine.

Chapter Two

1. Cited in Wyndham B. Blanton, *Medicine in Virginia in the Eighteenth Century* (Richmond: Garrett & Massie, Incorporated, 1931), p. 89.
2. George Logan to his brother Charles Logan, Edinburgh, 2 February 1777, Dr George Logan's Journal 1775–1779, Historical Society of Pennsylvania Mss, p. 167.
3. Alexander Lesassier [later Hamilton], 8 November 1805, Alexander Hamilton Collection, Box 11, Folder 72, Library of the Royal College of Physicians of Edinburgh, Edinburgh.
4. *Edinburgh Evidence*, p. 289.
5. *Ibid.*, p. 463.
6. Lesassier, 19 April 1806.
7. *Edinburgh Evidence*, p. 464.
8. The phrase is from a letter from Robert Saunders Dundas to Lord Minto, introducing Robert Blair, recently appointed a surgeon in the East India Company, 29 March 1809, Melville Castle, SRO GD51/4/1385/2. See the discussion of Sir David Wilkie's 1813 painting *The Letter of Introduction*, in Duncan Macmillan, *Painting in Scotland in the Golden Age* (Oxford: Phaidon Press Ltd. 1986), pp. 163–6.
9. James Rush to Benjamin Rush, Edinburgh, 23 Nov 1809, Rush Papers, Library Company of Philadelphia Mss, held in the Historical Society of Pennsylvania, Box 11, Yi2 7404 F21b.
10. Thomas Ismay, 'Letter from Thomas Ismay, Student of Medicine at Edinburgh, 1771, to his father', *University of Edinburgh Journal* 8 (1936–7): 60.
11. William Cullen, Mss. #33, 'Letter book, 1782,' RCPE Library. These letters are copies, and do not include the name of the person addressed.
12. *Edinburgh Evidence*, p. 288.
13. Rosalie Stott, 'The Incorporation of Surgeons and Medical Education and Practice in Edinburgh 1696–1755', (Ph.D. Dissertation, University of

Edinburgh, 1984), pp. 104–5, and Appendix VII, p. 371. Stott was able to trace 138 of the 564 apprentices.

14. RCSE papers, 'Indentures 1709–1811'. This collection contains records of thirty-eight indentures. It does not include the indenture for John Clerk, son of Sir John Clerk of Penicuik, Bart., discussed below.

15. Patricia Otto, 'Daughters of the British Aristocracy: Their Marriages in the Eighteenth and Nineteenth Century with Particular Reference to the Scottish Peerage' (Ph.D. Dissertation, Stanford University, 1974).

16. See T.C. Smout, 'Born Again at Cambuslang: New evidence on popular religion and literacy in eighteenth-century Scotland', *Past and Present* 97 (1982): 14–27.

17. There is, of course, no reason to think that he wished to, but his early education gives some idea of the obstacles involved for a son of a tenant farmer. David Daiches, *Robert Burns*, (New York: The Macmillan Company, 1966).

18. Comrie and Gardiner, Biographical Index of Graduates, EUL, s.v. 'Marshall, Andrew'.

19. Thomas Beddoes, Preface to *Elements of Medicine*, by John Brown, trans. by Thomas Beddoes (Portsmouth, N.H.: Oracle Press, 1803), p. xxii.

20. *Dictionary of National Biography*, s.v. 'Thomson, John'.

21. James Rush, Notes on back of class cards, American Philosophical Library Mss B R893.

22. RCSE papers, 'Indentures 1709–1811', See # 9/7, 9/11, 9/16 respectively.

23. Anthony La Vopa, *Grace, Talent, and Merit. Poor Students, Clerical Careers, and Professional Ideology in Eighteenth-Century Germany* (Cambridge: Cambridge University Press, 1988), especially pp. 19–57; Sheldon Rothblatt found a similar preference among mid-nineteenth-century Cambridge dons. *The Revolution of the Dons. Cambridge and Society in Victorian England* (Cambridge: Cambridge University Press, 1981), pp. 88–91.

24. Tobias Smollett, *Roderick Random* (New York: New American Library, 1964), p. 109.

25. Dorothy and Roy Porter, *Patient's Progress. Doctors and Doctoring in Eighteenth-Century England* (Stanford: Stanford University Press, 1989), pp. 122–125; see below, Chapter Ten.

26. Irvine Loudon gives several examples of 'gentlemen farmers and gentlemen of the cloth' who practiced medicine among the poor without formal training, presumably relying on their social position for authority, rather than their expertise. 'The Vile Race of Quacks with which this Country is Infested', in *Medical Fringe & Medical Orthodoxy 1750–1850*, ed. by W.F. Bynum and Roy Porter (London: Croom Helm, 1986), p. 107.

27. Dorothy Porter and Roy Porter, pp. 57–63.

28. Adam Murray to his brother, 29 January (1729?), Murray of Polmaise, SRO GD189/2/94A. Adam Murray was not related to John Murray, mentioned earlier.

29. 'Hints to Young Practitioners, and Observations for the Benefit of those whom they may concern', *Edinburgh Medical and Surgical Journal* 5 (1809): 338.

30. James Gregory, *Conspectus Medicinae Theoreticae. Ad usum academicum* (Edinburgh: Elliot, 1788). This was the textbook based on Professor James Gregory's course.

31. C.J. Lawrence, 'Medicine as Culture: Edinburgh and the Scottish Enlightenment', (Ph.D. Dissertation, University of London, 1984).
32. *A Comparative View of the Schools of Physic of Dublin and Edinburgh* (Dublin: Hodges & McArthur, 1818), p. 41.
33. See below, Chapter Five.
34. David Skene to his father, Dr Andrew Skene, Edinburgh, Nov. 1751, Skene Papers. Mss # 40. Aberdeen University Library.
35. The most accessible map is in A.J. Youngson, *The Making of Classical Edinburgh* (Edinburgh: Edinburgh University Press, 1966), p. 68. The University was frequently referred to as the College in the eighteenth century, and is so designated on maps.
36. Review of 'Sir John Carr's *Caledonian Sketches*', *Monthly Review* series 2, 60 (September–December 1809): 16.
37. 'Observations on Medical Reform, By a Member of the University of Oxford', *Pamphleteer* (May 1814): 419.
38. *Edinburgh Evidence*, p. 454.
39. *Ibid.*, p. 245.
40. David Skene to his father, Edinburgh, Nov. 1 1751, Skene Papers.
41. David Skene to his father, Edinburgh, 9 February 1752, Skene Papers. 'Pottage' is of course porridge. James Buchanan, *Linguae Britannicae Vera Pronunciatio: or, A New English Dictionary* (London: A. Millar, 1757; reprint ed., Menston, England: The Scolar Press Limited, 1967), s.v. 'Pottage'.
42. George Skene to David Skene, Edinburgh, 13 November 1768, Skene Papers.
43. Ismay, p. 59.
44. *Ibid.*
45. Blanton, p. 89.
46. David Freeman Hawke, *Benjamin Rush, Revolutionary Gadfly* (New York: Bobbs-Merrill Co., Inc., 1971), p. 54.
47. Job Harrison to his father, 8 October 1775, Chester City Record Office Ref. G/H.S. 99.
48. Expenses of Robert Whytt, eldest son of Dr Robert Whytt, Edinburgh, April 1766, Balfour of Pilrig, SRO GD69/298.
49. Sylas Neville, *The Diary of Sylas Neville, 1767–1788*, ed. by Basil Cozens-Hardy (London: Oxford University Press, 1950), pp. 191, 213–4.
50. James Gray, *History of the Royal Medical Society 1737–1937* (Edinburgh: Edinburgh University Press, 1952), p. 31.
51. George Logan to his brother Charles Logan, Edinburgh, 13 February 1779, Dr George Logan's Journal 1775–1779, Historical Society of Pennsylvania for the Season, see Rosalind K. Marshall, *Women in Scotland* (Edinburgh: The Trustees of the National Galleries of Scotland, 1979), pp. 63–72.
52. Benjamin Rush to James Rush, Philadelphia, 28 May 1810, Rush Papers, Yi2, Box 11, 7404, F25a.
53. David Skene to Dr Andrew Skene, Edinburgh, 9 February 1752, Skene Papers.
54. George Logan to Charles Logan, Edinburgh, 2 March, 1778, Dr George Logan's Journal 1775–1779.
55. Neville, p. 146.
56. George Logan to Charles Logan, Edinburgh, 2 May 1777, Dr George Logan's Journal 1775–1779.

57. Blanton, p. 89.
58. Anthony P. Coxon and Charles L. Jones, *The Images of Occupational Prestige* (New York: St. Martin's Press, 1978), p. 55, referring to work by J.H. Barkow, 'Prestige and Culture', *Current Anthropology* 16 (1975): 553–565.
59. Neville, p. 148.
60. See Chapter Seven.
61. William Thornton Papers, Film 724, Reel 1, American Philosophical Society, Philadelphia. Thorton never practiced; he is chiefly remembered for having designed the Capitol building in Washington DC. *Dictionary of American Biography*, s.v. 'Thornton, William'.
62. David Skene to Dr Andrew Skene, [November 1751], Skene Papers.
63. The following section owes a great deal to Sheldon Rothblatt, *Tradition and Change in English Liberal Education. An Essay in History and Culture* (London: Faber and Faber, 1976), pp. 13–101, and E.G.W. Bill, *Education at Christ Church Oxford 1660–1800* (Oxford: Clarendon Press, 1988), pp. 1–16.
64. Buchanan, s.v. 'Liberal'.
65. Rothblatt, *Tradition and Change*, p. 46.
66. Samuel Johnson, *A Dictionary of the English Language*, 2 vols. (London: J. Knapton, C. Hitch and L. Hawes, A. Millar, R. and J. Dodsley, and M. and T. Longman, 1756), s.v. 'Liberal'. Rothblatt, *Tradition and Change*, pp. 23–31.
67. William Whewell, *Of Liberal Education in General* (London: John W. Parker, 1850), p. 1.
68. Bill, p. 14–15.
69. Rothblatt, p. 26.
70. 'Advice by Sir John Clerk to his son, John, when he went to serve his apprenticeship as chirurgeon under Adam Drummond and John Campbell, 1745', Clerk of Penicuik, SRO GD18/2331.
71. See, for example, Celsus, *De re medica, accessurus index vocabulorum omnium, et cujuscunque ad rem pertinentis more dictionarii. In usum humanitatis et medicinae studiosorum.* (Glasgow: Foulis, 1766). The vocabulary was both an index to important 'medicinal words and phrases' used by Celsus and a dictionary of their English meaning.
72. Sir John Clerk, 'Advice'.
73. John Rutherford, 'Clinical Lectures 1749–53', EUL Dc.3.90.
74. William Cullen, 'Clinical Lectures' [1770?], College of Physicians of Philadelphia Mss. These are incorrectly labeled 'Clinical Lectures', since they give the substance of Cullen's course on Medical Practice.
75. *Edinburgh Evidence*, p. 203.
76. Antoine–Laurent Lavoisier, *Traité Elémentaire de Chimie, Présenté dans un ordre nouveau et d'après les découvertes modernes*, (Paris: Cuchet, 1793); Henry Guerlac, *Antoine-Laurent Lavoisier, Chemist and Revolutionary* (New York: Scribner, 1975); Robert Fox, *Caloric Theory of Gases from Lavoisier to Regnault* (Oxford: Clarendon Press, 1971).
77. For an analysis of the divorce between classical studies and science from a different perspective, see Bill, pp. 307–326, and Rothblatt, *Tradition and Change*, pp. 117–132.
78. Neville, p. 20.
79. See below, Chapter Eight.
80. John Bard to Samuel Bard, New York 14 October 1763, Bard Papers.

81. The distinction between liberal and servile stemmed from Aristotle. Rothblatt, *Tradition and Change*, pp. 23–4; Bill, p. 1–7.
82. John Gregory, 'Notes from Dr Gregory's Clinical Lectures in the Royal Infirmary 1771', RMS Mss, pp. 3–4. A note on the front cover incorrectly attributes the lectures to James Gregory.
83. *Guide*, p. 24.
84. The published version of Ismay's letters mentions a Dutchman named 'Cadonx', but this was probably a transcription error. A Mathieu Cadoux appears in the matriculation records and in the Royal College of Surgeons indenture lists.
85. Ismay, p. 60.
86. See below, Chapter Seven. Rothblatt, *Tradition and Change*, pp. 59–74, 102–116.
87. Ismay, p. 58.
88. James Rush, 10 Oct 1809, Diary during part of a stay in Scotland, Box 13, 7406 f. 46, Library Company of Philadelphia Mss held in the Historical Society of Pennsylvania.
89. Neville, p. 241. There is also anti-Irish and anti-Scottish graffiti in John Brown, *Elements of Medicine* (London: J. Johnson, 1788) and in William Cullen, *First Lines of the Practice of Physic, for the Use of Students in the University of Edinburgh* 2 vols., (Edinburgh: William Creech, 1777, 1779), in the Edinburgh University Library Rare Books Room. At the University of Pennsylvania medical school in the early 19th century, the particularly despised group were the 'Ginnie' (Virginia) students, applied to anyone from the southern states. George Corner, *Two Centuries of Medicine. A History of the School of Medicine, University of Pennsylvania* (Philadelphia: J.B. Lippincott Company, 1965), p. 72.
90. Job Harrison to his father, Edinburgh, Oct 30 1774, Letters of Job Harrison.
91. The phrase is from John Fothergill, *Chain of Friendship: Selected Letters of Dr. John Fothergill of London, 1735–1780*, ed. by B.C. Corner and C.C. Booth (Cambridge, MA: Harvard University Press, 1971). For Quaker connections in action in Edinburgh, see Bell, 'Thomas Parke'.
92. Job Harrison to his father, Edinburgh, Oct 30 1774, Letters of Job Harrison.
93. Charles Camic, *Experience and Enlightenment. Socialization for Cultural Change in Eighteenth–century Scotland* (Chicago: University of Chicago Press, 1983), pp. 181–185.
94. Neville, pp. 139–40; Rush, Diary, 7 October 1809; Lesassier, 10 November 1805, 4 April 1806.
95. Lesassier, 20 May 1805.
96. Lesassier, 28 May 1805, Journal 28 May–21 June 1805.
97. Neville, p. 138.
98. *Ibid.*, p. 215.
99. *Ibid.*, p. 224.
100. Lesassier, 10 June 1805.
101. Erik Erametsa, *A Study of the Word 'Sentimental' and of other Linguistic Characteristics of Eighteenth Century Sentimentalism in England* (Helsinki, University of Helsinki, 1951).
102. Neville, p. 151.
103. One example from Neville is p. 151, but there are many others; Lesassier, 25 December 1805; Jean de Carro, *Letters of Jean de Carro to Alexandre Marcet*,

1794–1817, ed. by Henry E. Sigerist (Baltimore: Johns Hopkins Press, 1950), p. 20.
104. Neville, p. 154.
105. *Ibid.*, p. 193.
106. Rush, Diary, 30 October 1809.
107. Lesassier, 24 April 1806.
108. Rush, Diary, 30 October 1809. For a discussion of modern medical students putting private life 'on hold' until it is professionally convenient to attend to it, see Robert S. Broadhead, *The Private Lives and Professional Identity of Medical Students* (New Brunswick: Transaction Books, 1983).
109. Lesassier, 24 April 1806.
110. Neville, p. 143.
111. *Ibid.*
112. Rush, Diary, 18 October 1809.
113. *Ibid.* For other examples of reactions to operations, see John M.T. Ford, ed., *A Medical Student at St. Thomas's Hospital, 1801–1802. The Weekes Family Letters* (London: Wellcome Institute for the History of Medicine, 1987), pp. 51–52.
114. Neville, p. 143.
115. Alexander Monro, Lectures on Anatomy and Surgery, ca. 1770, 6 vols, 5:139, College of Physicians of Philadelphia Mss 10A/91.
116. Alexander Monro, *secundus*, 'Lectures on Surgery', c. 1774–5, Royal College of Physicians of Edinburgh (RCPE) Alexander Monro, *secundus* Mss # 13, p. 237.
117. *Ibid.*
118. *Ibid.*
119. Neville, p. 143.
120. John Gregory, p. 53.
121. *Ibid.*
122. *Ibid.*
123. Ismay, p. 59.
124. *Ibid.*
125. *Medical Commentaries* 5 (1777): 333–4. Charles Darwin would have been the maternal uncle of the biologist Charles Darwin.

Chapter Three

1. David Skene to Dr Andrew Skene, Edinburgh, 5 November 1751, Skene Papers. Mss # 40. Aberdeen University Library. 'College' was an older word for lecture.
2. Whitfield J. Bell, Jr., 'Thomas Parke's Student Life in England and Scotland, 1771–1773', *The Pennsylvania Magazine of History and Biography* 75 (1951): 250; Alexander Morgan, ed, *University of Edinburgh, Charters, Statutes, and Acts of the Town Council and the Senatus, 1583–1858* (Edinburgh: Oliver and Boyd, 1937), p. 241.
3. Morgan, p. 224.
4. Edinburgh University Library (EUL) Matriculation Album, vol. I, 1766–7.
5. EUL Matriculation Album, vol. I, 1773–4.

6. Morgan, p. 244.
7. See Appendix A.
8. There was a similar unwritten rule at the University of Pennsylvania that students who attended lectures given by a professor twice did not have to pay if they attended a third course of lectures. The faculty proposed to the Board of Trustees of the University that the matriculation fee be dispensed with for third and subsequent years as well. Graduation at the University of Pennsylvania required attendance for only two years. Minutes of the Medical Faculty, 14 November 1815, University of Pennsylvania Archives Ms 1475.
9. Peter Mark Roget to his uncle, Edinburgh, 31 December 1893, cited in D.L. Emblen, *Peter Mark Roget. The Word and the Man* (New York: Thomas Y. Crowell Company, 1970), p. 22. Roget was at this point only fifteen and not yet studying medicine, but he occasionally attended Monro's lectures during the week–long vacation between Christmas and the New Years.
10. EUL Matriculation Album, vol. I, 1771–2.
11. *Edinburgh Evidence*, Appendix, p. 107.
12. The amount of work involved in this becomes apparent when the Matriculation Albums are compared with the General and Medical Registers. EUL Da. See Appendix A.
13. Glasgow University kept careful records from 1803, following the reorganization of medical teaching, but they were not as detailed or consistent as Edinburgh's. Derek Dow and Michael Moss make a similar assumption in 'The Medical Curriculum at Glasgow in The Early-Nineteenth Century', *History of Universities* 7 (1988): 227–257. The University of Pennsylvania, which modelled its medical faculty on that of Edinburgh, kept records of student enrollment consistently from 1806, but did not record the courses they attended. Ledgers of Medical Matriculation, 1806–1815, University of Pennsylvania Archives, Ms 1571; Medical Matriculation Book 1816–1834, University of Pennsylvania Archives, Ms 1576.
14. On record-keeping at the Royal Infirmary, see Michael Barfoot, 'Reading Records and Writing Hospital History', unpublished manuscript. The manuscript collection of the Royal College of Physicians of Edinburgh contains extensive records of the College's activities. For references to the Royal College of Surgeons' minutes, see Chapter Five.
15. For a few of numerous examples, see Andrew Duncan senior, *An Address to the Students of Medicine at Edinburgh* (Edinburgh, 1776); James Russell, *Remarks on the Utility and Importance of Clinical Lectures of Surgery* (Edinburgh: J&C Muirhead, 1824; James Syme, *Letter to the Right Hon. the Lord Provost, Magistrates, and Town-Council of Edinburgh, in regard to the Chair of Pathology in the University of Edinburgh* (Edinburgh, 1837); David Boswell Reid, *A Memorial to the Patrons of the University on the Present State of Practical Chemistry* (Edinburgh, 1834).
16. *Annals of Medicine 4 (1799): 532)*; These figures were printed in L.R.C. Agnew, 'Scottish Medical Education', in *The History of Medical Education*, ed. by C.D. O'Malley (Berkeley: University of California Press, 1970), p. 258.
17. Thomas Ismay, 'Letter from Thomas Ismay, Student of Medicine at Edinburgh, 1771, to his father', *University of Edinburgh Journal* 8 (1936–7): 58.
18. I have taken the schedule for the following courses from *Edinburgh Evidence*, Appendix, p. 107, but it remained the same throughout the period, though

some classes were added. See David Hosack's schedule in C.C. Robbins, *David Hosack, Citizen of New York* (Philadelphia: American Philosophical Society, 1964), p. 24.

19. Mary Hewson to her son, Thomas Tickell Hewson, 9 July 1795 Hewson Papers, B H492, vol. 2, # 32, American Philosophical Society Library, Philadelphia.

20. David Skene to Dr Andrew Skene, Edinburgh, 5 November 1751, Skene Papers.

21. Botany was only supposed to cost two guineas, but George Logan complained of the Botany Professor that 'such is his meanness that he will take three guineas not only the first but the second year'. Logan to Charles Logan, Edinburgh, March 2, 1778, Letter Book, Historical Society of Pennsylvania, cited in Whitfield J. Bell, Jr., 'Philadelphia Medical Students in Europe, 1750–1800', *The Pennsylvania Magazine of History and Biography* 67 (1943): 11. The price of all courses had risen to four guineas by 1822. Alexander Bower, *The Edinburgh Student's Guide: Or an account of the classes of the University arranged under the four faculties; with a detail of what is taught in each* (Edinburgh: Waugh and Innes, 1822), p. xxiv.

22. J. Johnson, *A Guide for Gentlemen Studying Medicine at the University of Edinburgh* (London: J. Robinson, 1792). Both of the Hamiltons were outspoken in their opposition to the medical faculty, and the *Guide* criticized certain professors severely; it also claimed that Midwifery was unfairly kept from being a requirement for the MD. J.D. Comrie, *History of Scottish Medicine*, 2 vols. (London: The Wellcome Historical Medical Museum, 1932), 1:305; *Dictionary of National Biography*, s.v. 'Hamilton, James, the Younger'.

23. Students frequently obtained information about courses from other students, but the information was not always reliable, since it was filtered through their own or their informer's perceptions. This chapter provides many examples, but see especially the cases of William Black and James Mosely, Chapter Four.

24. *Guide*, p. 5.

25. Comrie, 1:320; R.E. Wright-St.Clair, *Doctors Monro: A Medical Saga* (London: The Wellcome Historical Medical Library, 1964).

26. A. Logan Turner, *Story of a Great Hospital. The Royal Infirmary of Edinburgh* (Edinburgh: Oliver and Boyd, 1937), p. 144; Alexander Grant, *The Story of the University of Edinburgh during its First Three Hundred Years* 2 vols. (London: Longmans, Green, and Co., 1884), 1:321–2.

27. *Guide*, p. 5.

28. *Ibid.*, p. 6.

29. Logan to Charles Logan, Edinburgh, 2 March 1778, cited in Bell, 'Philadelphia Medical Students', p. 11.

30. Alexander Monro, Lectures on Anatomy and Surgery, ca. 1770, 6 vols, College of Physicians of Philadelphia Mss 10A/91. John Bell, discussed in Chapter Five, was a more receptive student than Logan.

31. Cited in Bell, 'Philadelphia Medical Students', p. 11.

32. Comrie, 2:628.

33. Dow and Moss, p. 244.

34. R.B. McDowell and D.A. Webb, *Trinity College Dublin 1592–1952* (Cambridge: Cambridge University Press, 1982), p. 89.

35. See below, Chapter Nine.
36. *Edinburgh Evidence*, Appendix, p. 266.
37. List of Students of Anatomy and Surgery 1814/15–1821/32, Ms. Department of Anatomy, Edinburgh University, courtesy of Dr. Michael Barfoot. Practical Anatomy was listed in the matriculation album for 1804, but systematic records were not kept of student attendance. C.J. Lawrence, 'The Edinburgh Medical School and the End of the "Old Thing" 1790–1830' *History of Universities* 7 (1988): 265–268, gives an excellent analysis of the interaction between Monro *tertius'* course and extra-academical anatomy classes.
38. For a discussion of the relationship between Cullen and Black, see Arthur L. Donovan, *Philosophical Chemistry in the Scottish Enlightenment: The Doctrines and Discoveries of William Cullen and Joseph Black* (Edinburgh: Edinburgh University Press, 1975), especially pp. 165–182.
39. Thomas Parke's journal, Pemberton Papers, LVII, 93–98, Historical Society of Pennsylvania, cited in Whitfield J. Bell, Jr., 'Thomas Parke's Student Life in England and Scotland, 1771–1773', *The Pennsylvania Magazine of History and Biography* 75 (1951): 249.
40. John Gregory, *Observations on the Duties and Offices of a Physician; and on the Method of Prosecuting Inquiries in Philosophy* (London: W. Strahan, 1770), p. 69. For a detailed discussion of Gregory's philosophy, see C.J. Lawrence, 'Medicine as Culture: Edinburgh and the Scottish Enlightenment' (Ph.D. Dissertation, University of London, 1984), pp. 253–311.
41. *Guide*, p. 17.
42. Logan to Charles Logan, Edinburgh, 2 March 1778, cited in Bell, 'Philadelphia Medical Students', p. 11.
43. Sylas Neville, *The Diary of Sylas Neville, 1767–1788*, ed. by Basil Cozens-Hardy (London: Oxford University Press, 1950), p. 216.
44. For chemistry as a fashionable subject, see J.B. Morrell, 'Practical Chemistry in the University of Edinburgh', *Ambix* 16 (1969): 66–80; and Steven Shapin, 'The Audience for Science in Eighteenth Century Edinburgh, *Hist. of Science* 12 (1974): 95–110.
45. *Guide*, p. 32.
46. James Ford, 'What is the best method for studying medicine considering its different branches in order . . . so as to obtain the greatest advantage possible, considering also their mutual dependency and necessary collateral sciences?' Royal Medical Society (RMS) Dissertations, November 1778, 11:158.
47. David Skene to Andrew Skene, Edinburgh, November 1751, Skene papers. Albrecht Haller (1708–77) was a prominent physiologist, and his textbook, *First Lines of Physiology*, went through many editions.
48. Cited in Bell, 'Thomas Parke', p. 249.
49. As he was described by Richard Kentish Jr, 'On Gout', Dissertations, 1783–4, 15:432, and Thomas Parke and Benjamin Rush, respectively, cited in Bell, 'Philadelphia Medical Students', p. 13.
50. Comrie, 1:314. The letter, signed by 160 students, is cited by John Thomson, *An Account of the Life, Lectures, and Writings of William Cullen, MD*, 2 vols. (Edinburgh: William Blackwood and Sons, 1859), 1:155–8.
51. Lisa Rosner, 'Students and Apprentices: Medical Education at Edinburgh

University 1760–1805' (Ph.D. Thesis, The Johns Hopkins University, 1985), p. 82; EUL Matriculation Album, vol 1, 1769–1772.
52. *Ibid.*
53. Ismay, p. 58.
54. For a discussion of Cullen's Nosology, see Lawrence, 'Medicine as Culture' pp. 347–371.
55. *Dictionary of Scientific Biography*, s.v. 'Linnaeus, Carl', by Sten Lindroth.
56. William Cullen, 'Clinical Lectures' [1770?], College of Physicians of Philadelphia Mss 10a/247, Lecture Five.
57. Ford, p. 158.
58. James Gregory, 'Notes from Dr Gregory's Lectures on practice of Physic 1817–18', College of Physicians of Philadelphia. Mss 10a/249, pp. 1–15; *Guide*, p. 33, for the persistence of nosologies in teaching see Thomas Young, *An Introduction to Medical Literature, including A System of Practical Nosology. Intended as a Guide to Students, and an Assistant to Practitioners.* (London: W. Phillips, 1823).
59. Neville, p. 198.
60. Comrie, 1:311.
61. Lawrence, 'Medicine as Culture'.
62. *Guide*, p. 20.
63. William Cullen, *Works of William Cullen, MD*, John Thomson, ed., 2 vols. (Edinburgh: William Blackwood, 1827), 1:3.
64. *Dictionary of National Biography*, s.v. 'Duncan, Andrew, The Elder;' Lisa Rosner, 'Andrew Duncan MD, FRSE, 1744–1828', *Scottish Men of Medicine Series*, Edinburgh: History of Medicine and Science Unit, 1981.
65. See below, Chapter Nine.
66. In 1792, when David Hosack studied, Duncan taught Medical Theory at 8 am, and James Home taught Materia Medica at 11 am, but that seems to have been an unusual schedule. Robbins, p. 24, but see Ismay, p. 58.
67. Not all did. Professors Cullen and John Gregory gave the clinical lectures for several years; James Gregory and James Home did as well. *Edinburgh Evidence*, p. 200. Michael Barfoot, 'Clinical Medicine at the Edinburgh Royal Infirmary in the Eighteenth Century', Paper presented at the Wellcome Seminar, 27 March, 1985; Guenther Risse, *Hospital Life in Enlightenment Scotland: Care and Teaching at the Royal Infirmary of Edinburgh* (Cambridge: Cambridge University Press, 1986), p. 242–6.
68. *Guide*, p. 37.
69. See Risse, pp. 240–278, for a detailed description of the mechanics of clinical teaching. Historians have generally ascribed the success of the medical school to the clinical facilities at the Royal Infirmary. L.R.C. Agnew, 'Scottish Medical Education', in *The History of Medical Education*, ed by C.D. O'Malley (Berkeley: University of California Press, 1970), p. 259; David Hamilton, *The Healers. A History of Medicine in Scotland* (Edinburgh: Canongate, 1981), p. 125.
70. P.M. Eaves Walton, 'The Early Years in the Infirmary', in *The Early Years of the Edinburgh Medical School*, ed by R.G.W. Anderson and A.D.C. Simpson (Edinburgh: Royal Scottish Museum, 1976), p. 77.
71. David Skene to Andrew Skene, Edinburgh, 13 November 1751, Skene Papers.
72. Josef Frank, *Reise nach Paris, London, und Einem Grossen Theile des Uebrigen*

England und Schottlands in Bezeihung auf Spitaeler. Versorgunghaeuser, und Gefaengnisse (Vienna: Camesina, 1804), part 2:228.

73. See below, Chapter Five.
74. Samuel Powell Griffitts to Benjamin Rush, London, 10 Aug. 1783, Rush Mss, cited in Bell, 'Philadelphia Medical Students', p. 15. Many Americans came to Edinburgh for the lectures, but went to London for practical experience. Jane Rendall, 'The Influence of the Edinburgh Medical School on America in the Eighteenth Century', in Anderson and Simpson, p. 103.
75. Howard S. Becker, Blanche Geer, Everett C. Hughes, Anselm L. Strauss, *Boys in White. Student Culture in Medical School* (New Brunswick, NJ: Transaction Books, 1977), pp. 221–254, 329–331.
76. Neville, p. 208.
77. Gregory's lectures began with a discussion of the importance of practical bedside experience. See Chapter Two, above.
78. Samuel Lewis to Mrs. W.P. Hinds, Edinburgh, 12 October 1837, Samuel Lewis Correspondence, Edinburgh University Library GEN 1429/8.
79. Ismay, p. 60.
80. *Guide*, pp. 26–7.
81. *Edinburgh Almanack*, 1793.
82. *Guide*, p. 26.
83. Ismay, p. 58.
84. *Guide*, p. 24.
85. Neville, p. 152.
86. *Guide*, p. 24.
87. Neville, p. 203.
88. Job Harrison to his father, Edinburgh, 2 July 1775, Chester City Record Office Ref. G/H.S. 99.
89. *Guide*, p. 14.
90. Comrie does not mention the course, and no professor is listed in the Matriculation Album.
91. Samuel Bard to John Bard, Edinburgh, 7 February 1764, Bard Papers, New York Academy of Medicine Library.
92. *Ibid.*
93. Neville, p. 205.
94. *Ibid.*
95. Robbins, p. 24.
96. Neville, p. 189.
97. *Dictionary of National Biography*, s.v. 'Duncan, Andrew, the Elder'.
98. Morrell, pp. 66–80.
99. EUL Matriculation Album, vol. I, 1776–7; *Medical Commentaries* 4 (1776): 355.
100. *Medical Commentaries* 5 (1777): 220–223; *Medical Commentaries* 6 (1779): 353–355.
101. James Hamilton to Lord and Lady Balgonie, Edinburgh, 31 March 1802, Leven and Melville, SRO GD26/13/846.
102. On the demand for certification, see Chapter Eight.
103. James Rush to Benjamin Rush, 23 October 1809, Rush Papers, Yi2, Box 11, 7404, F25a, Historical Society of Pennsylvania.
104. David Skene to Andrew Skene, Edinburgh, Nov. 1751, Skene Papers.
105. Letters from George Skene to Dr. David Skene, Skene Papers.

106. Neville, pp. 134, 137–8.
107. Ismay, p. 57.
108. Neville, p. 137–8; *Edinburgh Evidence*, p. 263.
109. Ismay, pp. 57–9.
110. *Ibid.*, p. 60. 'Dr Innis' was John Innes.
111. E.G.W. Bill, *Education at Christ Church Oxford 1600–1800* (Oxford: Claren-
     don Press, 1988), pp. 218–223, 245–326, has found that serious study
     increased in the late 18th century, but student schedules were still not nearly
     as rigorous as at Edinburgh. For further comparison see L.W. Brockliss,
     *French Higher Education in the Seventeenth and Eighteenth Centuries. A Cultural
     History* (Oxford: Oxford University Press, 1987), pp. 63–4, 95–109.
112. Benjamin Rush, *Letters of Benjamin Rush*, ed. by L.H. Butterfield, 2 vols.
     (Princeton: Princeton University Press, 1951), 1:40.
113. For example, Neville, pp. 155, 171, 217.
114. Alexander Lesassier [later Hamilton], 13 December 1805, Alexander Hamil-
     ton Collection, Box 11, Folder 77, Library of the Royal College of Physicians
     of Edinburgh, Edinburgh.
115. Neville, p. 155; *Edinburgh Evidence*, Appendix, p. 204.
116. *Edinburgh Evidence*, p. 204.
117. David Skene to Andrew Skene, Edinburgh, 13 November 1751, Skene
     papers.
118. Mary Hewson to her son, Thomas Tickell Hewson, 7 July 1795 Hewson
     Papers.

Chapter Four

1. Sylas Neville, *The Diary of Sylas Neville, 1767–1788*, ed. by Basil Cozens-
   Hardy (London: Oxford University Press, 1950), p. 226.
2. Taken from the '*Sponsio Academicae Edinburgenae nunc ad Gradum in Medicina
   Doctoralem capessendum*', the oath required of all graduates in medicine,
   printed in *List of the graduates in medicine in the University of Edinburgh from
   MDCCV to MDCCCLXVI* (Edinburgh: Neill & Co., 1867), p. iv.
3. Alexander Morgan, ed, *University of Edinburgh, Charters, Statutes, and Acts of
   the Town Council and the Senatus, 1583–1858* (Edinburgh: Oliver and Boyd,
   1937), p. 174. J.B. Morrell has suggested, however, that the Town Council
   intended from the first to link teaching with graduation. J.B. Morrell, 'The
   Edinburgh Town Council and its University, 1717–1766', in *The Early Years
   of the Edinburgh Medical School*, ed. by R.G.W. Anderson and A.D.C.
   Simpson (Edinburgh: Royal Scottish Museum, 1976), pp. 50–1. The Town
   Council minute cited by Morgan was omitted in 1726, but inserted on 26
   August 1747. Rosalie Stott, 'The Incorporation of Surgeons and Medical
   Education and Practice in Edinburgh 1696–1755' (Ph.D. Dissertation,
   University of Edinburgh, 1984), p. 137, implies that it was inserted to
   provide a precedent for the appointment by the Town Council of Robert
   Whytt as Professor of Medicine.
4. Morgan, p. 248. Translated in Alexander Grant, *The Story of the University
   of Edinburgh during Its First Three Hundred Years*, 2 vols. (London: Longman,
   Green & Co., 1884), 1:248; John Thomson, *An Account of the Life, Lectures,*

and Writings of William Cullen, MD, 2 vols.(Edinburgh: William Blackwood and Sons, 1859), 1:464.

5. Morgan, p. 253, translated in Grant, 1:330.
6. Morgan, p. 254.
7. Thomson, 1:463. Thomson was citing John Coakley Lettson's biography of Fothergill.
8. Thomson, 1–463–472.
9. EUL Matriculation Albums, vol. I, 1764–5, 1765–6. David Hamilton, *The Healers. A History of Medicine in Scotland* (Edinburgh: Canongate, 1981), p. 144, based his account of the incident on Thomson.
10. Samuel Bard to John Bard, Edinburgh, 4 September 1764, Bard Papers, New York Academy of Medicine Library.
11. Journal of George Logan, 2 March 1778, Historical Society of Pennsylvania, cited in Jane Rendall, 'The Influence of the Edinburgh Medical School on America in the Eighteenth Century', in Anderson and Simpson, p. 102.
12. Lisa Rosner, 'Students and Apprentices: Medical Education at Edinburgh University 1760–1805' (Ph.D. Thesis, The Johns Hopkins University, 1985), Table 5.1, p. 150.
13. Samuel Bard to John Bard, Edinburgh, 2 June 1764, Bard Papers.
14. Thomas Ruston Papers, College of Physicians of Philadelphia, Hirsch #931, Folder 1, Item 2.
15. This incident is discussed in Juanita G.L. Burnby, *A Study of the English Apothecary from 1660 to 1760*, (London: Wellcome Institute for the History of Medicine, 1983), pp. 88–89. For a later example of student concern over unsuitable persons obtaining Edinburgh degrees, see Neville, p. 218.
16. William Black, *A State of Facts, relative to William Black, Student of Medicine* (Edinburgh, 1770), p. 7.
17. *Ibid.*, p. 13.
18. *Ibid.*, p. 23.
19. Morgan, p. 254. Grant refers to the 1783 notice as a new regulation, 1:331.
20. Adam Smith to William Cullen, London, 20 September 1774, cited in Thomson, 1:477–8.
21. *Ibid.*, 1:486.
22. Neville, p. 217. See William Pulteney Alison's account of this, in *Edinburgh Evidence*, p. 192.
23. Joseph Black to Worthington, 1792, EUL Gen 875/111/251*F. Black was in part responding to J. Johnson, *A Guide for Gentlemen Studying Medicine at the University of Edinburgh* (London: J. Robinson, 1792), which, he said, implied that students did have to pay the professor of a given course in order to graduate even if they had taken the course elsewhere.
24. Rendall, p. 102.
25. See the description of graduation examinations, below.
26. J.B. Morrell, 'The Edinburgh Town Council'; J.R.R. Christie, 'The Origins and Development of the Scottish Scientific Community, 1680–1760', *History of Science* 12 (1974): 122–141; George W. Corner, *Two Centuries of Medicine. A History of the School of Medicine, University of Pennsylvania* (Philadelphia: J.B. Lippincott Company, 1965), pp. 1–48.
27. Samuel Bard to John Bard, Edinburgh, 4 September 1764, Bard Papers.
28. Robert Christison, 'Memorial To The Principal and Professors of the

University of Edinburgh', 13 Oct 1824, EUL P.470/26, p. 4. This letter
was presented to the Royal Commission, and included in *Edinburgh Evidence*,
pp. 321–325.

29. Howard S. Becker, Blanche Geer, Everett C. Hughes, Anselm L. Strauss,
Boys in White. Student Culture in Medical School (New Brunswick, NJ:
Transaction Books, 1977), pp. 65–184.

30. Becker et al, pp. 107–134.

31. Christison, p. 8.

32. See above, Chapter Three.

33. George Logan's Journal, cited in Rendall, p. 102.

34. Neville, p. 138.

35. David MacLagan, Dedication to *De sanitate tuenda* (Edinburgh: A. Neill &
Co., 1805).

36. James Vernon, Dedication to *Dissertatio medica inauguralis de diabete* (Edinburgh: R.Allen, 1796).

37. James Chew, Dedication to *Dissertatio medica inauguralis de animi affectionibus*
(Edinburgh: G. Mudie & Sons, 1795).

38. Neville, p. 167.

39. The Dean was 'generally the youngest member of the Medical Faculty, having
more trouble than any other', according to Professor William Pulteney
Alison. *Edinburgh Evidence*, p. 191. The Dean took care of all the paperwork
required for graduation such as checking class tickets, arranging the time
and place of examination and keeping the medical faculty minutes.

40. Morgan, p. 262. See Chapter Nine.

41. Neville, p. 217.

42. For examples, see Neville, pp. 170, 214.

43. *Ibid.*, p. 217.

44. *Ibid.*, p. 20.

45. *Ibid.*, p. 219.

46. Other Edinburgh university regulations had been written in English from
the late seventeenth century. See Morgan, p. 216, and Grant, 1:330.

47. George Jardine, *Outlines of Philosophical Education, Illustrated the Method of
Teaching the Logic Class in the University of Glasgow* (Glasgow: University Press,
1825), p. 469. Jardine's book was extremely influential; see below, Part
Two.

48. Robert Christison, *The Life of Sir Robert Christison, Bart.* 2 vols. (Edinburgh:
William Blackwood and Sons, 1885), 1:157–161, cited in J.D. Comrie,
History of Scottish Medicine, 2 vols. (London: The Wellcome Historical Medical
Museum, 1932), 2:476.

49. Edinburgh Evidence, p. 208. Giving grinders official status as medical tutors
was frequently recommended, especially as a way of getting around the
problem of professors not having time to examine students in large classes,
pp. 288, 346, 453, 459, 568.

50. Archibald Robertson, *Colloquia Anatomica, Physiologica atque Chemica, Quaestionibus et Responsis, ad usum Ingenuae Juventutis Accommodata* (Edinburgh: C.
Stewart, 1814). p. iv. According to his preface, Robertson gave lectures on
medical subjects. *Colloquia Anatomica*, p. iv. For similar books aimed at
surgeons, see below, Chapter Eight.

51. William Cullen. *Synopsis Nosologiae Methodicae, exhibens clariss. virorum
Sauvagesii, Linaei, Vogelii, Sagari et Macbridii, systemata nosologica: edidit*

suumque proprium systema, nosologicum adjecit Gulielmus Cullen, MD (Edinburgh: William Creech, 1803). This is one of many editions, and included an English translation of the Nosology.

52. *Edinburgh Evidence*, p. 203.

53. Hippocrates' aphorisms were no longer proposed by the 1820s.

54. See the requirements for entrance to the Royal College of Physicians of Edinburgh, discussed in R.P. Ritchie, *The Early Days of the Royall Colledge of Phisitians, Edinburgh* (Edinburgh: George P. Johnston, 1899), pp. 93–98, and degree requirements for Leyden discussed in G.A. Lindeboom, 'Medical Education in the Netherlands 1575–1750', in *The History of Medical Education*, ed by C.D. O'Malley (Berkeley: University of California Press, 1970), p. 203. See also 'Commentaries on Selected Aphorisms of Hippocrates, by Sir John Pringle and D.A. Foulis . . . for membership in the Royal College of Physicians of Edinburgh', Library of the Royal College of Physicians of Edinburgh (RCPE), Hippocrates Mss # 1. Commentaries on an aphorism of Hippocrates and a case history were graduation requirements in Italy at the end of the 16th century. Richard Palmer, *The Studio of Venice and its Graduates in the Sixteenth Century* (Padua: Edizioni LINT, 1983), pp. 37–8.

55. Minutes and Proceedings of the Medical Faculty 1776–1811, EUL M. Dup 171; Minutes of the Medical Faculty 1811–1831, EUL.

56. Morgan, p. 255.

57. See the account of Neville's examination, below.

58. Samuel Bard to John Bard, Edinburgh, 15 May 1765, Bard Papers.

59. *Ibid.*

60. Celsus, *De re medica, accessurus index vocabulorum omnium, et cujuscunque ad rem pertinentis more dictionarii. In usum humanitatis medicinae studiosorum.* (Glasgow: Foulis, 1766), p. 1.

61. Celsus, *Of Medicine, In Eight Books*, trans. James Grieve (London: D. Wilson & T. Durham, 1756).

62. William Cullen, 'Clinical Lectures' [1770?], College of Physicians of Philadelphia Mss 10a/247.

63. Neville, p. 218.

64. Jones' view of the case is contained in Robert Jones, *An Inquiry into the State of Medicine, on the Principles of Inductive Philosophy*, (Edinburgh: C. Elliot, 1781). Andrew Duncan senior's view is in *A Letter to Dr. Robert Jones of Caermarthenshire, in Answer to the Account which he has published of the case of Mr. John Braham Isaacson Student of Medicine, and to the Injurious Aspersions which He Has Thrown Out Against the Physicians who Attended Mr. Isaacson* (Edinburgh: C. Elliot, 1782). See also Michael Barfoot, 'Brunonianism under the bed: an alternative to university medicine in Edinburgh in the 1780s,' in *Brunonianism in Britain and Europe*, ed. by W.F. Bynum and Roy Porter (London: Wellcome Institute for the History of Medicine, 1988), pp. 22–45.

65. Minutes and Proceedings of the Medical Faculty 1776–1811.

66. Samuel Bard to John Bard, 15 May 1765, Bard Papers.

67. Neville, p. 218.

68. Cullen, *Synopsis Nosologiae Methodicae*, Class, Ord. III, Genus 62., p. 313.

69. Samuel Bard to John Bard, 15 May 1765, Bard Papers.

70. Thomas Ruston to Mr. De Berdt, Edinburgh, 18 August 1765, Thomas Ruston Papers, folder 1, item 1.

71. List, n.d., Thomas Ruston Papers, folder 3. There is no guarantee that the list was drawn up by Ruston, since it is neither signed nor dated.
72. Christison, *Life*, cited in Comrie, 2:478.
73. Neville, p. 219.
74. In 1823 John Wilson Anderson, Professor Thomas Charles Hope's assistant, offered courses on practical chemistry within the University buildings. There were extra-academical courses from 1800. Since they were not taught by medical faculty, they do not appear in the matriculation albums, and we do not know how many students attended them. J.B. Morrell, 'Practical Chemistry in the University of Edinburgh', *Ambix* 16 (1969): 66–80.
75. Joseph Black, *De humore acido a cibis orto, et Magnesia Alba*, (Edinburgh: Balfour and Smellie, 1754).
76. Arthur L. Donovan, *Philosophical Chemistry in the Scottish Enlightenment: The Doctrines and Discoveries of William Cullen and Joseph Black* (Edinburgh: Edinburgh University Press, 1975), pp. 168–80.
77. *Edinburgh Evidence*, p. 204. For similar discussion, see the pamphlet included in the Minutes of the Medical Faculty of the University of Pennsylvania, 1800-1811, University of Pennsylvania Archives Ms. 1475.
78. Donovan, pp. 168–180.
79. Daniel Rutherford, *De Aere Fixo Dicto, Aut Mephitico* (Edinburgh: Balfour and Smellie, 1772).
80. William Meade, *De Aquis Mineralibus* (Edinburgh: Balfour and Smellie, 1790.
81. William Meade, *An experimental inquiry into the chemical properties and medicinal qualities of the principal mineral waters of Ballston and Saratoga; in the state of New-York (Philadelphia: Harrison Hall, 1817).*
82. *Benjamin Rush, De Coctione Ciborum in Ventriculo* (Edinburgh: Balfour and Smellie, 1768); Benjamin Rush, *The Autobiography of Benjamin Rush, his 'Travels Through Life' together with his Commonplace Book for 1789–1813*, ed. by George W. Corner, (Princeton: Princeton University Press, 1948), p. 434.
83. George Kellie, *De Electricitate Animali Complectans* (Edinburgh: Alex. Smellie, 1803).
84. Alexander Philip Wilson, *De Dyspepsia* (Edinburgh: Balfour and Smellie, 1792).
85. Lisa Rosner, 'Eighteenth-Century Medical Education and the Didactic Model of Experiment', in *The Literary Structure of Scientific Knowledge: Historical Studies*, ed. by Peter Dear (Philadelphia: University of Pennsylvania Press, 1991), pp. 182–194.
86. Hugh Owen, 'De Contagione', *Thesaurus Medicus Edinburgensis Novis: sive, dissertationum in Academia Edinensi, ad rem medicam pertinentium, ab anno 1759 ad annum 1785, delectus, ab illustri Societate Regia Medica Edinensi habitus*, 4 vols. (Edinburgh: G. Elliot, 1785), 3:365.
87. Neville, p. 220.
88. *Ibid.*
89. Minutes and Proceedings of the Medical Faculty 1776–1811.
90. Neville, p. 221.
91. *Ibid.*, p. 222.
92. *Ibid.*, p. 223.
93. Thomas Beddoes, Biographical Preface to *Elements of Medicine of John Brown*

(Portsmouth, New Hampshire: Oracle Press, 1803), p. xlix. Professor William Pulteney Alison also thought most students wrote their theses in English, and had help translating them into Latin. *Edinburgh Evidence*, p. 204.

94. *Ibid.* Beddoes was trying to discredit Brown, who he claimed had paid his way through Edinburgh in part by translating and writing theses.
95. Neville, p. 223.
96. *Ibid.*, p. 225. Neville had his erstwhile friend Baker in mind.
97. James Jeffray to William Hamilton, Professor in Glasgow, Edinburgh, 2 January 1783, Letters to Thomas and William Hamilton, RCPE, Hamilton, Family of, Mss # 1, 'Letters to Thomas Hamilton, and to his son William, c. 1778–9'. Jeffray became Professor of Anatomy at Glasgow University.
98. Taken from Samuel Allvey, 'Erysepelas', RMS Dissertation, 1786–7, 20:279, but the idea found frequent expression at Edinburgh.
99. John Wainman, *De Epilepsia* (Edinburgh: Balfour and Smellie, 1781).
100. Cited in Jones, p. 270.
101. *Ibid., p. 371.*
102. *Ibid., p. 371. Edinburgh Evidence*, p. 259.
103. Jones., p. 371.
104. James Jeffray to William Hamilton, Edinburgh, 8 May 1783, Hamilton, Family of, Mss. # 1.
105. Morgan, p. 255.
106. Neville, p. 223.
107. George Logan's Journal, 2 March 1778, cited in Rendall, p. 102.
108. Minutes and Proceedings of the Medical Faculty 1776–1811.
109. Daniel Rutherford, 'Essays by Students on Medical Subjects Proposed by Daniel Rutherford ca. 1788–90', EUL Mss DC 5.10.
110. Robert Christison, *The Life of Sir Robert Christison, Bart.*, 2 vols. (Edinburgh: William Blackwood and Sons, 1885), cited in Comrie, 2:478.
111. Hippocrates, *The Aphorisms of Hippocrates and the Sentences of Celsus with Explanations and References to the most considerable writers in Physic and Philosophy, both Ancient and Modern, 2nd edition*, e.d. by Sir Conrad Sprengel (London: R. Wilkin, 1735), Book 1, Aphorism 17, p. 15. During examinations, aphorisms were proposed and commented on in Latin. All translations of the aphorisms in the text are taken from Sprengel's edition. This work seems to have been a translation of one of the editions of *Hippocratis Aphorismi, variorum auctorum, maxime Hippocratis et Celsi, locis parallelis illustrati, subjiciuntur Celsi Sententiae*, trans. and ed. by Theodore Jansson van Almeloveen. The earliest edition I have seen is Amsterdam: Henric Wetsten, 1685. It was reprinted frequently throughout the eighteenth century, and contained a handy index to the subjects treated in Hippocrates' aphorisms for students and other writers, who wished to be able to cite an appropriate aphorism in their work. For a late example of the continued adaptation of the *Aphorisms* to medical teaching, see Elias Marks, *The Aphorisms of Hippocrates, from the Latin of Verhoofd, with a Literal Translation on the Opposite Page and Explanatory Notes. The Work Intended as a Book of Reference to the Medical Student* (New York: Collins and Co., 1817).
112. James Gregory, *Conspectus Medicinae Theoreticae. Ad usum academicum* (Edinburgh: Elliot, 1788).

113. Sprengel, *Hippocrates Aphorisms*, Book 2, Aphorism 29, p. 31.

114. The citation from Celsus in Harries' essay appears van Almeloveen, *Hippocratis Aphorismi*, 'Celsi Sententiae', which suggests it had had a long history of use in medical teaching.

115. Rutherford, EUL DC 5.10, Nicholas Bindon, 1788; Sprengel, *Hippocrates Aphorisms*, Book 2, Aphorism 2, p. 21.

116. Rutherford, EUL DC 5.10, Joseph Redhead, 1789; Sprengel, *Hippocrates Aphorisms*, Book 2, Aphorism 33, p. 41.

117. Rutherford, EUL DC 5.10, Henry Stanistreet, 1787, George Kittsom, 1788; Sprengel, *Hippocrates Aphorisms*, Book 2, Aphorism 13, p. 27.

118. Rutherford, EUL DC 5.10, Henry Stanistreet, 1787.

119. *Ibid.*

120. William Cullen, *First Lines of the Practice of Physic, for the use of Students in the University of Edinburgh*, 2 vols. (Philadelphia: Edward Parker, 1820).

121. Rutherford, EUL DC 5.10, Henry Stanistreet, 1787; Cullen, *First Lines*, 1: para. 49, pp. 118–9.

122. Rutherford, EUL DC 5.10, George Kittsom, 1788. These and subsequent translations of questions are my own.

123. Rutherford, EUL DC 5.10, Andrew Mitchell, 1789.

124. Rutherford, EUL DC 5.10, James Fletcher, 1790.

125. Rutherford, EUL DC 5.10, Robert McCausland, 1789.

126. Rutherford, EUL DC 5.10, John Eiston, 1788.

127. This case was recorded as being proposed by James Gregory. Rutherford, EUL DC 5.10, Thomas Trotter, 1788.

128. Rutherford, EUL DC 5.10, Thomas Trotter, 1788; Cullen, *Synopsis Nosologiae Methodicae*, Class II, Ord. I, Gen. 42, p. 274.

129. Cullen, *Synopsis Nosologiae Methodicae*, English translation included in volume, p. 98.

130. Rutherford, EUL DC 5.10, Thomas Trotter, 1788: Cullen, *First Lines*, 2: para. 1094–1097, pp. 66–7.

131. Rutherford, EUL DC 5.10, Thomas Trotter, 1788.

132. Cullen, *First Lines*, 2: para. 1099–1100, pp. 68–74.

133. Neville, p. 225.

134. *Ibid.*

135. Printed in the *List of graduates*, p. vi. Quakers could swear a separate oath that did not mention God.

136. Neville, p. 226.

137. See below, Chapter Seven.

138. Neville, p. 225.

139. *Ibid.*, p. 227.

140. *Ibid.*, p. 226.

Chapter Five

1. Fellow of the Royal College of Surgeons of Edinburgh. 'Mr. Brown on Surgical Apprenticeships' *Edinburgh Medical and Surgical Journal* 26 (1826): 82–3.

2. For my analysis of course attendance patterns I am consider 'apprentices' to be students who are listed in the Minutes of the Royal College of Surgeons

of Edinburgh as indentured to Fellows, in order to maintain consistency over the period. Unfortunately, this means that my own list of apprentices is too low by approximately twenty, since relatives of Fellows who were indentured sometimes evaded the booking fee and thus did not appear in the RCSE Minutes. For the course attendance of Fellows between 1763 and 1805, see Lisa Rosner, 'Students and Apprentices: Medical Education at Edinburgh University 1760–1805' (Ph.D. Thesis, The Johns Hopkins University, 1985), Table 6.1, p. 212, Table III.2 and III.3, p. 401. Information on Fellows comes from *List of the Fellows of the Royal College of Surgeons of Edinburgh from the year 1581 to 31st December 1873* (Edinburgh: George Robb, 1874), and on apprentices and Fellows from RCSE Minutes, vols 4–9, 1708–1828.

3. Oswei Temkin, 'The Role of Surgery in the Rise of Modern Medical Thought', *Bulletin of the History of Medicine* 25 (1951): 252–3.
4. Temkin, p. 253.
5. There is a substantial literature on the 'rise of the surgeons'. Erwin H. Ackerknecht, *Medicine at the Paris Hospital* (Baltimore: Johns Hopkins University Press, 1967): Toby Gelfand, *Professionalizing Modern Medicine. Paris Surgeons and Medical Science and Institutions in the 18th Century* (Westport, Conn.: Greenwood Press, 1980): Michael B. Burke, *The Royal College of San Carlos. Surgery and Spanish Medical Reform in the Late Eighteenth Century*, (Durham, N.C.: Duke University Press, 1977). On pathological anatomy see Russell Maulitz, *Morbid Appearances. The Anatomy of Pathology in the Early Nineteenth Century* (Cambridge: Cambridge University Press, 1987): Susan Lawrence, 'Science and Medicine at the London Hospitals. The Development of Teaching and Research 1750–1815' (Ph.D. Thesis, University of Toronto, 1985); John Lesch, *Science and Medicine in France: The Emergence of Experimental Physiology, 1790–1855* (Cambridge, MA: Harvard University Press, 1984).
6. Guenther Risse, *Hospital Life in Enlightenment Scotland: Care and Teaching at the Royal Infirmary of Edinburgh* (Cambridge: Cambridge University Press, 1986), pp. 291–2; Michael Barfoot, 'Reading Records and Writing Hospital History', pp. 29–30: see Temkin, pp. 256–259.
7. Clarendon Hyde Creswell, *The Royal College of Surgeons of Edinburgh. Historical Notes from 1505 to 1905* (Edinburgh: Oliver & Boyd, 1926), p. 122; Rosalie Stott, 'The Incorporation of Surgeons and Medical Education and Practice in Edinburgh 1696–1755' (Ph.D. Dissertation, University of Edinburgh, 1984), p. 85.
8. Rosalie Stott, 'The Battle for Students: Medical Teaching in Edinburgh in the First Half of the Eighteenth Century', in *Edinburgh's Infirmary* (Edinburgh: Scottish Society of the History of Medicine, 1979), p. 3.
9. See below, Chapter Eight. For a good discussion of Dundas' influence, see Alexander Murdoch, *The People Above. Politics and Administration in Mid-Eighteenth Century Scotland* (Edinburgh: John Donald Publishers Ltd., 1980), and Alexander Murdoch, 'The Importance of Being Edinburgh: Management and Opposition in Edinburgh Politics, 1746–1784', *Scottish Historical Review* 173 (1983): 1–16. Ronald M. Sunter, *Patronage and Politics in Scotland 1707–1832* (Edinburgh: John Donald Publishers Ltd, 1986) gives a detailed picture of the unreformed patronage system at work.
10. RCSE papers, 'Indentures 1709–1811'.
11. RCSE Minutes, 6:210, 1 May 1782.

12. Taken from RCSE Minutes, 6:447, 12 September 1793, but apparently in effect from the 1780s.
13. John Bell to Lord Kames, 1780, Abercairny, SRO GD24/1/590. Bell graduated MD in 1779. Probably some of the nine years were spent in Arts courses, because he later extolled the value of a classical education. John Bell, *Letters on Professional Character and Manners: on the Education of a Surgeon, and the Duties and Qualifications of a Physician: addressed to James Gregory, M.D* (Edinburgh: John Muir, 1810), p. 355.
14. John Bell, *Answer for the junior members of the Royal College of Surgeons of Edinburgh to the Memorial of Dr. James Gregory* (Edinburgh: Peter Hill, 1800), section 2, p. 12.
15. RCSE minutes, 6:210, 1 May 1782.
16. Stott, 'Incorporation of Surgeons', p. 102.
17. Indenture between Messrs Thomas and Charles Anderson, and William Bremner, # 9/23, 1805. RCSE Papers, 'Indentures 1709–1811'. This is not a complete list of all indentures. John Clerk's, for example, does not appear on it. Sir John Clerk, 'Advice by Sir John Clerk to his son, John, when he went to serve his apprenticeship as chirurgeon under Adam Drummond and John Campbell, 1745', Clerk of Penicuik, SRO GD18/2331.
18. Bell, *Answer*, section 2, p. 10.
19. Contemporary descriptions of apprenticeship can be found in James Lucas, *A Candid Inquiry into the Education, Qualifications, and Offices of a Surgeon-Apothecary* (Bath: S. Hazard, 1800); William Chamberlaine, *Tirocinium Medicum, or a Dissertation on the Duties of Youth Apprenticed to the Medical Profession* (London: Sherwood, Neely & Jones, 1812). One reviewer called Lucas' book 'a sensible tract'. *Monthly Review* series 2, 36 (Sept.–Dec. 1801): 432–433. See also Joan Lane, 'The role of apprenticeship in eighteenth-century medical education in England', in *William Hunter and the Eighteenth-Century Medical World* ed. by William Bynum (Cambridge: Cambridge University Press, 1985), pp. 57–104.
20. James Parkinson, *The Hospital Pupil; or Observations Addressed to the Parents of Youths Intended for the Profession of Medicine and Surgery* (London: Sherwood, Neely, & Jones, 1817), p. 37–8. See Irvine Loudon, *Medical Care and the General Practitioner 1750–1850* Oxford: Clarendon Press, 1986), pp. 34–49.
21. Alexander Lesassier [later Hamilton], 1 January 1805, Alexander Hamilton Collection, Box 11, Folder 72, Library of the Royal College of Physicians of Edinburgh, Edinburgh.
22. This was the precipitating cause of their final quarrel. Lesassier, 20 March 1805.
23. *Ibid.*, 27 February 1804.
24. *Ibid.*, 24 April 1804.
25. RCSE Minutes, 5:509, 18 April 1770.
26. RCSE Minutes, 5:506, 4 April 1770.
27. RCSE Minutes, 5:509, 18 April 1770. According to Stott, 'Incorporation of Surgeons', p. 222, this practice had been going on for some time, but the increasing numbers of students in Edinburgh may have made it more of an issue in the 1770s. Gelfand, p. 47, describes a similar practice among Paris surgeons.
28. This regulation was later repealed: as we will see in Chapter Eight, the

College developed other mechanisms for dealing with students who wished to learn surgery.

29. This was 'Lang Sandy Wood', a good friend of Andrew Duncan Senior. J.D. Comrie, *History of Scottish Medicine*, 2 vols. (London: The Wellcome Historical Medical Museum, 1932), 1:302, 329.

30. Andrew Duncan junior, 'The English Apothecaries' Act', *Edinburgh Medical and Surgical Journal* 25 (1826): 414.

31. *Ibid.*

32. Duncan was one of the few men to receive an MA from Edinburgh University in the eighteenth century *Dictionary of National Biography*, s.v. 'Duncan, Andrew, Junior'.

33. Sheldon Rothblatt, *The Revolution of the Dons. Cambridge and Society in Victorian England* (Cambridge: Cambridge University Press, 1981), pp. 33–60. Though Dissenting academies may have catered to would-be medical students: see the description of Warrington Academy in *Medical Register for the Year 1779* (London: J. Murray, 1779), pp. 102–103.

34. Lesassier, 12 September 1803.

35. *Ibid.*, 13 September 1803.

36. Parkinson, p. 56.

37. *Ibid.*, p. 79.

38. *The Complete Letter-Writer, containing Familiar Letters on the most common Occasions in Life*, (Edinburgh: T. Ross, 1796), p. 67.

39. Alexander Wemyss to George Lindsay of Wormiston, Kirkcaldy, 30 November 1757, SRO GD203/8/11/99.

40. Katherine Wemyss to Lady Wormiston, Kirkcaldy, 9 March 1757, Lindsay, SRO GD203/8/11/99.

41. Lesassier, 26 March 1804.

42. Stott, 'Incorporation of Surgeons', p. 137.

43. See Stott, 'Incorporation of Surgeons', pp. 138–9; R.E. Wright-St Clair, *Doctors Monro. A Medical Saga* (London: Wellcome Historical Medical Museum, 1964), pp. 47–48.

44. RCSE Minutes 5:323, 14 Jan. 1756.

45. RCSE Minutes, 5:411, 17 Nov. 1762.

46. See Chapter Eight.

47. RCSE Minutes, 5:504, 7 Feb. 1770.

48. RCSE Minutes, 6:150, 20 May 1778.

49. RCSE Minutes, 6:155–6. 10 August 1778.

50. *Ibid.*

51. RCSE Minutes, 6:158, 10 August 1778.

52. RCSE Minutes, 6:211, 2 February 84.

53. Bell, *Letters*, p. 406.

54. Sir John Clerk, 'Advice'.

55. Bell, *Letters*, p. 556. This corresponds to the surgical view of disease described in Temkin, p. 256–8.

56. 35 out of 148 did not sign the matriculation albums. It is possible that they attended classes without signing, but it still is noteworthy that after 1780 apprentices consistently did sign.

57. See Alexander Lesassier's comments, Chapter Six.

58. Benjamin Bell, who entered the College in 1771, was no relation to John

Bell. Andrew Wardrop and James Russell both entered in 1777. George
Bell, Benjamin's son, took over his share of the partnership after Benjamin
died in 1806.

59. One hundred and fifty-four out of 426. There were thirty-two Fellows of the
Royal College of Surgeons active in 1779, according to *Medical Register for
the Year 1779*. (London: J. Murray, 1779), p. 158–9; if we assume the
number practicing at any one time was roughly the same throughout the
period, Bell, Wardrop and Russell were obviously attracting a disproportion-
ate number of apprentices.

60. See Chapter Eight, below.

61. Bell, *Letters*, pp. 140–3, 291.

62. Brown, p. 82.

63. *Ibid.*

64. *Ibid.*, p. 83.

65. See Chapters Three and Ten.

66. There was similar movement between being a lecturer's apprentice or private
pupil and attending his lectures in other tie where there were large numbers
of students, like London and Philadelphia. Susan Lawrence, 'Entrepreneurs
and private enterprise: the development of medical lecturing in London,
1775–1820', *Bulletin of the History of Medicine* 63 (1988): 171–192; James E.
Gibson, 'Benjamin Rush's Apprenticed Students', *Transactions and Studies of
the College of Physicians of Philadelphia* 14:127–132; James Rush, 'Notices of
the Names and Characters of the Private pupils of Doctor James Rush. Begun
in the year 1813', James Rush Section, 24, Rush Papers, Library Company
of Philadelphia.

67. Brown, p. 85.

68. Howard S. Becker, Blanche Geer, Everett C. Hughes, Anselm L. Strauss,
Boys in White. Student Culture in Medical School (New Brunswick, NJ:
Transaction Books, 1977), pp. 351–61.

69. James Rush, 'Notices'. See below, Chapter Seven, for interaction between
older and younger students.

70. Brown, p. 82.

71. Note attached to Brown, p. 86.

72. RCSE Minutes, 4:118, 7 Feb. 1712.

73. The phrase is taken from 1804 regulations. RCSE Minutes 7:510, 19 June
1804.

74. RCSE Minutes, 12 Feb. 1782.

75. All the examinations in vol. 5 fit this pattern.

76. Trepan, for example, was assigned to Joseph Robertson in 1768, Benjamin
Bell in 1771, both Edward Inglis and Andrew Duncan in 1772, William
Rae and Andrew Wardrop in 1777, James Arrott in 1783, James MacDowall
in 1784, John Bell in 1786, James Hamilton in 1788, John Walker in 1791,
James Clark and Walter Harkness in 1792, John Henderson in 1797, George
Bell in 1798, William Newbigging and John Cheyne in 1799, Lewis
Flanagan in 1800, James Brown Johnston and James Bremner in 1802, and
John Jack Gibson in 1803. As a point of comparison, Professor James
Russell's entire eight volumes of surgical cases from 1786–1792 gives only
one unambiguous case of trepan, for head injuries caused by a fall. James
Russell, 'Surgical Cases', 1784–92, RCPE James Russell Mss # 1.

77. RCSE Minutes, 6:243, 2 Feb. 1784, 6:447, 12 September 1793.

78. RCSE Minutes 7:553, 6 November 1804.
79. RCSE Minutes, 7:508, 19 June 1804.
80. *Edinburgh Evidence*, p. 335. Wood became a Fellow in 1805.
81. RCSE Minutes, 7:508, 19 June 1804.
82. RCSE Minutes, 9:101, 4 July 1823. Mackintosh had been an army surgeon; he received his MD from Marischal College, Aberdeen, in 1820. P.J. Anderson, ed. *Fasti Academiae Mariscallanae Aberdonensis. Selections from the Records of the Marischal College and University MDXCIII – MDCCCLX*, 3 vols. (Aberdeen: New Spalding Club, 1898). Vol. 2: *Officers, Graduates, and Alumni*, p. 153.
83. Cited in Robert Jones, *An Inquiry into the State of Medicine, on the Principles of Inductive Philosophy*, (Edinburgh: C. Elliot, 1781), p. 270.
84. RCSE Minutes, 8:238–9, March 1816.
85. See below, Chapter Eight. RCSE Minutes, 8, 3 April 1817. The records of Licentiate examinations stated whether the candidate was a student or apprentice, because apprentices paid no fee.

Chapter Six

1. Alexander Lesassier [later Hamilton], 25 October 1805, Alexander Hamilton Collection, Box 11, Folder 72, Library of the Royal College of Physicians of Edinburgh, Edinburgh.
2. See below, Chapter Ten.
3. Both meanings are given by James Buchanan, *Linguae Britannicae Vera Pronunciatio: or, A New English Dictionary* (London: A. Millar, 1757; reprint ed., Menston, England: The Scolar Press Limited, 1967), s.v. 'Occasional'.
4. Sylas Neville, *The Diary of Sylas Neville, 1767–1788*, ed. by Basil Cozens-Hardy (London: Oxford University Press, 1950), p. 216.
5. J. Johnson, *A Guide for Gentlemen Studying Medicine at the University of Edinburgh.* (London: J. Robinson, 1792), p. 15.
6. *Guide*, p. 17.
7. *Ibid.*, p. 15.
8. *Ibid.*, pp. 54–5.
9. Whitfield Bell, 'Thomas Parke's Student Life in England and Scotland, 1771–1773', *The Pennsylvania Magazine of History and Biography* 75 (1951): 237–59.
10. Jane Rendall, 'The Influence of the Edinburgh Medical School on America in the Eighteenth Century', in *The Early Years of the Edinburgh Medical School*, ed. by R.G.W. Anderson and A.D.C. Simpson (Edinburgh: Royal Scottish Museum, 1976), p. 102.
11. James Rush to Benjamin Rush, Edinburgh, 23 November 1809 and 24 May 1810, Rush Papers, Library Company of Philadelphia Mss, held in the Historical Society of Pennsylvania, Box 11, Yi2 7404 F21b.
12. The phrase is from Sir Henry Halford, Great Britain, Parliament, House of Commons, *Report from the Select Committee on Medical Education: With the Minutes of Evidence, and Appendix.* 1834 (602, I, II, and III), Part 1: Royal College of Physicians, London) p. 17. See Chapter One.
13. See Chapter One. It is likely that this group studied at the London hospitals as well.

14. *Guide*, pp. 54–5.
15. Irvine Loudon, *Medical Care and the General Practitioner 1750–1850* (Oxford: Clarendon Press, 1986).
16. *Medical Register for the Year 1779*. London: J. Murray, 1779. This is a useful list, but it is certainly not a complete listing of all practitioners in Scotland or England. Ian E. McCracken, using a variety of sources, estimated that there were approximately seventeen practitioners in Roxburghshire between 1750–1770, but the county is not even mentioned in the *Medical Register*. Ian E. McCracken, 'Eighteenth Century Medical Care: A Study of Roxburghshire', *Proceedings of the Royal Society of Medicine* 42 (1949): 415. A writer for the *Monthly Review* noted that parts of it were 'defective and erroneous', but that other parts 'appear to be executed with sufficient accuracy and judgment'. *Monthly Review*, series 1, 61 (July–December 1779): 61.
17. *Medical Register*, pp. 163–167.
18. Of 178 practitioners without MDs listed, 32 had signed the matriculation albums. *Medical Register*, pp. 142–149.
19. 33 of 59 practitioners without MDs listed. *Medical Register*, pp. 69–71.
20. 'Letter from Andrew Marshall recommending the course of study necessary for becoming a doctor, 1796', Leven and Melville, SRO GD26/13/779. Marshall was 'much honoured', at his lordship's thought that the young man might work with him, but could not avail in himself of the honour, 'for various reasons, which it would be impertinent to intrude on your Lordship's attention'.
21. See John M.T. Ford, ed., *A Medical Student at St. Thomas's Hospital, 1801–1802. The Weekes Family Letters* (London: Wellcome Institute for the History of Medicine, 1987).
22. Alexander Lesassier, 12 September 1803. See Chapter Five, above.
23. Thomas Ismay, 'Letter from Thomas Ismay, Student of Medicine at Edinburgh, 1771, to his father'. *University of Edinburgh Journal* 8 (1936–7): 61.
24. James Lucas, *A Candid Inquiry into the Education, Qualifications, and Offices of a Surgeon-Apothecary* (Bath: S. Hazard, 1800), p. 18.
25. *Medical Register*, p. 144.
26. Alexander's father Peter (Pierre) had studied in Edinburgh from 1782–6 and later set up practice there. He married Professor James Hamilton's sister in 1786; she died in 1790. Joy Pitman, 'Alexander (Le Sassier) Hamilton: An Eventful Life,' *Proceedings of the Royal College of Physicians of Edinburgh* 17 (October 1987): 286–290.
27. David Skene to Dr Andrew Skene, [November 1751], Skene Papers, Mss # 40, Aberdeen University Library.
28. Ismay, p. 57.
29. Rendall, p. 102.
30. *Guide*, p. 5.
31. Lucas, p. 57.
32. *Ibid.*, p. 57.
33. See below, Chapter Eight.
34. Lucas, p. 66.
35. *Ibid.*
36. *Guide*, p. 65.
37. John Gregory, *Observations on the Duties and Offices of a Physician; and on the*

Method of Prosecuting Inquiries in Philosophy (London: W. Strahan, 1770), p. 69.

38. Lucas, pp. 63–4.
39. *Guide*, p. 65.
40. Ismay, p. 58.
41. Lucas, p. 65.
42. *Ibid.*, p. 70.
43. *Guide*, p. 20.
44. *Ibid.*, p. 65.
45. Irvine Loudon, 'The Nature of Provincial Medical Practice in Eighteenth-Century England', *Medical History* 29 (1985): 27–28.
46. Job Harrison to his father, 2 July 1775, 8 October 1775, Chester City Record Office Ref. G/H.S. 99. See Chapters One and Two.
47. William Cullen, *Works of William Cullen, MD*, eb. by John Thomson, 2 vols. (Edinburgh: William Blackwood, 1827), 1:440.
48. *Ibid.*
49. Ismay, p. 58. See Chapter Three, above.
50. *Ibid.*, p. 59.
51. Benjamin Rush, *The Autobiography of Benjamin Rush. His 'Travels Through Life' together with his Commonplace Book for 1789–1813*, George W. Corner, ed. (Princeton: Princeton University Press, 1948), p. 42.
52. *Edinburgh Evidence*, Appendix, p. 266. The medical faculty was protesting against the Royal Commission's recommendation that both classes be given at 9 am.
53. See the discussion of attendance at Midwifery, Chapter Four.
54. James Rush to Benjamin Rush, Edinburgh, 23 December 1809, Rush Papers.
55. Lesassier, 25 October 1805.
56. See Chapter Two.
57. James Rush to Benjamin Rush, Edinburgh, 24 May 1810, Rush Papers.
58. James Rush to Benjamin Rush, Edinburgh, 28 January 1810, Rush Papers.
59. James Rush to Benjamin Rush, Edinburgh, 23 November 1809, Rush Papers.
60. At least he spent less time complaining. James Rush to Benjamin Rush, London, 4 March 1811, Rush Papers.
61. Lesassier, 1 January 1806.
62. *Ibid.*, 25 Jan 1806.
63. *Ibid.*, 25 October 1805.
64. Ismay, p. 57.
65. Lesassier, 17 November 1805.
66. *Ibid.*, 11 November 1805.

Chapter Seven

1. Gilbert Blane, 'Address to the Medical Society of Students at Edinburgh, upon laying the Foundation of their Hall, 21st April 1775', cited in William Stroude, 'History of the Royal Medical Society', in *List of Members, Laws and Library-Catalogue, of the Medical Society of Edinburgh* (Edinburgh: William Aitken, 1820), p. xiii–xiv. It is also cited in the more recent history of the

Society, James Gray, *History of the Royal Medical Society 1737–1937* (Edinburgh: Edinburgh University Press, 1952), p. 41.

2. My use of 'keywords' comes from Raymond Williams, 'they are significant, binding words in certain activities and their interpretation; they are significant, indicative words in certain forms of thought'. Raymond Williams, *Keywords, A Vocabulary of Culture and Society* (New York: Oxford University Press, 1976), p. 13.

3. The phrase is from Susan Lawrence, ' "Desirous of Improvements in Medicine,': Pupils and Practitioners in the Medical Societies at 'Guy's and St. Bartholomew's Hospitals, 1795–1815', *Bulletin of the History of Medicine* 59 (1985): 89–104.

4. John Aitken, *An Address to the Chirurgo-Obstetrical Society: Delivered at their first meeting* (Edinburgh: J. McKenzie, 1786), p. 7.

5. Hugh Blair, *Lectures on Rhetoric and Belles-Lettres* (Philadelphia: James Kay, Jun. & Brother, 1846), pp. 169–170.

6. There is a substantial literature on Edinburgh clubs. See Davis D. McElroy, *Scotland's Age of Improvement. A Survey of 18th Century Literary Clubs and Societies* (Washington State: Washington State University Press, 1969), pp. 131–5; N.T. Phillipson, 'Culture and Society in the 18th Century Province: The Case of Edinburgh and the Scottish Enlightenment', in Lawrence Stone (ed.) *The University and Society*, 2 vols., (Princeton: Princeton University Press) 2:407–448; for a discussion of a student literary society in this period, see James McLachlan, 'The *Choice of Hercules*: American Student Societies in the Early 19th Century', in Stone, 2:449–94.

7. Cited in Phillipson, 2:433. The Rankenian Club was not a student society, but Phillipson notes that a large part of its membership were young men. Howard S. Becker Blanche Geer, Everett C. Hughes, Anselm L. Strauss, *Boys in White, Student Culture in Medical School* (New Brunswick, NT: Transaction Books, 1977), pp. 138–79, discuss the role of student interaction in reinforcing attitudes towards medical study.

8. They also discussed philosophical issues, where relevant. See C.J. Lawrence, 'Medicine as Culture: Edinburgh and the Scottish Enlightenment' (Ph.D. Dissertation, University of London, 1984), p. 204–6.

9. James Ford, 'What is the best method of studying medicine?' Royal Medical Society (RMS) Dissertations, 1778, 11:156. Both dissertations and minute books are currently held in the library of the Royal Medical Society, Student Centre, Bristo Square. A microfilm of all dissertations is also available at the National Library of Medicine, Bethesda, MD.

10. Lisa Rosner, 'Eighteenth-Century Medical Education and the Didactic Model of Experiment', in *The Literary Structure of Scientific Knowledge: Historical Studies*, ed. by Peter Dear (Philadelphia: University of Pennsylvania Press, 1991), pp. 182–94.

11. John Bard to Samuel Bard, New York, 11 December 1765, Bard Papers, New York Academy of Medicine Library. For the negative connotations of 'pedantry' in this period see Sheldon Rothblatt, *Tradition and Change in English Liberal Education. An Essay in History and Culture* (London: Faber and Faber, 1976), pp. 80–83.

12. Cited in Stroude, p. xiii.

13. John Bard to Samuel Bard, New York, 11 December 1765, Bard Papers.

14. Cited in Stroude, p. xiii.

15. Cited in Stroude, p. xiv.
16. J. Johnson, *A Guide for Gentlemen Studying Medicine at the University of Edinburgh*, (London: J. Robinson, 1792) p. 48. Several of these societies were discussed briefly in McElroy, pp. 136–9.
17. The *Edinburgh Almanack* for 1785, p. 59, lists Professor John Walker as honorary president.
18. 'List of the Members of the Chemical Society 1785,' EUL Mss. GEN 875/11/246–7; see J. Kendall, 'The First Chemical Society', *University of Edinburgh Journal* 16 (1951–3): 346–58, 385–400; Gwen Averley, 'The "Social Chemists": English Chemical Societies in the Eighteenth and Early Nineteenth Century', *Ambix* 33 (1986): 99–100.
19. The *Edinburgh Almanack* for 1785, p. 59, stated that the Natural History Society 'consists of about 100 members, who, in rotation, write papers on some subject of natural history'. See also *Dissertations read before the Chemical Society, Instituted in the Beginning of the Year 1785*, Chemical Library Mss., Edinburgh University.
20. *Edinburgh Almanack*, 1789, p. 63.
21. The four presidents were Henry Bowles, William Lecky, Peter Ashton, and William Forbes. *Edinburgh Almanack*, 1787, p. 105. The first three went on to graduate. That does not, of course, preclude their being interested in surgery and obstetrics.
22. Dr George Logan to his brother Charles Logan, Edinburgh, 2 March 1778, Dr George Logan's Journal 1775–1779, Historical Society of Pennsylvania Mss.
23. He wrote on Dyspepsia and Ulceration for the Chirurgo-Medical Society, and Innoculation for both Societies. Although ulcertation and innoculation might be considered surgical subjects, Logan discussed the medical, not surgical, treatment.
24. For the Annual Presidents of the Natural History Society, see *Edinburgh Almanack*, 1785–1797; members of the Royal Medical Society are printed in *List of the Members, Laws, and Library-Catalogue of the Medical Society of Edinburgh, instituted 1737; incorporated by Royal Charter Dec. 14, 1778* (Edinburgh: Printed for the Society by William Aitken, 1820).
25. *Guide*, p. 53.
26. After spending two years researching his thesis on gout, according to Robert Christison. Robert Christison, *The Life of Sir Robert Christison, Bart.*, 2 vols (Edinburgh: William Blackwood and Sons, 1885), cited in J.D. Comrie, *History of Scottish Medicine*, 2 vols. (London: The Wellcome Historical Medical Museum, 1932) 2:478. See above, Chapter Five. Stroude may have also read every book in the Royal Medical Society library.
27. J. Pettigrew, *Life and Writings of J.C. Lettsom*, vol. III, pp. 288–291, cited in Gray, p. 16. Much of Gray's information concerning the Society up to 1820 is taken from Stroude's history.
28. Hugh Arnot, *History of Edinburgh* (1779), p. 430, cited in Gray, p. 43.
29. RMS Minutes, 7 February 1800.
30. *Edinburgh Almanack*, 1785, p. 57.
31. Stroude, p. lxii.
32. *Laws of the Medical Society of Edinburgh, Instituted 1737, incorporated by Royal Charter 1778* (Edinburgh, 1796), p. 46. The earliest record of the laws of the Society is a manuscript volume held in the Society library, entitled

'Regulations of a Society instituted at Edinburgh for improvement in medical knowledge 1737'. It is not clear when these regulations were drawn up. Several versions of the laws were published. In addition to the 1796 *Laws*, I will refer primarily to those published in 1788, *Laws of the Medical Society of Edinburgh* (Edinburgh: Printed by William Smellie, for the Society, 1788).

33. Gray, p. 75.
34. *Laws*, 1788, pp. 19–22.
35. *Ibid.*, 1788, p. 24.
36. Andrew Duncans, junior, 'Extracts from the correspondence of Andrew Duncan, Junior, MD, FRCPE, Professor of Materia Medica in the University of Edinburgh from 1821 until 1832', ed. by W.A. MacNaughton, *Journal of the Caledonian Medical Society* (1912): 204.
37. *Edinburgh Evidence*, p. 489. Andrew Duncan junior was Librarian in 1826.
38. *Laws* 1788, p. 32.
39. Stroude, p. lxvii.
40. RMS Minutes, 1778–1784, 1797–1805, 1805–1811. Royal Medical Society Library, Edinburgh.
41. *Laws*, 1788, p. 34.
42. Stroude, p. lxvi.
43. *Ibid.*, p. lxvii.
44. *Laws*, 1796. No mention of the aphorisms was made in the description of public business, p. 46.
45. It is not clear when the dissertations were bound in the form in which they are today, with the essays for each year bound in a separate volume. Volume 1 of the essays is dated 1751, though it appears to have been collected and bound later. Volume 8 contains the report of the Experimental Committee, set up in 1785, which apparently lasted only one year. Volumes 9 (1777) and 10 (1794) are labelled *Medical News*. These are essays on medical subjects, which appear to have been written by non-members, and collected by the Society, perhaps with the intention of publishing them. See Gray, pp. 66–8, for a discussion of the Society's unsuccessful attempts to collect papers for publication. The rest of the volumes contain the cases, questions, and aphorisms written by members. Volumes 2–6 date from the 1770s, but do not follow chronological order; from Volume 11, for 1778, however, the essays were arranged more or less chronologically, each volume containing either cases, questions, or aphorisms. The best guess as to when the earlier volumes were bound in their present form is the 1790s, since otherwise it is hard to explain how Medical News from 1794 could be bound as Volume 10, while dissertations from 1778–1793 are bound as Volume 11–31.
46. Stroude, p. xxi.
47. Samuel Bard to John Bard, Edinburgh, 6 Sept. 1763, Bard Papers.
48. Samuel Bard to John Bard, Edinburgh, May 15, 1765, Bard Papers.
49. These were the case histories collected in RMS Dissertations, November 1780–1781, vol. 7.
50. *Index Alphabeticus Morborum de quibus agitur in eorum dissertationibus inauguralibus qui, in Academia Edinensi, ad gradum MD admissi fuerunt, ab anno 1726, usque ad annum 1799*, (Edinburgh: D.Schaw & Co., 1800).
51. Twenty-seven essays were written on various aspects of the blood, twenty-one on digestion, eight on Peruvian Bark, and eight on Air, that is,

pneumatic chemistry. For a discussion of students' interest in chemistry and experiment, see Rosner, 'Eighteenth Century Medical Education'.

52. Aitken, p. 11.
53. Stroude, p. xxi.
54. Aitken, p. 12. This raises the intriguing question as to whether students ever came unprepared, and simply sat without anything to say.
55. Lawrence Nihel, 'Pneumonia', RMS Dissertations, 1778, 11:342.
56. William Withering, 'Apoplexy', RMS Dissertations, 1799, 38:338–348.
57. Stroude, p. xiii.
58. Samuel Allvey, 'Erysepelas', RMS Dissertations, 1786–7, 20:279. See Chapter Five.
59. See above, Chapter Four.
60. See Chapter Two.
61. *Guide*, p. 50.
62. Stroude, p. lxiv.
63. Gray, p. 31.
64. *Ibid.*, p. 110.
65. *Ibid.*
66. *Ibid.*, pp. 109, 110.
67. Stroude, p. lxv.
68. James Rush to Benjamin Rush, Edinburgh, 23 October 1809, Rush Papers, Library Company of Philadelphia Mss, held in the Historical Society of Pennsylvania, Box 11, Yi2 7404 F21b.
69. Sylas Neville, *The Diary of Sylas Neville, 1767–1788*, Basil Cozens-Hardy, ed. (London: Oxford University Press, 1950), p. 148.
70. *Ibid.*, p. 143.
71. *Ibid.*, p. 200.
72. *Ibid.*, p. 243. See below.
73. Samuel Bard to John Bard, Edinburgh, September 1763, Bard Papers.
74. Neville stayed in Edinburgh the year after he graduated. Neville, p. 236–243.
75. *Edinburgh Evidence*, p. 489.
76. Alexander Lesassier [later Hamilton], 25 October 1805, Alexander Hamilton Collection, Box 11, Folder 72, Library of the Royal College of Physicians of Edinburgh, Edinburgh.
77. Cited in Wyndham B. Blanton, *Medicine in Virginia in the Eighteenth Century* (Richmond: Garrett & Massie, Incorporated, 1931), p. 89.
78. John Bard to Samuel Bard, New York, 11 Dec. 1765, Bard Papers.
79. Stroude, p. xii.
80. Sheldon Rothblatt, 'The Student Sub-culture and the Examination System in Early 19th Century Oxbridge', in Stone 1:247–304.
81. *Laws*, 1796, p. 42.
82. Aitken, p. 15.
83. James Rush to Benjamin Rush, Edinburgh, 23 October 1809, Rush papers.
84. George Sutherland, RMS Dissertations, 1751, 1:68.
85. *Ibid.*
86. Neville, p. 240.
87. *Ibid.*, p. 241.
88. The most recent work on Brown is in W.F. Bynum and Roy Porter, eds.,

Brunonianism in Britain and Europe (London: Wellcome Institute for the History of Medicine, 1988). For the Edinburgh context of Brown's ideas, and their political implications, see especially Michael Barfoot, 'Brunonianism under the Bed: An alternative to University of Medicine in Edinburgh in the 1780s', pp. 22–45. See also Guenther Risse, 'The History of John Brown's Medical System in Germany During the Years 1790–1806' (Ph.D. Dissertation, University of Chicago, 1971).

89. Marginalia in John Brown, *Elements of Medicine* (London: J. Johnson, 1788), copy held by the Edinburgh University Library Rare Books Room, p. 37. This is signed 'Cambrianus,' and so could have been written by Robert Jones. See Chapter Four.

90. William Cullen, *First Lines of the Practice of Physic, for the Use of Students in the University of Edinburgh* 2 vols., (Edinburgh: William Creech, 1777, 1779), 1:237, copy held in the Edinburgh University Library Rare Books Room. Even this is temperate compared with some of the marginalia.

91. Stroude, p. lxxxi.

92. This was presented in 'Medical Intelligence', published in the *Edinburgh Evening Post*, # 290, 292, and 300, February–March 1783. The articles were printed in the appendix of an action filed by Robert Cullen on behalf of the Society for damages, a copy of which is held by the Royal Medical Society. 'The Petition of the Presidents, and other Members of the Medical Society of Edinburgh,' 27 February 1783. See Gray, pp. 58–60. Lord Cullen made the case that publication of the account of the meeting infringed on the Society's sole right to publish its own proceedings, but the judge in the case ruled that 'it was lawful for every one to publish an account of the enquiries and debates of a Society instituted for the purpose of free enquiry and debate, concerning matters of science'. Gray, p. 60.

93. William Cullen, 'Clinical Lectures', 1771–2, RCPE William Cullen Mss # 4, vol. 1, p. 52.

94. Thomas Pemberton, 'Is the duration of fevers capable of being shortened by the exhibition of medicines?' RMS Dissertations, 1776, 3:335.

95. Benjamin Rush, cited in Whitfield J. Bell Jr. 'Philadelphia Medical Students in Europe, 1750–1800,' *The Pennsylvania Magazine of History and Biography* 67 (1943): 13.

96. John Watson Howell, 'What are the likliest [sic] means of rescuing, or at least relieving the art of medicine, from its present state of uncertainty and error,' RMS Dissertations, 1778, 12:69.

97. Mary Hewson to Thomas Tickell Hewson, Philadelphia, 9 July 1795, Hewson Papers, B H492, vol. 2, # 32, American Philosophical Society Library, Philadelphia. See Chapter Three.

98. James Jeffray to William Hamilton, Professor in Glasgow, Edinburgh, November 1783, Letters to Thomas and William Hamilton, RCPE, Hamilton, Family of, Mss # 1, 'Letters to Thomas Hamilton, and to his son William, c. 1778–9'. See above, Chapter Four.

99. Richard Kiernan, 'Dysentery', RMS Dissertations, 1780, 13:433.

100. RMS Mss, 'Regulations of a Society instituted at Edinburgh for Improvement in Medical Knowledge 1737'.

101. Richard Pew, 'Rheumatism', RMS Dissertations, 1772, 5:248–254.

102. Thomas Girdleston, 'Hepatitis', RMS Dissertations, 1786–7, 20:2.

103. Thomas Blackburn, 'Diabetes', RMS Dissertations, 1772, 5:188.

104. Francis Home, *Clinical Experiments, Histories, and Dissections* (Edinburgh: William Creech, 1780), p. 296–326; *Catalogue of the Library of the Medical Society of Edinburgh* (Edinburgh: Printed for the Society by A. Balfour & Co., 1832), p. 104.

105. William Cullen, *Synopsis Nosologiae Methodicae, exhibens clariss. virorum Sauvagesii, Linaei, Vogelii, Sagari et Macbridii, systemata nosologica: edidit suumque proprium systema, nosologicum adjecit Gulielmus Cullen, MD* (Edinburgh: William Creech, 1803).

106. William Spooner, 'Gonorrhea', RMS Dissertations, 1784–5, 16:237. For a discussion of Fyfe's role in Royal Medical Society experiments, see Rosner, 'Eighteenth-Century Medical Education'.

107. Twentieth-century students have been known to do as well. Becher *et al.* argue throughout their book that students responded to the pressures of medical school by adopting attitudes and study habits that got them through school, rather than always keeping in mind what they may need for practice.

108. Charles Throckmorton, 'Enteritis', RMS Dissertations, 1784–5, 46.

109. See, for example, William Withering's essay on 'Apoplexy', RMS Dissertations, vol. 39, 1798–9, pp. 338–348.

110. Edmund Goodwyn, 'Colica Pictonum', RMS Dissertations, 1785–7, 18:162.

111. Herbert Packe, 'Phthisis Pulmonalis', RMS Dissertations, 1790, 25:10–19.

112. John Thomson, 'Hectic Fever,' RMS Dissertations, 1790, 25:102. By the time Thomson wrote his biography of Cullen forty years later, his opinion of Brown was highly unfavorable, as Christopher Lawrence notes in 'Cullen, Brown, and the Poverty of Essentialism', in Bynum and Porter, pp. 14–23. One factor contributing to the change was that in 1790 Thomson was a young extra-academical teacher like his friend John Allen, who also was influenced by Brown; both may have been drawn to a doctrine which had developed in opposition to the University medical faculty. By the 1830s Thomson was a well-established University professor himself and had adopted Cullen as his model.

113. Stroude, pp. lxxxii–lxxxiii.

114. The letter is not signed, but the author apparently expected his recommendation to be sufficient. 10 November 1784, William Thornton Papers, American Philosophical Mss Film 724, reel 1.

115. I am here explicitly dissenting from Michael Barfoot's analysis of Brunonianism as an alternative to University medicine, though I agree that followers of Brown picked up on many of the points of opposition to the medical faculty current in Edinburgh. For a comparison with more obviously radical student societies, see James C. McClelland, *Autocrats and Academics. Education, Culture and Society in Tsarist Russia* (Chicago: University of Chicago Press, 1979), pp. 96–106; Samuel D. Kassow, *Students, Professors, and the State in Tsarist Russia* (Berkeley, California: University of California Press, 1989).

116. See below, Chapter Eight.

Introduction to Part Two

1. George Jardine, *Outlines of Philosophical Education, illustrated by the Method of Teaching the Logic Class in the University of Glasgow* (Glasgow: University Press, 1825), p. 460.

2. There is some lag time in figures, both because I calculated figures from first year of study and because many students would not have received their commissions until two to four years later. William Johnston, *Roll of Commissioned Officers in Medical Service of the British Army* (Aberdeen: Aberdeen University Press, 1917).

3. Robert Hamilton, *The Duties of a Regimental Surgeon Considered: with observation on his General Qualifications; and hints relative to a more respectable practice, and better regulation of that department*, 2 vols. (London: J. Johnson, [1787]).

4. Robert Jackson, *A System of Arrangement and Discipline for the Medical Department of Armies* (London: John Murray, 1805).

5. William Turnbull, *The Navy Surgeon; comprising the entire duties of professional men at sea*. (London: Richard Phillips, 1806).

6. Neil Cantlie, *A History of the Army Medical Department* 2 vols. (Edinburgh: Churchill Livingston, 1974), 1:180–2.

7. *Ibid.*, 1:201.

8. See Chapter One.

9. Sheldon Rothblatt, *Tradition and Change in English Liberal Education. An Essay in History and Culture* (London: Faber and Faber, 1976), pp. 105–6, 120–1.

10. Lord Kellie to Robert Saunders Dundas, 21 Oct. 1820, Melville Castle, SRO GD51/4/1579. For the assumptions behind this kind of patronage in Scotland, see Ronald M. Sunter, *Patronage and Politics in Scotland 1707–1832* (Edinburgh: John Donald Publishers Ltd, 1986).

11. E.G.W. Bill, *Education at Christ Church Oxford 1600–1800* (Oxford: Clarendon Press, 1988), pp. 218–220.

12. *Gradus ad Cantabrigiam; or New University Guide to the Academica Customs, and Colloquial or Cant Terms peculiar to the University of Cambridge; observing wherein it differs from Oxford* (London: John Hearne, 1834), p. 119. It is not clear, though, that the authors felt particularly inclined to strive for that honor, since their description of a 'reading-man', p. 91 is not altogether appealing. Then again, neither is their definition of a 'non reading-man', p. 77.

13. Sheldon Rothblatt, 'The Student Sub-culture and the Examination System in Early 19th Century Oxbridge', in Lawrence Stone (ed.) *The University and Society*, 2 vols. (Princeton: Princeton University Press, 1974) 1:247–304.

14. See below, Chapter Ten.

15. For a summary of this process, see Rothblatt, *Tradition and Change*, pp. 119–127.

16. Jardine, p. 24.

17. *Ibid.*, pp. 459–60.

18. 'Outlines of Philosophical Education', *Blackwood's Magazine* 3 (April–Sept 1818): 420–4; it was also reviewed in connection with the Royal Commission in 'State of the Universities', *Quarterly Review* 36 (June–October 1827): 216–268. See Chapter Ten.

19. A.J. Youngson, *The Making of Classical Edinburgh* (Edinburgh: Edinburgh University Press, 1966).

20. George Logan to his brother Charles Logan, Edinburgh, 2 March 1778, Dr. George Logan's Journal 1775–1779, Historical Society of Pennsylvania Mss.

21. Youngson, p. 200–202.

22. Peter Mark Roget and his family lodged in Rose Street in 1793. D.L. Emblen, *Peter Mark Roget. The Word and the Man* (New York: Thomas Y. Crowell Company, 1970), p. 20. After 1810, more students in James Hamilton's

Midwifery lecture had addresses in the New Town. James Hamilton, 'Lists of Students Attending Lectures in Obstetrics', 1802–1831, 3 vols. RCPE Mss. Hamilton, James, # 10.

23. Bruce Lenman, *Integration, Enlightenment, and Industrialization* (London: Edward Arnold, 1981).
24. Youngson, p. 260–2.
25. Henry Cockburn, *Memorials of His Time*, (Edinburgh: T.N. Foulis, 1856), p. 97–99.
26. John Ramsay, *Letters of John Ramsay of Ochtertyre, 1799–1812*, ed. Barbara L.H. Horn (Edinburgh: T. & A. Constable Ltd. 1966), p. 43. This was a common theme in his letters.
27. Alexander Lesassier [later Hamilton], 5 November 1805, Alexander Hamilton Collection Box 11, Folder 72, Library of the Royal College of Physicians of Edinburgh.
28. Professor John Leslie wrote that, when finished, 'it would unquestionably be the boast of our northern metropolis'. Cited in Youngson, p. 197.

Chapter Eight

1. *The Medical Calendar: a Student's Guide to the Medical Schools in Edinburgh, London, Dublin, Paris, Oxford, Cambridge, Glasgow, Aberdeen, and St. Andrews.* (Edinburgh: MacLachlan and Stewart, 1828), pp. 46–7.
2. RCSE Minutes, 5:504, 7 Feb. 1770.
3. RCSE Minutes, 6:13, 3 July 1772.
4. [William Taplin], *The Aesculapian Labyrinth Explored; or, Medical Mystery Illustrated. A Series of Instructions to Young Physicians, Surgeons, Accouchers, Apothecaries, Druggists, and Practitioners of Every Denomination, in Town and Country* (Dublin: Zachariah Jackson, 1789), p. 14.
5. RCSE Minutes, 6:85, 1 May 1777.
6. RCSE Minutes, 6:151–2, 22 May 1778. In 1781, the price for the surgeon's mate diploma was set at two guineas, instead of the full £5/11/1/3. RCSE Minutes, 6:190, 7 March 1781.
7. See above, Chapter Five.
8. RCSE Minutes, 6:255, 13 Nov 1784.
9. RCSE Minutes, 6:301, 2 February 1787.
10. The Incorporation had, in the 17th century, given certificates of skill for navy surgeons, but I have found no trace of this practice in the 18th century. Rosalie Stott, 'The Incorporation of Surgeons and Medical Education and Practice in Edinburgh 1696–1755', (Ph.D. Dissertation, University of Edinburgh, 1984), p. 102.
11. RCSE Minutes, 8:276, 18 June 1816; *List of Licentiates of the Royal College of Surgeons of Edinburgh from 1815 to 1859, and of Fellows of the College at 1st August 1859* (Edinburgh: Robert Hardie & Co. 1859).
12. For parallel developments on the part of the Royal College of surgeons of Dublin, see J.D.H. Widdiss, *The Royal College of Surgeons in Ireland and its Medical School, 1784–1984*, (Dublin: Royal College of Surgeons of Dublin, 1984), pp. 9–67.
13. Robert Christison, 'Letter to the Principal and Professors of the University of Edinburgh', October, 1824, p. 8. See Chapter Four.

14. RCSE Minutes, 7:514, 19 June 1804.
15. 'Regulations to be observed by candidates desirous of obtaining diplomas from the Royal College of surgeons of Edinburgh', 15 March 1808, Melville Castle, SRO GD 51/5/670/3. This sentence appeared in every set of regulations issued by the Royal College through 1828. 'Secretary's Copy, Regulations, &c,' RCSE; *Medical Calendar.*
16. 'Regulations to be observed by candidates, previous to their being taken on trials for obtaining diplomas from the Royal College of Surgeons of Edinburgh, Surgeons' Hall, Edinburgh, September 1826', RCSE.
17. *Ibid.*
18. This appears in every set of regulations up to 1828, and in *Medical Calendar*, p. 45.
19. *Medical Calendar*, pp. 46–7.
20. The phrase was routinely used; this example was taken from RCSE Minutes 9:63, 3 February 1823. For others examples see 9:10, 14 June 1822, 9:31, 1 August 1822, 9:63, among many others.
21. See above, Chapter Five.
22. J. Johnson, *A Guide for Gentlemen Studying Medicine at the University of Edinburgh* (London: J. Robinson, 1792), pp. 54–5. See Chapter Six.
23. This information is taken from the matriculation albums, EUL Da.
24. David Birrel to his parents, Edinburgh, 14 Nov 1807, Kinross, SRO GD 1/58/2/4/14/5.
25. Birrel fell under the pre-1808 regulations, which did not specifically require many classes. After 1808, he would have had to attend Medical Theory and Clinical Lectures as well. 'Regulations, 1808'.
26. *Edinburgh Evidence*, p. 450.
27. RCSE Minutes, 5:85, 11 August 1748.
28. See, for example, David Skene to Andrew Skene, 22 Dec. 1751, Skene Papers, Aberdeen University Library (AUL) # 40, and Chapter Two.
29. A. Logan Turner, *Story of a Great Hospital, The Royal Infirmary of Edinburgh* (Edinburgh: Oliver and Boyd Lt., 1937), p. 143; Guenther Risse, *Hospital Life in Enlightenment Scotland: Care and Teaching at the Royal Infirmary of Edinburgh* (Cambridge: Cambridge University Press, 1986), pp. 266–9.
30. RCSE Minutes, 6:17, 27 Aug. 1772.
31. *Ibid.*
32. J.D. Comrie, *History of Scottish Medicine*, 2 vols. (London: The Wellcome Historical Medical Museum, 1932), 1:328.
33. RCSE Minutes, 5:323, 14 January 1756. See Chapter Five.
34. Turner, p. 144.
35. RCSE Minutes, 6:281, 2 Feb. 1786.
36. *Guide*, p. 44.
37. Alexander Monro, *secundus*, 'Lectures on Surgery', c. 1774–5, RCPE, Alexander Monro *secundus* Mss # 13, p. 21.
38. *Ibid.*
39. *Guide*, p. 44.
40. *Ibid.*
41. Oswei Temkin, 'The Role of Surgery in the Rise of Modern Medical Thought', Bulletin of the History of Medicine 25 (1951): 248–259.
42. A set of Russell's case notes survive from the years 1786–91. They may have been used in his lectures, since they are carefully copied out and bound, and

fit the *Guide*'s description of the course as illustrating the practice of surgery, in the same manner as the clinical lectures illustrated the practice of physic. James Russell, 'Surgical Cases', 1784–1792, RCPE James Russell Mss # 1.

43. Russell, 2:3–4.
44. Russell, 5:3.
45. *Dictionary of National Biography*, s.v. 'Russell, James'.
46. Alexander Bower, *The Edinburgh Student's Guide: Or an account of the classes of the University arranged under the four faculties; with a detail of what is taught in each* (Edinburgh: Waugh and Innes, 1822), pp. 73–6.
47. Only 6 per cent of one–year auditors attended it, however.
48. RCSE Minutes, 7:388, 15 May 1802.
49. *Ibid.*
50. *Ibid.*
51. John Thomson, 'Lectures on Practice of Surgery', 1809–1810, RCPE John Thomson Mss # 2, Lecture 4, 1 Nov., unpaginated.
52. *Ibid.*
53. *Ibid.*
54. *Ibid.*
55. RCSE Minutes, 7:616, 1 July 1806.
56. Comrie, 2:629.
57. *Edinburgh Evidence*, p. 452.
58. Archibald Robertson, *Conversations on Anatomy, Physiology, and Surgery* (Edinburgh: Robert Buchanan, 1827), p.v. For Robertson, see Chapter Four.
59. William Gordon, *Academical Examinations on the Practice of Surgery, intended for the use of students* (Edinburgh: Maclachlan and Stewart, 1828). Gordon was a licentiate.
60. David Birrel to his parents, Edinburgh, 19 May 1808, Kinross, SRO GD 1/58/2/4/14/5.
61. RCSE Minutes, 7:709–11, 21 April 1809.
62. *Ibid.*
63. *Ibid.* This incident is briefly discussed in Clarendon Hyde Creswell, *The Royal College of Surgeons of Edinburgh. Historical Notes from 1505 to 1905* (Edinburgh: Oliver & Boyd, 1926), pp. 186–7.
64. RCSE Minutes, 9:330–331, 4 March 1826.
65. RCSE, Secretary's Copy, Regulations, &c.
66. RCSE Minutes, 6:237, 25 July 1783.
67. Zachary Cope, *The History of the Royal College of Surgeons of England* (London: Anthony Blond Ltd., 1959), p. 7.
68. The transformation of an old regime institution is a theme of John Gascoigne, *Cambridge in the Age of the Enlightenment. Science, Religion, and Politics from the Restoration to the French Revolution* (Cambridge: Cambridge University Press, 1988). Also see Ian R. Christie, *Stress and Stability in Late Eighteenth-Century Britain. Reflections on the British Avoidance of Revolution* (Oxford: Clarendon Press, 1984).
69. For an excellent survey of the conflict between the upper branches of all the professions, based in traditional corporations, 'heavily entrenched behind generations of custom and usage', and the lower branches' insistence on specialized qualifications, see W.J. Reader, *Professional Men. The Rise of the Professional Classes in Nineteenth-Century England* (London: Weidenfeld and Nicolson, 1966), pp. 44–58.

70. RCSE Minutes, 6:347, 10 Oct. 1789.
71. RCSE Minutes, 6:205, 21 October 1799.
72. RCSE Minutes, 7:78, 18 March 1797; 7:471, 1 Nov. 1803; 7:577, 15 May 1805. Medical ranks in the army were reorganized in 1805: surgeon's mates, formerly warrant officers, were raised to assistant surgeons, and made commissioned officers.
73. RCSE Minutes, 8:112, 7 May 1813.
74. The phrase is from Lord Kellie to Robert Saunders Dundas, 21 October 1820, Melville Castle, SRO GD51/4/1579. See the Introduction to Part Two. Fifteen per cent of the licentiates appear in Dirom Grey Crawford's *Roll of the Indian Medical Service* (London: W. Thacker & Co, 1930); 12% appear in William Johnston's *Roll of Commissioned Officers in the Medical Service of the British Army* (Aberdeen: Aberdeen University Press, 1917).
75. *Edinburgh Evidence*, p. 450.
76. RCSE Minutes, 9:12–13, 2 July 1822.
77. RCSE Minutes, 9:131–2, 25 November 1823.
78. *Edinburgh Evidence*, p. 215.
79. Andrew Wardrop, 'Can the advantages expected arise from methodical nosology?' RMS Dissertations, 1776, 3:128.
80. James Russell, 'On the theory of vision', RMS Dissertations, 1776, 3:36; 'Combination of epilepsy and hysteria', 1776, 3:189.
81. For example, James Law, 'Opthalmia', RMS Dissertations, 1780, 13:440; James Hamilton, 'By what power is the digestion performed in man?', 1786–7–8, 21:447; John Herdman, 'In what manner are we to account for the effects of cold bathing in those diseases in which it has been found useful?', 1794–5, 32:400; Robert Robertson, 'Scorbutics', 1795, 33:381.
82. John Thomson, RMS Dissertations, 'Hectic Fever', 1790–1–2, 25:486; 'Catarrh', 1790–1–2, 25:102.
83. See *Index Alphabeticus Morborum de quibus agitur in eorum dissertationibus inauguralibus qui, in Academia Edinensi, ad gradum MD admissi fuerunt, ab anno 1726, usque ad annum 1799*, (Edinburgh: D.Schaw & Co., 1800).
84. George Bell, 'Fistula Lachrymalis', 1798–9, 39:302.
85. James Wardrope, 'Popliteal Aneurism', RMS Dissertations, 1801–2, 45:176; William Wood, 'What are the comparative methods of the operations of extracting and depressing the cataract', 1804–5, 52:347; James Bremner, Hydrocele', 1800, 43:19; John William Turner, 'Hydrocele', 1809–10, 62:443; Thomas Lothian, 'What are the causes which render amputation necessary?' 1805–6, 54:114; John Gordon, 'What is the process of nature in the healing of wounds?' 1805–6, 54:1; James Keith, 'What is the process by which nature heals up wounds?' 1811–12, 66:150; David Hay, 'What are the occasional bad consequences of venaesection at the bend of the arm?' 1811–12, 66:140.
86. A modern example of the impact of visibility was reported by Paul Rodenhauser and Amanda M. Romero, who found that the mere presence of a medical student psychiatry club at Wright State University School of Medicine led to increased interest in psychiatry generally, and to more students choosing psychiatric residencies. *Journal of Medical Education* 63 (December 1988): 925–6.
87. James Baillie Pender, 'What are the circumstances who render amputation preferable to an attempt to preserve the limb in compound Fracture', RMS

Dissertations, 1802–3, 48:37; Thomas Lothian, 'What are the causes which render amputation necessary', 1805–6, 54:114; Thomas Haines Banning, 'On Amputation', 1808–9, 74:17; Edmund Lyon, 'In cases of compound fracture', 1814–15, 71:369; Anthony Pringle, 'In injuries to the extremities where the limb is to be removed, are we to amputate immediately or wait untill [sic] the inflammatory symptoms subside?' 1816–17, 74:17; Thomas Woodforde, 'Amputation', 1824–5, 85:194. Pender was an apprentice and a licentiate, Lothian was an apprentice and Fellow, and Anthony Pringle was an apprentice and licentiate as well as an MD. Banning, Lyon, and Woodforde were all MDs with no affiliation with the College of Surgeons.

88. They were William Wood, 'What are the comparative merits of the operations of extracting and depressing the cataract?' RMS Dissertations, 1804–5, 52:347; John Foster Drake Jones, 'Cataract', 1801–2, 45:348; John W. Stirk, 'Cataract,' 1809–10, 62:223; Thomas Becher, 'Whether is depression or extraction of the cataract the preferred operation?' 1821, 80:107; Francisco de Souza, 'Cataract', 1806–7, 55:186; Henry Fisher, 'Cataract,' 1809–10, 62:39; Henry Jeffrays, 'Cataract', 1808–9, 60:197.

89. They were William Wood, 'Hydrocele. What are the comparative merits of the operations which have been employed for its cure?' RMS Dissertations, 1805–6, 54:302; John Williamson Turner, 'Hydrocele', 1809–10, 62:443; Peter J. Skerratt, 'Hydrocele', 1814–15, 71:251; James Bremner, 'Hydrocele', 1800, 43:19; Henry Harris, 'Hydrocele', 1803–5, 51:381; Anthony Musgrave, 'How is Hydrocele of the Tunica vaginalis to be distinguished from other diseases affecting the same part? and what is the best method of eradicating the disease,' 1813–14, 70:85. Turner became a licentiate before entering the College as a Fellow.

90. George Meek, 'On Gun-Shot Wounds', RMS Dissertations, 1802–3, 49:49.

91. James Robertson, 'On Incised Wounds', RMS Dissertations, 1798–9, 41:200.

92. Thomas Haines-Banning, 'On Amputation', RMS Dissertations, 1808–9, 61:79–107.

93. Gordon, p. 23.

94. The phrase is from John Bell, *Letters on Professional Character and Manners: on the Education of a Surgeon, and the Duties and Qualifications of a Physician: addressed to James Gregory, M.D* (Edinburgh: John Muir, 1810), p. 534.

95. Pender, p. 372.

96. Humphrey Herbert Jones, 'On Gun–Shot Wounds', RMS Dissertations, 1807–8, 57:256.

97. Meek, p. 53.

98. *Ibid.*

99. Jones, p. 256.

100. Lothian, p. 115.

101. William Stroude, 'History of the Royal Medical Society', in *List of Members, Laws and Library-Catalogue, of the Medical Society of Edinburgh*, (Edinburgh: William Aitken, 1820), p. lxxxiii. See Chapter Seven.

102. Sir John Clerk, 'Advice by Sir John Clerk to his son, John, when he went to serve his apprenticeship as chirurgeon under Adam Drummond and John Campbell, 1745', Clerk of Penicuik, SRO GD18/2331.

103. RCSE Minutes, 6: 1, 7 January 1771.

104. RCSE Minutes, 6:76, 18 February 1777.

105. *Medical Calendar*, p. 47.
106. Jacques Barzun, ed., *Burke and Hare: The Resurrection Men* (Metuchen, N.J.: Scarecrow Press, 1974); Robert Christison, *Life of Sir Robert Christison, Bart.* (Edinburgh: William Blackwood and Sons, 1885), 1:175–80, 305–11.

Chapter Nine

1. *The Medical Calendar: a Student's Guide to the Medical Schools in Edinburgh, London, Dublin, Paris, Oxford, Cambridge, Glasgow, Aberdeen, and St. Andrews* (Edinburgh: MacLachlan and Stewart, 1828), pp. 37–40.
2. D.E. MacDonnel, *Dictionary Quotations in Most Frequent Use*, (London: G. Wilkie and J. Robinson, 1811), s.v. 'Quieta non movere'.
3. Henry Cockburn, *Memorials of His Time* (Edinburgh: T.N. Foulis, 1856), p. 42.
4. Cockburn, p. 52.
5. As C.J. Lawrence has said, 'The Rutherfords, Monros, Humes, Gregorys, Hopes, Duncans, and Hamiltons virtually carved up the University's medical chairs in the period 1780–1830'. 'The Edinburgh Medical School and the End of the "Old Thing" 1790–1830', *History of Universities* 7 (1988): 263.
6. Alexander Bower, *The Edinburgh Student's Guide: Or an account of the classes of the University arranged under the four faculties; with a detail of what is taught in each* (Edinburgh: Waugh and Innes, 1822), p. 72.
7. Robert Christison, 'Memorial To The Principal and Professors of the University of Edinburgh', Oct 1824, EUL P.470/26, p. 3.
8. Eric G. Forbes, ed., *Index of Fellows of the Royal Society of Edinburgh Elected from 1783 to 1882* (Edinburgh: Manpower Services Commission (STEP) Project for the preservation of Scotland's Cultural Heritage, [1980].
9. Andrew Duncan junior, 'Medical Education', *Edinburgh Medical and Surgical Journal* 28 (1826): 218.
10. The rumor is repeated in J.D. Comrie, *History of Scottish Medicine*, 2 vols, (London: The Wellcome Historical Medical Museum, 1932), 2:493.
11. James Rush to Benjamin Rush, Edinburgh, 23 Nov 1809, Rush Papers, Library Company of Philadelphia Mss, held in the Historical Society of Pennsylvania, Box 11, Yi2 7404 F21b.
12. Robert Christison, *Life of Sir Robert Christison, Bart.*, 2 vols. (Edinburgh: William Blackwood and Sons, 1885), 1:54–5, 160.
13. Prince Adam Constantine Czartoryski to his uncle Prince Adam George Czartoryski, Edinburgh, 27 January 1823, Edinburgh University Library Mss. Dc.2.48.
14. 'Medical Schools of Dublin and Edinburgh', *Blackwood's Magazine* 4 (October 1818–March 1819): 439–441; *A Comparative View of the Schools of Physic of Dublin and Edinburgh* (Dublin: Hodges & McArthur, 1818).
15. J.B. Morrell, 'Practical Chemistry in the University of Edinburgh,' *Ambix* 16 (1969): 66–70, and 'The Chemical Breeders: The Research Schools of Liebig and Thomas Thomson,' *Ambix* 19 (1972): 1–35; for opportunities in Paris, see *Medical Calendar*, p. 150.
16. *Medical Calendar*, pp. 53–113, 150–160.
17. 'American Medical Schools,' *Edinburgh Medical and Surgical Journal* 26 (1826): 210.

18. James Coutts, *A History of the University of Glasgow from its Foundation in 1451 to 1909* (Glasgow: James Maclehose and Sons, 1909), pp. 511–520; *Comparative View*, p. 63; from 1809, the *Edinburgh Medical and Surgical Journal* regularly printed the lectures offered in Edinburgh, Glasgow, and London.
19. Coutts, pp. 519–510. These disputes are discussed in great detail in *Glasgow Evidence*.
20. See the advertisement in the *Edinburgh Medical and Surgical Journal* 2 (1806): 507–9.
21. Susan Lawrence, 'Science and Medicine at the London Hospitals. The Development of Teaching and Research 1750–1815' (Ph. D. Thesis, University of Toronto, 1985), pp. 635–636.
22. William Pulteney Alison discussed this with the Commissioners in *Edinburgh Evidence*, pp. 211.
23. Irvine Loudon, *Medical Care and the General Practitioner 1750–1850* (Oxford: Clarendon Press, 1986), pp. 129–151, 208–223, has especially noted a rise in the number of dispensing druggists, which intensified competition for the General practitioners.
24. E.A. Wrigley and R.S. Schofield, *The Population History of England 1541–1871* (Cambridge: Cambridge University Press, 1981), pp. 210–211.
25. *Medical Calendar*, p. 208.
26. *Medical Calendar*, pp. 211–13.
27. John Thomson, 'Lectures on Practice of Surgery', 1809–1810, RCPE John Thomson Mss # 2, Lecture 4, 1 Nov., unpaginated.
28. Oswei Temkin, 'The Role of Surgery in the Rise of Modern Medical Thought', *Bulletin of the History of Medicine* 25 (1951): 248–259; Toby Gelfand, *Professionalizing Modern Medicine. Paris Surgeons and Medical Science and Institutions in the 18th Century* (Westport, Conn.: Greenwood Press, 1980); M.J. Peterson, *The Medical Profession in Mid-Victorian London* (Berkeley: University of California Press, 1978); for a description of the many conflicts remaining between the different branches of all the professions by mid-century, see W.J. Reader, *Professional Men. The Rise of the Professional Classes in Nineteenth-Century England* (London: Cox and Wyman Ltd., 1966), pp. 59–72.
29. T.C. Speer, *Thoughts on the Present Character and Constitution of the Medical Profession* (Cambridge: J. Smith, 1823), p. 92.
30. *Ibid.*, p. 97.
31. *Ibid.*, p. 98.
32. Alexander Pope, *Poetry and Prose of Alexander Pope*, ed. by Aubrey Williams (Boston: Houghton Mifflin Company, 1969), p. 141–2.
33. Isaac Kramnick, *Bolingbroke and His Circle, The Politics of Nostalgia in the Age of Walpole* (Cambridge, MA: Harvard University Press, 1968).
34. Loudon, pp. 147–151.
35. [Edward Barlow,] 'An Attempt to develope [sic] the Fundamental Principles which should guide the Legislature in regulating the Profession of Physic', *Edinburgh Medical and Surgical Journal* 14 (1818): 1–26. This was cited with approval by Thomas Alcock, 'An Essay on the Education and Duties of the General Practitioner in Medicine and Surgery', *Transactions of the Associates Apothecaries and Surgeon-Apothecaries* 1 (1823): 1–135.
36. 'Medical Reform', *Quarterly Review* 33 (December 1840–March 1841): 58.

37. *Ibid.*, p. 59.

38. He changed his name to Hamilton in hopes of being adopted as his uncle's successor. *List of the graduates in medicine in the University of Edinburgh from MDCCV to MDCCCLXVI* (Edinburgh: Neill & Co., 1867).

39. Speer, p. 40. Speer had studied in Edinburgh from 1810–12, during the wars.

40. *Ibid.*, p. 41.

41. *Glasgow Evidence*, p. 131.

42. Speer, p. 97.

43. Medico-Chirurgus, *A Letter addressed to the Medical Profession, on the encroachments on the practice of the surgeon-apothecary, by a new set of physicians* (London: John Anderson, 1826), p. 5. This was published in 1826, and the author may well have been promoted to write it by the convening of the Royal Commission. It should therefore be taken as expressing perceptions of the Scottish Universities, rather than as depicting the reality.

44. 'Letter to the Editor of the Edinburgh Medical and Surgical Journal, explaining the Object of the Society of Physicians of the United Kingdom', *Edinburgh Medical and Surgical Journal* 25 (1826): 325.

45. Joseph Kett, 'Provincial Medical Practice in England, 1730–1815', *Journal of the History of Medicine* 19 (1964): 17–29; P.J. Anderson, ed. *Fasti Academiae Mariscallanae Aberdonensis. Selections from the Records of the Marischal College and University MDXCIII – MDCCCLX*, 3 vols. (Aberdeen: New Spalding Club, 1898). Vol. 2: *Officers, Graduates, and Alumni*, pp. 111–159; P.J. Anderson, ed. *Officers and Graduates of University and King's College, Aberdeen MDV–MDCCCLX*, (Aberdeen: New Spalding Club, 1893) pp. 131–160.

46. The disputes are discussed at great length in Great Britain, Parliament, House of Commons, *Report from the Select Committee on Medical Education: With the Minutes of Evidence, and Appendix*. 1834 (602, I, II, and III), Part 1: Royal College of Physicians, London). The position of the Fellows is presented in A.H.T. Robb-Smith, 'Medical Education at Oxford and Cambridge Prior to 1850', in *The Evolution of Medical Education in Britain*, ed. by F.N.L. Poynter (Baltimore: The Williams and Wilkins Company, 1966), and in G. Clark, *The Royal College of Physicians of London*, 3 vols. (Oxford: Clarendon Press, 1966) 2:552–573, 614–632.

47. 'Medical Reform', p. 53.

48. Dorothy Porter and Roy Porter, *Patient's Progress. Doctors and Doctoring in Eighteenth-Century England* (Stanford: Stanford University Press, 1989). See Chapter Two.

49. In 1825 an amendment to the Apothecaries Act was proposed, and Andrew Duncan junior commented on the original act and the amendment in 'The English Apothecaries Act', *Edinburgh Medical and Surgical Journal* 25 (1826): 407–424.

50. 'Observations on Medical Reform, by a member of the University of Oxford', *Pamphleteer* (May, 1814): 414–431.

51. *Ibid.*, p. 421–3.

52. *Ibid.*, p. 423–4.

53. Andrew Duncan junior, 'English Apothecaries Act', p. 418.

54. Lawson Whalley, *A Vindication of the University of Edinburgh (As a School of Medicine,) from the aspersions of 'A member of the University of Oxford', with remarks on medical reform* (Lancaster: in C. Clark, 1816), p. 37.

55. 'Society of Physicians', pp. 323–4.
56. 'Observations on Medical Reform', p. 420.
57. Robert Heller, '*Officier de Santé*: The second-class doctors of nineteenth-century France,' *Medical History* 22 (1978): 25–43; Russell Maulitz, *Morbid Appearances. The Anatomy of Pathology in the Early Nineteenth Century* (Cambridge: Cambridge University Press, 1987), pp. 85–94, has found that the examiners responsible for certifying *officiers de santé* were besieged with requests for exemptions from students and practitioners. See also Matthew Ramsay, *Professional and Popular Medicine in France, 1770–1830, The Social World of Medical Practice* (Cambridge: Cambridge University Press, 1988).
58. Review of 'Institutions for the Education of *Empirical Practitioners*, necessary in the present state of Society. By Professor Reil,' *Edinburgh Medical and Surgical Journal* 2 (1806): 472.
59. *Ibid.*, p. 473.
60. Professor James Hamilton, *Edinburgh Evidence*, p. 313.
61. *Edinburgh Evidence*, pp. 240–1; Professor James Hamilton claimed it was impossible for 'a man in extensive medical practice' to examine the candidates for degrees, p. 313.
62. *Edinburgh Evidence*, p. 241.
63. *Ibid.*, p. 259.
64. Sylas Neville, *The Diary of Sylas Neville, 1767–1788*, ed. by Basil Cozens-Hardy (London: Oxford University Press, 1950), p. 226.
65. *Edinburgh Evidence*, p. 448.
66. *Ibid.*, p. 193.
67. *Ibid.*, p. 299.
68. *Ibid.*, p 277.
69. Andrew Duncan senior, 'Intended Proposal by Dr Duncan senior to the Senatus Academicus of the University of Edinburgh, for granting Diplomas in Surgery', 1824, EUL P. 470/20. This was formulated in opposition to the degree regulations actually adopted, but gives an indication of some of the issues under consideration.
70. This was discussed by several professors in *Edinburgh Evidence*, pp. 199, 235, 283.
71. Alexander Morgan, ed, *University of Edinburgh, Charters, Statutes, and Acts of the Town Council and the Senatus. 1583–1858* – (Edinburgh: Oliver and Boyd, 1937), p. 264.
72. *Ibid.*, p. 266.
73. 'New Regulations for obtaining Medical Degrees, enacted by the Universities of Aberdeen and St. Andrews', *Edinburgh Medical and Surgical Journal* 26 (1826): 209–210.
74. *Medical Calendar*, p. 181; *St. Andrews Evidence*, pp. 16–17.
75. Andrew Duncan junior, 'English Apothecaries Act', p. 424.

Chapter Ten

1. Great Britain. House of Commons. *Report Made to His Majesty by a Royal Commission of Inquiry into the State of the Universities of Scotland*. October, 1830, p. 59.
2. *Edinburgh Evidence*, Appendix, p. 253.

3. 'State of the Universities', *Quarterly Review* 36 (June–October 1827): 216.
4. *Report*, p. 5.
5. *Edinburgh Evidence*, Appendix, p. 253.
6. The Medical Faculty commented on the proposals at great length 'Considerations,' *Edinburgh Evidence*, Appendix, pp. 259–271.
7. *Glasgow Evidence*, Appendix, pp. 562–565.
8. R.D. Anderson, *Education and Opportunity in Victorian Scotland. Schools and Universities*. (Oxford: Clarendon Press, 1983), p. 49.
9. *Report*, p. 13.
10. Anderson, pp. 27–69.
11. *Ibid.*, p. 48.
12. See the letter signed by Thomas Thomson, among others, in *Glasgow Evidence*, Appendix, p. 564.
13. *Edinburgh Evidence*, p. 199; also cited in *Report*, p. 188. Alison was Dean of the Faculty during the Commission.
14. L.J. Saunders, *Scottish Democracy 1815–1840. The Social and Intellectual Background* (Edinburgh: Oliver and Boyd, 1950); G.E. Davie, *The Democratic Intellect. Scotland and Her Universities in the Nineteenth Century* (Edinburgh: Edinburgh University Press, 1961).
15. Anderson, pp. 38, 46.
16. 'Admission of Dissenters to Degrees in the English Universities', *Blackwood's Magazine* 35 (January–June, 1834): 716.
17. *Glasgow Evidence*, p. 153.
18. *Edinburgh Evidence*, p. 304.
19. 'Paper . . . presented on the 18th of August, 1829, and ordered to be printed,' *Edinburgh Evidence*, Appendix, p. 144.
20. *Report*, p. 7.
21. 'State of the Universities', p. 218. The author claimed this was a quotation from Francis Bacon.
22. *Ibid.*, p. 217.
23. *Report*, p. 8.
24. *Ibid.*, p. 56.
25. *Ibid.*
26. *Edinburgh Evidence*, p. 193.
27. Howard S. Becker, Blanche Geer, Everett C. Hughes, Anselm L. Strauss, *Boys in White. Student Culture in Medical School* (New Brunswick, NJ: Transaction Books, 1977), pp. 341–51.
28. Adam Smith to William Cullen, London, 10 September 1774, cited in John Thomson, *An Account of the Life, Lectures, and Writings of William Cullen, MD*, 2 vols. (Edinburgh: William Blackwood and Sons, 1859), 1:477–8. See above, Chapter Four.
29. *Report*, p. 12.
30. Cited in Andrew Duncan junior, 'Medical Education,' *Edinburgh Medical and Surgical Journal* 28 (1827): 219.
31. Anderson, pp. 38–9.
32. *Report*, p. 11.
33. Sir William Hamilton, 'Review of *Report made to His Majesty . . . into the State of the Universities of Scotland*', *Edinburgh Review* 59 (April–June 1834): 196–226; for a recent discussion of the impact of patronage on the universities, see Roger L. Emerson, 'Lord Bute and the Scottish Universities

1760–1792', in *Lord Bute: Essays in Reinterpretation*, ed. Karl W. Schweizer (Leicester: Leicester University Press, 1988) pp. 147–179.

34. *Edinburgh Evidence*, Appendix, p. 269.
35. *Glasgow Evidence*, p. 567.
37. 'Considerations' *Edinburgh Evidence*, Appendix, p. 155. The Glasgow faculty made a similar point. *Glasgow Evidence*, p. 564.
38. Glasgow Evidence, p. 563.
39. *Report*, p. 11.
40. Charles Badham's letter, *Glasgow Evidence*, p. 566.
41. *Edinburgh Evidence*, p. 192.
42. *Report*, p. 57.
43. Adam Smith to William Cullen, London, 20 September 1774, cited in Thomson, 1:475. See above, Introduction.
44. *Report*, p. 64.
45. *Report*, p. 167. The Commissioners used the numbers provided by the medical faculty, which had been obtained by counting the number of students who signed the matriculation albums each year. For a discussion of the problems this method causes in estimating the ratio of graduates to matriculates, see Appendix A. It is possible that the faculty had provided the Commissioners with the figures as a deliberate strategy to show their high enrollments.
46. Edinburgh Evidence, p. 194; cited in *Report*, p. 188.
47. *Report*, p. 64.
48. 'State of the Universities', p. 235.
49. This memorial was included in *Edinburgh Evidence*, Appendix, p. 145, with no author given. 'Brummingham' was a slang word meaning cheap imitation, a corruption of Birmingham, where they were allegedly made.
50. This motive for the General Medical Council is discussed by Ivan Waddington, *The Medical Profession in the Industrial Revolution* (Dublin: Gill and Macmillan Humanities Press, 1984), pp. 139–52.
51. *Glasgow Evidence*, p. 129.
52. *Ibid.*, p. 152.
53. *Ibid.*, p. 155.
54. *Edinburgh Evidence*, p. 237. I have rearranged the order of the questions.
55. George Crabb, *English Synonyms Explained, in Alphabetical Order; with Copious Illustrations and Examples Drawn from the Best Writers*, 3rd ed. (London: Baldwin, Cradock, and Joy, 1824), s.v. 'Education'.
56. George Jardine, *Outlines of Philosophical Education, illustrated by the Method of Teaching the Logic Class in the University of Glasgow* (Glasgow: University Press, 1825), p. 460.
57. Adam Smith, *Wealth of Nations*, cited by the Medical Faculty in *Edinburgh Evidence*, Appendix, p. 262.
58. *Edinburgh Evidence*, Appendix, p. 262.
59. Thomas Ismay, 'Letter from Thomas Ismay, Student of Medicine at Edinburgh, 1771, to his father', *University of Edinburgh Journal* 8 (1936–7): 59.
60. William Cullen, 'Lectures on Chemistry', c. 1755, RCPE MSS. Cullen, William, # 11.
61. 'Medical Reform', *Quarterly Review* 67 (December 1840–March 1841): 54.
62. 'State of the Universities', p. 217.

63. John Robison to Joseph Ewart, Edinburgh, 30 December 1790, EUL MSS PHOT 1727.
64. Cited in J.B. Morrell, 'Practical Chemistry in the University of Edinburgh', *Ambix* 16 (1969): 66.
65. 'The London University', *Quarterly Review* 33 (December 1825–March 1826): 266.
66. *Ibid.*, p. 260. For the concern about novelty in education, see Sheldon Rothblatt, 'The Student Sub-culture and the Examination System in Early 19th Century Oxbridge', in Lawrence Stone (ed.) *The University and Society*, 2 vols. (Princeton: Princeton University Press, 1974) 1:247–304.
67. William Whewell, *Of A Liberal Education in General and with Particular Reference to the Leading Studies of the University of Cambridge* (London: John W. Parker, 1850), p. 123.
68. *Ibid.*
69. *Report*, p. 10.
70. *Edinburgh Evidence*, p. 221.
71. *Report*, p. 62.
72. *Ibid.*, p. 63.
73. *Ibid.*, p. 39.
74. *Ibid.*
75. *Ibid.*, p. 60.
76. Thomas Turner, *Outlines of a System of Medico-Chirurgical Education, Containing Illustrations of the Application of Anatomy, Physiology, and other Sciences to the Principal Practical Points in Medicine and Surgery* (London: Thomas and George Underwood, 1824), p. i.
77. Robert Christison, 'Memorial To The Principal and Professors of the University of Edinburgh', 13 Oct 1824, EUL P.470/26, p. 4. See Chapter Four.
78. *Edinburgh Evidence*, p. 223.
79. *Ibid.*, p. 214.
80. *Ibid.*, p. 504; cited in the *Report*, p. 192.
81. *Edinburgh Evidence*, p. 504.
82. *Report*, p. 56.
83. *Edinburgh Evidence*, pp. 338, 457.
84. 'Advice of Sir John Clerk of Penicuik to his son, John, when he went to serve his apprenticeship as a chirurgeon under Adam Drummond and John Campbell', 16 April 1745, Clerk of Penicuik Mss, SRO GD18/2331.
85. *Edinburgh Evidence*, pp. 203, 238–9; Appendix, p. 262; see Chapter Two.
86. *Report*, p. 38.
87. So much so that no one saw any reason to explain how classical studies did this. For a history of this kind of rhetoric in favor of the classics, see Anthony Grafton and Lisa Jardine, *From Humanism to the Humanities. Education and the Liberal Arts in Fifteenth– and Sixteenth–Century Europe* (Cambridge, MA: Harvard University Press, 1986).
88. [Thomas Denman, Baron Denman], 'Review of *Essays on Professional Education*, by R.L. Edgeworth', *Monthly Review* Series 2, 62 (May–August 1810): 7.
89. 'State of the Universities', p. 223.
90. Henry Cockburn, *Memorials of His Time* (Edinburgh: T.N. Foulis, 1855), p. 388–9.

91. *Report*, p. 56.
92. *Glasgow Evidence*, p. 564.
93. *Report*, p. 66–68.
94. *Ibid.*, p. 10.
95. *Ibid.*, p. 9.
96. Lesassier did graduate in 1816, but only after a number of years as an army surgeon, so even if the Commissioners' regulations been in effect he could have requested that an exception be made because of his professional experience.
97. 'Considerations,' *Edinburgh Evidence*, Appendix, p. 260.
98. *Edinburgh Evidence*, p. 215. Andrew Duncan junior had used the same expression in 'Medical Education', *Edinburgh Medical and Surgical Journal* 28 (1827): 190.
99. 'State of the Universities', p. 223.
100. See Conclusion.
101. *Report*, p. 61.
102. *Edinburgh Evidence*, p. 235; Appendix, p. 262.
103. William Pulteney Alison, citing Mr. Lawrence, a London teacher, *Edinburgh Evidence*, p. 197.
104. *Edinburgh Evidence*, Appendix, p. 262.
105. *Ibid.*
106. *Ibid.*, Appendix, p. 263.
107. See the new regulations for medical degrees in 1833, which stayed in effect until 1861, in Alexander Morgan, ed, *University of Edinburgh, Charters, Statutes, and Acts of the Town Council and the Senatus, 1583–1858* (Edinburgh: Oliver and Boyd, 1937), pp. 185–188; Alexander Grant, *The Story of the University of Edinburgh during Its First Three Hundred Years*, 2 vols. (London: Longman, Green & Co., 1884), 2:111.

Conclusion

1. Samuel Lewis to Mrs. W.P. Hinds, Edinburgh, 28 July 1838, EUL GEN 1429/8.
2. Andrew Duncan junior, 'Medical Education', *Edinburgh Medical and Surgical Journal* 28 (1827): 216.
3. William Hamilton, Review of 'Report made to His Majesty, by a Royal Commission of Enquiry into the State of the Universities of Scotland . . .', *Edinburgh Review* 59 (April–June 1834): 196–226.
4. 'Regulations, &c', 1829, Secretary's Copy, RCSE.
5. Alexander Morgan, ed, *University of Edinburgh, Charters, Statutes, and Acts of the Town Council and the Senatus, 1583–1858* (Edinburgh: Oliver and Boyd, 1937), p. 187.
6. James Syme, *Papers in Connexion with the Letter of Professor Syme, Regarding the Present State and Future Prospects of the Medical School* (Edinburgh: H. & J. Pillans, 1840), p. 2.
7. Samuel Lewis to Mrs. W.P. Hinds, Edinburgh, 28 July 1838.
8. R.D. Anderson, *Education and Opportunity in Victorian Scotland. Schools and Universities.* (Oxford: Clarendon Press, 1983) makes this point against George Davie's interpretation in *The Democratic Intellect. Scotland and Her Universities in the Nineteenth Century* (Edinburgh: Edinburgh University Press, 1961).

9. Susan Lawrence, 'Science and Medicine at the London Hospitals. The Development of Teaching and Research 1750–1815' (Ph.D. Thesis, University of Toronto, 1985), pp. 635–636.
10. Ruth G. Hodkinson, 'Medical Education in Cambridge in the Nineteenth Century', in *Cambridge and its Contribution to Medicine*, ed. by Arthur Rook (London: Wellcome Institute of the History of Medicine, 1971), pp. 79–106.
11. *Edinburgh Evidence*, p. 450.
12. Alexander Grant, *The Story of the University of Edinburgh during Its First Three Hundred Years*, 2 vols. (London: Longman, Green & Co., 1884), 2:108–111.
13. Mary Hewson to her son, Thomas Tickell Hewson, 7 July 1795 Hewson Papers, B H492, vol. 2, # 31, American Philosophical Society Library, Philadelphia.
14. Andrew Duncan junior, 'The English Apothecaries Act', *Edinburgh Medical and Surgical Journal* 26 (1826): 424.
15. John Bell, *Letters on Professional Character and Manners: on the Education of a Surgeon, and the Duties and Qualifications of a Physician: addressed to James Gregory. M.D* (Edinburgh: John Muir, 1810), p. 544.

Appendix A

1. The matriculation records are kept in the Edinburgh University Library Rare Books Collection. The reference number is Da, but they are more easily found by volume and year. I have used the Matriculation Albums stamped 'Matriculation 1762–1786', 'Matriculation 1786–1805', 'Matriculation 1804–1816', and 'Matriculation 1816–1828'. From 1762 until 1808, the Albums listed the name of each student with the courses he attended that year. From 1811, the Matriculation Album gave the name of each student, the faculty he intended to study in (Law, Medicine, Theology, Arts), his place of origin, and his matriculation number. Other matriculation records are kept in leather-bound volumes titled 'Medical 1791–1795', 'Medical 1796–1800', 'Medical 1801–1805', 'Medical 1806–1810', and, from 1811 'General and Medical' with the academic year (for example, 'General and Medical 1811–1812'). These records also listed each student, with the courses he attended each year. For their explanation, see below. I am grateful to Mrs. J. Currie for calling these and other University records to my attention.
2. *Annals of Medicine* 4 (1799): 532.
3. *Edinburgh Evidence*, Appendix, p. 127–8.
4. Alexander Morgan, 'Matriculates in the Faculty of Medicine Prior to 1858', *University of Edinburgh Journal* 8 (1936–7): 124–5.

5. L.R.C. Agnew, 'Scottish Medical Education', in *The History of Medical Education*, ed. by C.D. O'Malley (Berkeley: University of California Press, 1970), pp. 251–262.
6. Information on graduates is taken from *List of the graduates in medicine in the University of Edinburgh from MDCCV to MDCCCLXVI* (Edinburgh: Neill & Co., 1867). For records of Fellows, I have used Volumes Four to Nine, 1708–1828, of the minute books of the Royal College of Surgeons of Edinburgh, as well as the *List of the Fellows of the Royal College of Surgeons of Edinburgh from the year 1581 to 31st December 1873* (Edinburgh: George Robb, 1874). Students receiving diplomas were listed in the minute books, and from 1816 were called Licentiates and published in *List of the Licentiates of the Royal College of Surgeons of Edinburgh from 1815 to 1859, and of Fellows of the College at 1st August 1859* (Edinburgh: Robert Hardie & Co., 1859). Information on apprentices, together with their masters, is taken from the minute books. Information on membership in the Royal Medical Society is taken from *General List of the Members of the Medical Society of Edinburgh* (Edinburgh: John Stark, 1835). Information on the East India Company comes from Dirom Grey Crawford, *Roll of the Indian Medical Service*, (London: W. Thacker and Co., 1930), and on the Army Medical Service from William Johnston, *Roll of Commissioned Officers in Medical Service of the British Army*, (Aberdeen: Aberdeen University Press, 1917).
7. Oskar Morgenstern, *On the Accuracy of Economic Observations* (Princeton: Princeton University Press, 1950), discusses the futility of calculating statistics with great precision when the methods used to obtain the data do not warrant it.
8. Lawrence Stone, 'The Size and Composition of the Oxford Student Body 1580–1909', in *The University in Society*, ed. by Lawrence Stone, 2 vols. (Princeton: Princeton University Press, 1974), 1:83–8.
9. Richard Kagan, *Students and Society in Early Modern Spain* (Baltimore: Johns Hopkins Press, 1974), pp. 260–1.
10. See Stone, pp. 83–8, and Kagan, pp. 260–1.
11. Kagan, p. 261.
12. Smith mentions attending classes in a letter to his wife, published in Emily A. Smith, *The Life and Letters of Nathan Smith, MB, MD* (New Haven: Yale University Press, 1914), p. 19. According to Emily Smith, Nathan Smith attended Alexander Monro's lectures on Anatomy and Surgery and Joseph Black's lectures on Chemistry.
13. Stone, 1:13.
14. I have used the 'Medical' and 'General and Medical' volumes as my main source of information on students' course attendance from 1809, since the Matriculation Albums stopped providing course information in 1808.
15. 'General and Medical 1813–1814', EUL Da.
16. Attached to 'General and Medical 1814–15', EUL Da.
17. These percentages come from 'peeling away' the students who attended Chemistry only, as in Chapter Six.
18. These figures exclude those students who attended Chemistry only.
19. This figure may be too low. Professor James Hamilton's own class lists for Midwifery are kept in the Library of the Royal College of Physicians of Edinburgh, but I have not been able to check them systematically against the 'General and Medical' lists.

Index

Note: Those marked with an * studied medicine at Edinburgh University. Professor indicates Professor of Medicine, Edinburgh University.